Primary Care
Ophthalmology

David A. Palay, M.D.

Associate Clinical Professor
Department of Ophthalmology
Emory University School of Medicine
Atlanta, Georgia

Jay H. Krachmer, M.D.

Professor and Chairman
Department of Ophthalmology
University of Minnesota Medical School
Minneapolis, Minnesota

Primary Care Ophthalmology

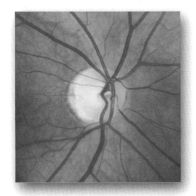 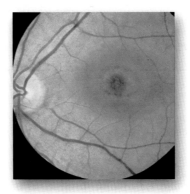 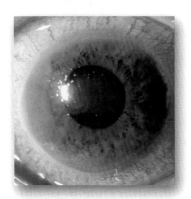

SECOND EDITION

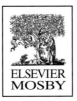

ELSEVIER
MOSBY

ELSEVIER
MOSBY

1600 John F. Kennedy Blvd.
Ste 1800
Philadelphia, PA 19103-2899

Primary Care Ophthalmology
Copyright © 2005, Mosby Inc.

ISBN 0-323-03316-4

Notice

Knowledge and best practice in this field are constantly changing. As new research and experience broaden our knowledge, changes in practice, treatment and drug therapy may become necessary or appropriate. Readers are advised to check the most current information provided (i) on procedures featured or (ii) by the manufacturer of each product to be administered, to verify the recommended dose or formula, the method and duration of administration, and contraindications. It is the responsibility of the practitioner, relying on their own experience and knowledge of the patient, to make diagnoses, to determine dosages and the best treatment for each individual patient, and to take all appropriate safety precautions. To the fullest extent of the law, neither the Publisher nor the Authors assume any liability for any injury and/or damage to persons or property arising out or related to any use of the material contained in this book.

Previous edition copyrighted 1997

Library of Congress Cataloging-in-Publication Data
Primary Care Ophthalmology / [edited by] David A. Palay, Jay H. Krachmer.—2nd ed.
    p. ; cm.
  Rev. ed. of: Ophthalmology for the primary care physician. c1997.
  ISBN 0-323-03316-4
    1. Eye—Diseases.   2. Ophthalmology.   3. Primary care (Medicine)   I. Palay, David A.
II. Krachmer, Jay H.   III. Primary Care Ophthalmology.
  [DNLM: 1. Eye Diseases—diagnosis.   2. Eye Diseases—therapy.   3. Primary Health Care. WW 140
O616 2006]
RE46.O655 2006
617.7′0232—dc22

2005041596

Acquisitions Editor: Rolla Couchman
Publishing Services Manager: Frank Polizzano
Project Manager: Jeff Gunning
Design Direction: Ellen Zanolle
Cover Designer: Ellen Zanolle

Printed in China

Last digit is the print number: 9   8   7   6   5   4   3   2   1

This book is dedicated to
my wife, Debra, *my children,* Sarah and Matthew,
my sister, Deborah, *and my parents,* Sandra and Bernard,
and is in memory of
Anne and Jacob Kingloff *and* Israel and Ida Palay.

DAVID A. PALAY

With great love and appreciation I dedicate this book to
my wife, Kathryn, *our children,* Edward, Kara, and Jill,
and our parents, Paul and Rebecca Krachmer
and Louis and Gertrude Maraist.

JAY H. KRACHMER

Consulting Editors

Douglas D. Brunette, M.D.
Associate Professor
Department of Emergency Medicine
University of Minnesota Medical
    School
Program Director
Department of Emergency Medicine
Hennepin County Medical Center
Minneapolis, Minnesota

Jonathan J. Masor
Associate Professor of Medicine
Department of Medicine
Emory University School of Medicine
Atlanta, Georgia

Timothy J. J. Ramer, M.D.
Assistant Professor
Department of Family Medicine and
    Community Health
University of Minnesota Medical School
Minneapolis, Minnesota

Robert M. Segal, M.D., M.P.H.
Clinical Associate Professor
Department of Pediatrics
University of Minnesota Medical School
Medical Director
Inpatient Medical/Surgical Services
Children's Hospitals and Clinics
Minneapolis, Minnesota

Contributors

Maria Aaron, M.D.
Assistant Professor of Ophthalmology
Residency Program Director
Emory University School of Medicine
Chief of Service, Ophthalmology
Crawford Long Hospital
Atlanta, Georgia

Allen D. Beck, M.D.
Associate Professor
Department of Ophthalmology
Emory University School of Medicine
Atlanta, Georgia

Michael D. Bennett, M.D.
Associate Professor
Department of Surgery
University of Hawaii John A. Burns
    School of Medicine
President
Retina Institute of Hawaii
Honolulu, Hawaii

Douglas M. Blackmon, M.D.
Assistant Clinical Professor of
    Ophthalmology
Duke University School of Medicine
Durham, North Carolina

Geoffrey Broocker, M.D.
Professor of Ophthalmology
Emory University School of Medicine
Chief of Service, Ophthalmology
Grady Memorial Hospital
Atlanta, Georgia

Emmett F. Carpel, M.D.
Adjunct Professor
Department of Ophthalmology
University of Minnesota Medical
    School
Consultant, Hennepin County Medical
    Center
Staff, Phillips Eye Institute
Staff, Health Partners
Minneapolis, Minnesota

Michael C. Diesenhouse, M.D.
Eye Associates of Tucson
Tucson, Arizona

Arlene V. Drack, M.D.
Associate Professor
Department of Ophthalmology
University of Colorado School of
    Medicine
University of Colorado Denver
    Hospitals and Clinics
Chief, Pediatric Ophthalmology
The Children's Hospital
Denver, Colorado

Jonathan H. Engman, M.D.
Resident
Department of Ophthalmology
University of Minnesota
Minneapolis, Minnesota

Andrew R. Harrison, M.D.
Assistant Professor
Department of Ophthalmology
University of Minnesota Medical School
Minneapolis, Minnesota

Terry Kim, M.D.
Associate Professor of Ophthalmology
Duke University School of Medicine
Associate Director
Cornea and Refractive Surgery Services
Duke University Eye Center
Durham, North Carolina

Jay H. Krachmer, M.D.
Professor and Chairman
Department of Ophthalmology
University of Minnesota Medical School
Minneapolis, Minnesota

Timothy J. Martin, M.D.
Associate Professor of Surgical
  Sciences/Ophthalmology
Wake Forest University School of
  Medicine/Baptist Medical Center
Winston-Salem, North Carolina

Timothy W. Olsen, M.D.
Associate Professor and William H.
  Knobloch Endowed Retina Chair
Department of Ophthalmology
University of Minnesota Medical School
Minneapolis, Minnesota

David A. Palay, M.D.
Associate Clinical Professor
Department of Ophthalmology
Emory University School of Medicine
Atlanta, Georgia

Wayne A. Solley, M.D.
Texas Retina Associates
Dallas, Texas

Ted H. Wojno, M.D.
Professor of Ophthalmology
Emory University School of Medicine
Director of Oculoplastic and Orbital
  Surgery
The Emory Clinic
Atlanta, Georgia

Preface

Patients frequently present to primary care practitioners for treatment of an eye problem. It is estimated that greater than half of all eye drops prescribed in the United States are prescribed by physicians other than eye care specialists. It is important that primary care practitioners be able to recognize ophthalmic disease and to treat the problem if necessary, or to refer the patient for further evaluation.

For this second edition we have made several changes and additions:

We have changed the title of the book from *Ophthalmology for the Primary Care Physician* to *Primary Care Ophthalmology*, to emphasize that it is intended for anyone involved in direct patient care, including residents, medical students, optometrists, physician assistants, nurses, and nurse practitioners.

We also have added a chapter on the "red eye." This chapter pulls together material presented throughout the book, to emphasize that a red eye is caused by a variety of conditions, not only by conjunctivitis.

As technology changes, so does the way information is disseminated and shared. This edition of the book contains software that can be downloaded to a personal digital assistant (PDA).

The format of the second edition is the same as that of the first. Most chapters begin with a brief discussion of anatomy, followed by a more detailed description of various diseases. Each disease is described in an outline format that covers symptoms, signs, etiology, workup, differential diagnosis, and treatment. The text describes the core information of each condition, without providing unnecessary details. The highlight of the book is the more than 300 quality color illustrations that accompany the text. Most of the figures underwent a variety of modifications, such as labeling and addition of magnified insets and schematic illustrations, to augment their educational value and to emphasize desired features.

To achieve our goal of providing a practical guide to eye care, we have necessarily omitted a wealth of information that is included in the training of ophthalmologists. Many diseases that are intrinsic to the eye were excluded because the diagnosis and treatment were felt to be outside the realm of the primary care practitioner. The information in this book should not be substituted for a proper referral when necessary.

We tried to be as specific as possible when recommending treatment options. Drug dosages have been checked carefully; however, the reader is urged to consult the *Physicians' Desk Reference* or other source when prescribing medications that are unfamiliar.

We hope that this book will continue to serve as a valuable reference to all practitioners involved in delivering primary eye care. We welcome your comments.

David A. Palay, M.D.

Jay H. Krachmer, M.D.

Acknowledgments

We are extremely grateful to our many colleagues, associates, and friends who helped with the preparation of this book. We would like to credit and thank the following sources of material:

Antonio Capone Jr., M.D., Beaumont, Michigan (Figs. 10–28, 10–32, and 15–29)

James Gilman, CRA, Atlanta, Georgia (Figs. 1–14 and 9–8)

Glaxo Wellcome (Fig. 1–1)

Harrington DO: *The Visual Fields: A Textbook and Atlas of Clinical Perimetry* (Fig. 12–1)

Edward J. Holland, M.D., Cincinnati, Ohio (Fig. 5–21)

Scott Lambert, M.D., Atlanta, Georgia (Fig. 15–10)

Mark J. Mannis, M.D., Sacramento, California (Fig. 4–16)

Daniel F. Martin, M.D., Atlanta, Georgia (Figs. 10–10 and 15–2)

Robert A. Myles, CRA, Atlanta, Georgia (Fig. 10–27)

Maria Alexandra Pernetz, B.S., RDCS, Atlanta, Georgia (Fig. 10–17)

Dante Pieramici, M.D., Santa Barbara, California (Fig. 9–5)

Spalton DJ, Hitchings RA, Hunter PA: *Atlas of Clinical Ophthalmology*, ed 2 (Figs. 1–5, 1–7, 1–13, 14–1, and 14–2)

Paul Sternberg Jr., M.D., Nashville, Tennessee (Fig. 10–29)

Ray Swords, CRA, Atlanta, Georgia (Figs. 10–1, 10–18, and 10–26)

Keith Walter, M.D., Winston-Salem, North Carolina (Fig. 5–10)

George O. Waring III, M.D., Atlanta, Georgia (Figs. 5–20, 9–2, and 9–9)

Watson PG, Ortiz JM: *Color Atlas of Scleritis* (Fig. 7–1)

Contents

CHAPTER 1   *General Eye Examination* 1
MARIA AARON • WAYNE A. SOLLEY •
GEOFFREY BROOCKER

CHAPTER 2   *Ophthalmic Differential Diagnosis* 25
DAVID A. PALAY

CHAPTER 3   *The Red Eye* 39
JAY H. KRACHMER

CHAPTER 4   *Eyelid Abnormalities* 67
TED H. WOJNO

CHAPTER 5   *Conjunctival Abnormalities* 89
DAVID A. PALAY

CHAPTER 6   *Corneal Abnormalities* 103
DAVID A. PALAY

CHAPTER 7   *Scleritis* 119
MICHAEL C. DIESENHOUSE

CHAPTER 8   *Lens Abnormalities* 127
JONATHAN H. ENGMAN • ANDREW R. HARRISON •
JAY H. KRACHMER

CHAPTER 9   *Uveitis* 139
TERRY KIM • DOUGLAS M. BLACKMON

CHAPTER 10   *Retina* 149
TIMOTHY W. OLSEN

CHAPTER **11**   *Glaucoma* *189*
ALLEN D. BECK

CHAPTER **12**   *Neuro-ophthalmology* *199*
TIMOTHY J. MARTIN

CHAPTER **13**   *Pediatric Ophthalmology* *229*
ARLENE V. DRACK

CHAPTER **14**   *Orbital Disease* *275*
TED H. WOJNO

CHAPTER **15**   *Systemic Disease and Therapies* *293*
EMMETT F. CARPEL

CHAPTER **16**   *Ocular Trauma* *329*
GEOFFREY BROOCKER • WAYNE A. SOLLEY

CHAPTER **17**   *Guide to Ophthalmic Medications* *369*
GEOFFREY BROOCKER • MICHAEL D. BENNETT

Index *387*

CHAPTER 1

General Eye Examination

MARIA AARON • WAYNE A. SOLLEY • GEOFFREY BROOCKER

A structured approach is crucial in the evaluation of patients with ophthalmic complaints. This chapter introduces the primary care physician to a general approach to the eye exam in adult ophthalmic patients. Adherence to these basic steps minimizes the possibility of overlooking a serious ocular problem. (See Chapter 13 for details on the pediatric eye exam.)

Related Anatomy

The cornea is located at the anteriormost aspect of the globe; along with the tear film, it is the major refracting surface of the eye (Fig. 1–1). Directly posterior to the cornea is the anterior chamber, a fluid-filled space (containing the aqueous humor) in which blood, white blood cells, or fibrin may collect in injury, inflammatory disease, and infection. The iris is a pigmented structure that lies just anterior to the crystalline lens and represents the posterior boundary of the anterior chamber. It consists of the sphincter and dilator muscles, connective tissue, and pigmented epithelium. The lens is surrounded by a thin capsule. In cataract surgery (crystalline lens extraction), the capsule usually is left intact posteriorly and houses the intraocular lens implant. The lens is supported by small filaments termed *zonules* that attach to the periphery of the lens capsule and anchor at the ciliary processes of the ciliary body.

Posterior to the lens is the vitreous body, a clear gel that is firmly attached to the inner eye at the area of the ora serrata (the anterior termination of the retina) and the optic nerve head (optic disc). The wall of the eye (posterior to the cornea) is composed of three layers: the sclera, choroid, and retina. The sclera is a firm collagenous layer that protects the intraocular structures, gives the globe its shape, and is the site

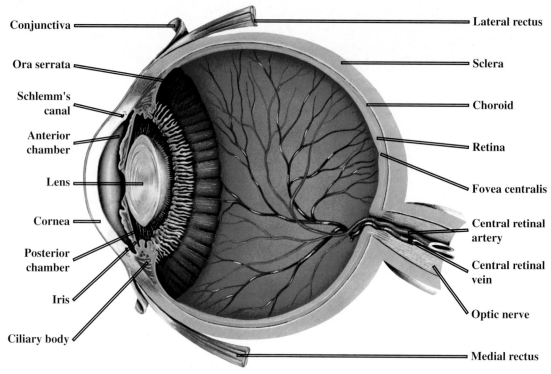

Conjunctiva

Ora serrata

Schlemm's canal

Anterior chamber

Lens

Cornea

Posterior chamber

Iris

Ciliary body

Lateral rectus

Sclera

Choroid

Retina

Fovea centralis

Central retinal artery

Central retinal vein

Optic nerve

Medial rectus

FIGURE 1–1   View of the globe, looking down on the right eye, showing major anatomic structures.

of attachment of the extraocular muscles. The choroid is a highly vascular layer forming part of the uveal tract (iris, ciliary body, and choroid) that lies just inside the sclera. The ciliary body controls accommodation, is the site of aqueous production, and lies posterior and lateral to the iris. The retina is located anterior to the choroid and posterior to the vitreous body; it is composed of photoreceptors and neural tissues. The optic nerve is a congregation of approximately 1.2 million axons from the entire retina, and it exits the globe posteriorly and slightly nasally.

The Ocular Examination

Vision

Visual acuity is the principal "vital sign" in ophthalmology. Often the status of the patient's visual acuity is the first question the ophthalmologist asks the examining physician when consulted. Evaluating the vision should be the first step in the exam, preceding any diagnostic maneuvers (e.g., pupil examination, direct ophthalmoscopy, dilation, intraocular pressure [IOP] evaluation). The examiner measures vision using a standardized visual acuity chart (Fig. 1–2) or near acuity card (Fig. 1–3). If these tools are unavailable, the examiner can use newsprint, the patient's chart, or an identification badge or a nameplate. The examiner monitors the patient to ensure that no

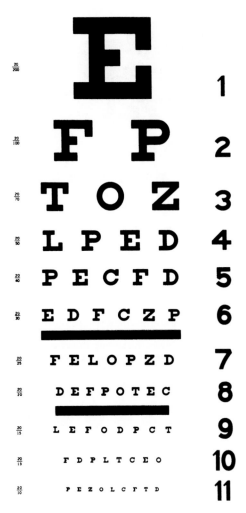

$\frac{20}{200}$	E
$\frac{20}{100}$	F P
$\frac{20}{70}$	T O Z
$\frac{20}{50}$	L P E D
$\frac{20}{40}$	P E C F D
$\frac{20}{30}$	E D F C Z P
$\frac{20}{25}$	F E L O P Z D
$\frac{20}{20}$	D E F P O T E C
$\frac{20}{15}$	L E F O D P C T
$\frac{20}{13}$	F D P L T C E O
$\frac{20}{10}$	P E Z O L C F T D

1
2
3
4
5
6
7
8
9
10
11

FIGURE 1–2 Snellen distance acuity chart.

peeking through fingers or around an occluder occurs in an attempt to perform well on the vision "test." The physician evaluates each eye individually, not only with respect to visual acuity but also in every step of the eye exam. This is especially essential if trauma is involved; occasionally the examining physician directs attention to the obviously injured eye and overlooks the "uninjured" eye.

When documenting visual acuity, the examiner should note whether optical correction (e.g., eyeglasses) was used and which eye was tested. The abbreviation *OD* (oculus dexter) represents the right eye; *OS* (oculus sinister), the left eye; and *OU* (oculus uterque), both eyes. If a standard eye chart is used, the physician notes acuity by the line where most characters are read correctly. The corresponding vision (e.g., 20/20, 20/400) is documented for each eye. This notation is based on a standardized system in which a letter subtends 5 minutes of arc on the retina at a specified distance. For example, a "20/20 E" on a distance chart is designed to subtend 5 minutes of arc on the retina at a distance of 20 feet. A "20/40 E" is designed to subtend an arc of

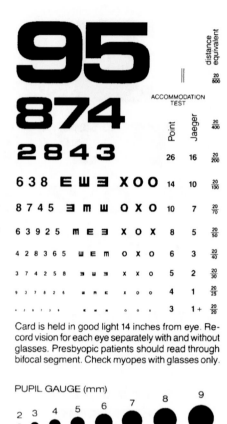

FIGURE 1–3   Snellen near acuity card.

5 minutes on the retina at 40 feet. A patient with 20/40 vision can discern at 20 feet what a patient with "normal," or 20/20, vision can discern at 40 feet. Near cards are designed for use at 14 to 16 inches, and these subtend the same distance as for the distance acuity charts. Patients older than 40 years of age may require reading glasses or bifocals to overcome *presbyopia,* the normal loss of focusing ability caused by hardening of the crystalline lens. For patients with less than 20/400 vision, the examiner can use the notations "count fingers" (CF), "hand motion" (HM), "light perception" (LP), and "no light perception" (NLP) vision.

Emmetropia, Myopia, Hyperopia, Astigmatism, and Pinhole Effect

Emmetropia is the refractive state of an eye in which parallel rays of light entering the eye are focused on the retina, creating an image that is perceived as crisp and in focus. Myopia, hyperopia, and astigmatism are abnormalities of this desired condition (Fig. 1–4). In *myopia,* or nearsightedness, the refractive power of the eye exceeds the refraction necessary for the axial length of the eye. As a result, the image is focused in front of the retina. Most commonly, this abnormality takes the form of axial myopia, in

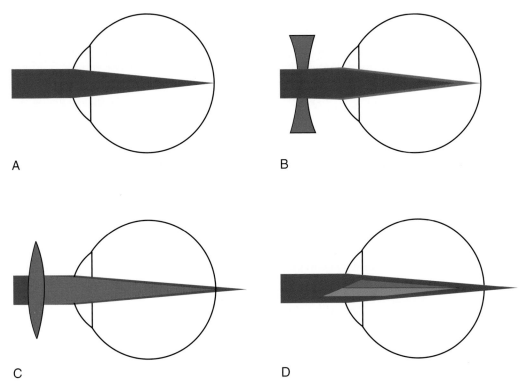

FIGURE 1–4   A, Emmetropia. Parallel light rays entering the eye are focused on the retina, providing a sharp image. **B,** Myopia. Parallel light rays entering the eye are converged anterior to the retina, and the image on the retina is perceived as blurred (*blue*). This is corrected by addition of a minus lens, which creates divergence in the rays and causes the image to focus on the retina (*red*). **C,** Hyperopia. Parallel light rays are focused posterior to the retina (*blue*). This is corrected by addition of a converging or plus lens to the eye, placing the image on the retina (*red*). **D,** Astigmatism. Parallel light rays are focused at two different planes because of unequal corneal or lenticular curvature in separate (usually perpendicular) meridians. This is corrected by addition of a cylindrical lens in the proper meridian.

which the eye is abnormally long, but other causes are an abnormally steep cornea and lens abnormalities (e.g., cataract), or a combination of these factors. Correction is obtained by placement of a "minus," or concave, lens in front of the eye, thus adding divergence to the incoming light rays and moving the focused image onto the retina.

Hyperopia, or farsightedness, is a refractive condition of the eye in which the axial length is too short, the cornea is too flat, or the lens has too little refractive power to focus the image on the retina. The image is therefore focused posterior to the retina. This condition is corrected by addition of a "plus," or convex, lens to the optical system, which provides additional convergence to the light rays entering the eye, thereby moving the image forward onto the retina.

In *astigmatism,* the refractive power of the eye in one plane (or meridian) is different from the refractive power in a different meridian. This results in essentially two focal planes from these two meridians, causing a blurred, distorted image. The disparity is corrected by placement of a cylindrical lens in front of the eye.

If the visual acuity is poor because of a refractive error, the patient's vision should improve on looking through a pinhole aperture. If a pinhole aperture is not available, a 3-inch by 5-inch card with several tiny holes (1 to 2 mm across) created with a sharp pencil may be used. Pinhole testing generally demonstrates correction of any uncorrected refractive errors. If correction is not seen, the examiner must ascertain whether a pathologic cause of decreased visual acuity such as unclear ocular media (e.g., a cataract), optic nerve disease, or retinal disease is present.

Pupils

The pupil exam is one of the most important determinants of the integrity of the anterior visual pathways. Too often the acronym PERRLA (*p*upils *e*qual, *r*ound, and *r*eactive to *l*ight and *a*ccommodation) is noted and substituted for an accurate assessment of pupil function. The first step in examining the pupils is to measure pupil size in dim light with the patient's gaze fixed on a distant object. The examiner directs a penlight at each pupil and notes the rapidity and amount of pupil constriction in each eye. *Anisocoria*, or a difference in pupil size, may be a normal finding (physiologic or essential anisocoria) but also may be a sign of ocular or neurologic disease (see Chapter 12). As a general rule, a pupil that reacts poorly to direct light is abnormal.

The relative afferent pupillary defect (RAPD), resulting in the so-called Marcus Gunn pupil, has both ocular and neurologic significance. The swinging flashlight test is an essential component of the pupillary evaluation (Fig. 1–5). In a dimly lit room, the patient fixates on a distant object. The examiner swings a penlight back and forth over the bridge of the nose and between both pupils. When the light focuses on one eye, the pupil constricts (direct response), as does the contralateral pupil because of the crossing fibers in the midbrain (consensual response). When the examiner swings

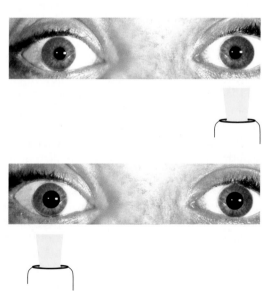

FIGURE 1–5 Right afferent pupillary defect. Stimulation of the left eye (*top*) produces bilateral pupillary constriction. Transfer of the light to the right eye (*bottom*) produces a relative dilation of the pupil in both eyes.

the light to the contralateral eye, this eye now manifests the direct response and the first eye constricts consensually. If a condition exists in one eye that markedly limits the amount of light the midbrain perceives, both direct and consensual responses are decreased, because the relative "input" to the system (the amount of light) is perceived to have decreased. In this case, shining the light in the "good" eye elicits a brisk, healthy pupillary response in both eyes. When swinging the light back and forth between the two eyes and observing the direct response of each eye, the examiner will find that the diseased eye reacts much less briskly or even dilates when the light shines in it. This reaction must not be mistaken for *hippus* (a rhythmically wavering pupil), which is a normal finding, particularly in young patients. In addition, in cases of severe bilateral disease, both eyes may react equally. In this case, no "relative" afferent pupillary defect exists.

External Examination

A general inspection of the periorbital region, eyelids, globe position, and lid margin is the next step in the ocular exam. The examiner who omits this inspection and instead proceeds to the slit lamp or fundus examination may miss key findings. For example, protrusion of the eye (known as *proptosis* or *exophthalmos*) alerts the examiner to possible orbital disease (e.g., Graves disease, orbital tumor or pseudotumor, orbital cellulitis, retrobulbar hemorrhage), and a sunken eye (known as *enophthalmos*) often is seen in fractures of the orbital floor. Both are noted during the general inspection.

The examiner inspects the conjunctiva superiorly and inferiorly and everts the upper lids for a better view of the superior cul-de-sac and examination of the superior eyelid conjunctiva. Both areas may hide a retained foreign body. To perform lid eversion, the examiner grasps the upper eyelashes, pulls the upper lid away from the globe, and uses a small, narrow object (such as an applicator stick) to press the region of the superior tarsal plate inferiorly (Fig. 1–6). The examiner also inspects the lids and especially the lid margins for any signs of disease such as erythema, crusting, lash loss, presence of chalazia, irregularity, and *ptosis* (drooping of the lids).

Motility, Position, and Extraocular Muscles

The six ocular muscles—superior, inferior, medial, and lateral recti and superior and inferior obliques—are responsible for movements of the globe (Fig. 1–7). Cranial nerve VI innervates the lateral rectus, which abducts (turns out) the eye. Cranial nerve IV innervates the superior oblique, which abducts, depresses, and intorts (rotates in) the eye. Cranial nerve III innervates the medial rectus, inferior rectus, superior rectus, and inferior oblique muscles. The medial rectus adducts (turns in) the eye, the inferior rectus depresses the eye, the superior rectus elevates the eye, and the inferior oblique abducts, elevates, and extorts (rotates out) the eye. Cranial nerve III also innervates the levator muscle, which is responsible for lid elevation. (The cardinal movements of the eye are shown in Fig. 1–8.)

The examiner must carefully note the position of the eyes and their excursions relative to each other in patients with complaints of diplopia, those with strabismus (misalignment of the eyes), and those with suspected neurologic or orbital disease. The extraocular movements involve complex coordination of frontomesencephalic and

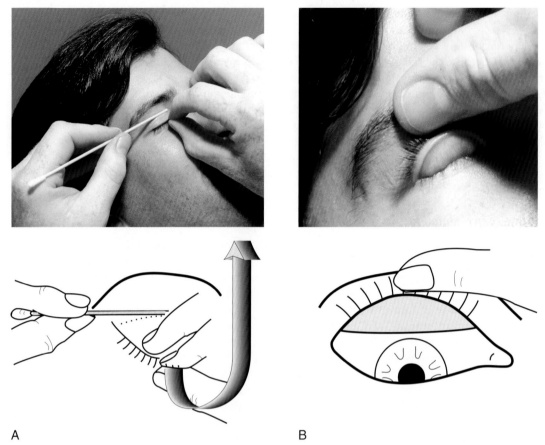

A   B

FIGURE 1–6 **A,** For eversion, the examiner places a wooden applicator stick at the superior edge of the superior tarsal plate, firmly grasps the lashes of the upper eyelid, and gently moves the applicator stick inferiorly while pulling up on the lashes slightly. **B,** The examiner removes the stick while holding the eyelid in place (often with the cotton-tipped end). Use of a topical anesthetic (proparacaine) may make this a slightly more comfortable procedure but is not essential.

cerebellomesencephalic interactions by the third, fourth, and sixth cranial nerves. Any disturbance in intracranial processing, midbrain or cranial nerve function, or intra-orbital muscle pathology may result in an ocular position imbalance. Abnormalities may be seen in the primary gaze (straight ahead) or congruity of gaze in the six cardinal positions: left, right, up and right, up and left, down and right, and down and left. The examiner can identify instances of esodeviation (as in cross-eye) or exodeviation (as in walleye) by position of the light reflex temporal to the central cornea (Fig. 1–9) or nasal to the central cornea (Fig. 1–10), respectively. A cover-uncover test can help document the presence of esodeviation, exodeviation, and hyperdeviation. In this test, the patient's gaze remains fixed on a distant object while the examiner covers and uncovers each eye. The deviated eye straightens when the normal eye is covered (opposite the direction of the original deviation). In esotropia (cross-eye), the

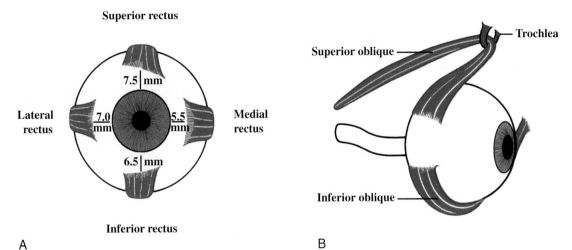

A   B

FIGURE 1–7   **A,** The four rectus muscles and their insertions into the right globe. **B,** The insertion of the oblique muscles into the right globe. The oblique muscles exert their action from the anteromedial part of the orbit. The superior oblique arises from the posterior orbit, and its tendon passes through the trochlea, the small, cartilaginous pulley on the frontal bone. The inferior oblique arises from the anteromedial orbit.

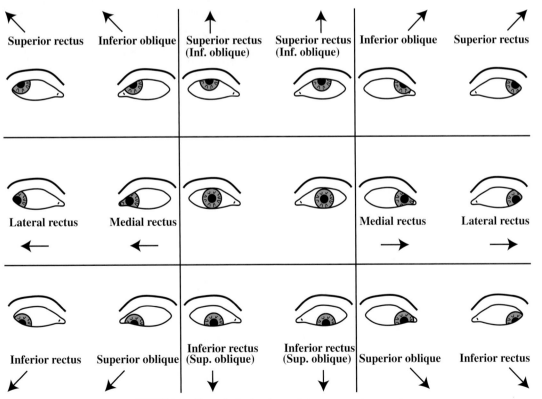

FIGURE 1–8   The principal actions of the extraocular muscles.

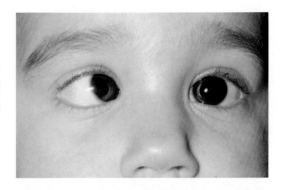

FIGURE 1–9 Esodeviation: cross-eye. Presence of esotropia (cross-eye) is most easily seen by observing the corneal light reflex differences in the two eyes. In an esotropic eye (turned in toward the nose), the corneal light reflex is temporally displaced.

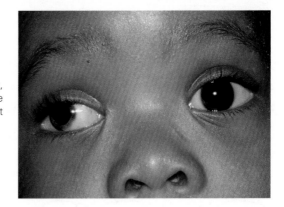

FIGURE 1–10 Exodeviation: walleye. As with esotropia, presence of exotropia (walleye) is seen by observing the corneal light reflexes. The nasal displacement of the light reflexes is diagnostic of an exodeviation.

eye moves temporally to pick up fixation when the straight, fixating eye is covered. In exotropia (walleye), the eye moves nasally when the straight, fixating contralateral eye is covered. The examiner also can identify vertical deviations using this method, with the higher eye labeled as hypertropic. Determining the origin of the motility disturbance may be challenging because the condition may be inherited, acquired, neural, muscular, or a combination of these factors.

Visual Fields

The examiner tests the integrated functioning of the separate parts of the visual system during the visual field evaluation. Defects in visual field testing can indicate injury at any point along the visual pathway from retinal damage to occipital lobe injury. Confrontation visual field testing provides gross evaluation of the integrity of the visual field. In this test, the patient covers one eye and the examiner faces the patient, positioned approximately 3 feet in front of the uncovered eye. The examiner then moves the fingers or uses a small red object to test the peripheral and central fields of each eye (Fig. 1–11). This method detects gross hemianopic defects (blindness in one half of the visual field that obeys the vertical midline) and isolated defects.

The examiner can use an Amsler grid to test the central 10 degrees of the visual field of each eye (Fig. 1–12). While the patient's gaze is fixed on the black central dot

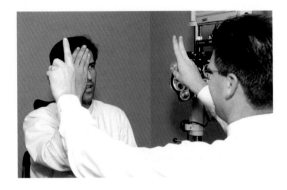

FIGURE 1–11 Confrontation visual fields. If the patient cannot see an object that is visualized in the examiner's field, a visual field defect probably is present.

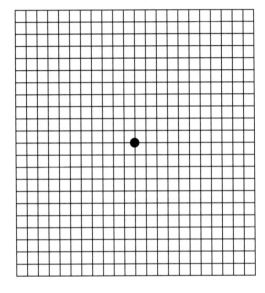

FIGURE 1–12 The Amsler grid.

of the white checkerboard, the grid is projected onto the central retina (macula). The patient maps wavy lines (metamorphopsia), blind spots (scotomata), and other irregularities in the checkerboard; these findings can help the examiner locate the disease process. In addition, Amsler grid testing can sometimes identify hemianopic defects.

Color Vision

Although formal color vision testing is not performed in the nonophthalmic setting, gross comparison of the two eyes can provide useful localizing information. Taken together, the macula and the optic nerve are essentially a color processing system. Defects in basic color sensitivity can localize disease to these anatomic locations. The most appropriate test in the primary care setting is the central red saturation-desaturation test. Using a penlight shining through the red cap of a bottle of a cycloplegic/mydriatic (dilating) agent, the examiner asks the patient to quantify the

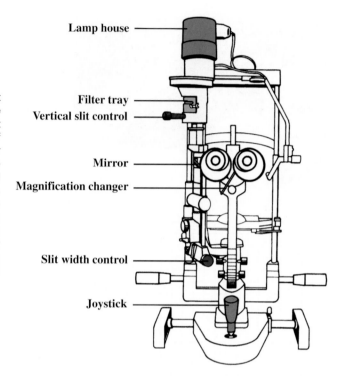

Lamp house

Filter tray
Vertical slit control

Mirror
Magnification changer

Slit width control

Joystick

FIGURE 1–13 A slit lamp and its optics. Light arising from a filament lamp in the lamp house passes through a condenser to a variable slit mechanism that allows the length and width of the slit to be altered. Below this is a tray for various filters to be inserted in the light path. The beam is directed into the eye by a mirror and focused so that the focal plane is the same as that for the viewing microscope. The angle between the illuminating beam and the viewing microscope can be varied at will. The microscope incorporates a two-stage magnification changer that alters the objective lenses without moving the focal plane. Height and focusing are altered by means of a joystick.

"degree" of redness seen by each eye. If the response indicates less than full saturation in one eye relative to that in the other, optic nerve or macular disease may be present.

Slit Lamp Examination

The anterior segment of the eye is best examined with the slit lamp biomicroscope (Fig. 1–13). This part of the examination is essential in any condition requiring an accurate and highly magnified view of the anterior and posterior segments of the eye. The patient places the chin on the chin rest and the forehead against the forehead rest. The examiner adjusts the height for comfort and for the appropriate range of excursion of the lamp, which is best accomplished by aligning the patient's eyes with the black line on the vertical pole next to the patient's face. The examiner who is wearing corrective lens or requires no correction should set the oculars (eyepieces) at zero and adjust their width to equal the examiner's interpupillary distance, such as with binoculars. With a hand on the base of the lamp, the examiner moves the chassis forward and backward and achieves fine focus with small forward-and-backward movements of the joystick. The light source is approximately 45 degrees to the patient/examiner axis, and the examiner adjusts the width of the beam from full (circular) to a very thin slit. Up-down control is on the joystick or a separate wheel, depending on the model of the slit lamp. The magnification is adjustable as well, usually beginning at low power and progressing to higher power if needed. With this setup, a thin beam can show the separate layers of the cornea and intraocular contents. The examiner must use a systematic approach to slit lamp examination, usually beginning with the eyelids and moving progressively posterior to examine the conjunctiva, cornea, anterior chamber, iris, lens, and anterior vitreous cavity.

Eyelids. The examiner inspects lid margins for lacerations, eversion (ectropion), inversion (entropion), abnormal lash growth toward the cornea (trichiasis), chalazia, meibomian gland dysfunction, and lash loss.

Conjunctiva. The examiner evaluates the conjunctiva for discharge, follicles, fluid accumulation (chemosis), and hyperemia. Conjunctival lacerations must be carefully examined to discover whether the underlying sclera also is injured. The slit lamp greatly facilitates foreign body removal, usually accomplished with use of topical anesthesia and a moistened cotton swab (see Chapter 16). For patients with foreign body sensation or corneal abrasions, eversion of the upper lid under slit lamp examination, although more difficult to achieve than on the external examination, allows a magnified view of the superior lid (tarsal) conjunctiva and cul-de-sac. Often a tiny foreign body can be found embedded in the conjunctiva in this location.

Cornea. The examiner inspects the epithelium for abrasions, edema, ulcers, and foreign bodies. A single drop of fluorescein stains areas of denuded epithelium. Once rotated into position, the cobalt blue filter highlights the stained areas. Tiny dots of green across the corneal surface signify punctate epithelial keratopathy (PEK), an indicator of diffuse epithelial disease (e.g., dry eyes, toxic epitheliopathy). Large areas of intense green staining indicate abrasions. The examiner evaluates the stroma for scars, edema (thickening), and foreign bodies. Keratic precipitates (collections of white blood cells and macrophages) on the endothelium, which is the internal layer of the cornea, are a hallmark of iritis and are easily seen with the slit lamp. The examiner also may find pigment and adhesions of iris to the cornea (anterior synechiae) in eyes subjected to prior trauma or surgery.

Anterior Chamber. The anterior chamber is an aqueous-filled chamber bounded by the iris posteriorly and the corneal endothelium anteriorly. The slit beam can identify inflammatory cells floating in the aqueous and flare (light scatter caused by inflammatory proteins in the aqueous) in iritis. Red or white blood cells may be present in the anterior chamber. Red blood cells usually originate from bleeding due to trauma, and the layering of these cells in the anterior chamber is a hyphema. The layering of white cells in iritis or infection is a hypopyon.

Iris and Lens. In the iris and lens exam, the examiner notes any pupil abnormalities, which may include traumatic tears in the iris sphincter and adhesions of the iris to the anterior lens capsule (posterior synechiae). The iris may plug corneal lacerations or be torn at its insertion (iridodialysis). Very few blood vessels normally are seen on the iris, and none usually are visible at the pupillary margin. Any fine blood vessels seen at the pupillary margin (rubeosis iridis) should prompt referral for ophthalmologic evaluation for possible neovascularization from retinal or ocular ischemic processes requiring treatment (e.g., proliferative diabetic retinopathy). Opacities of the lens (i.e., cataract) may result from aging or a number of secondary causes, including injury to the capsule of the lens in penetrating trauma, which causes the lens to hydrate rapidly and become densely white (mature cataract).

Vitreous. While the eye is dilated, the examiner focuses the slit beam posterior to the lens into the anterior vitreous. In inflammatory conditions involving the posterior segment of the eye, the examiner will note a cellular reaction in the vitreous, much like the cells seen in the anterior chamber in iritis. Vitreous hemorrhage is the presence of numerous red blood cells in the vitreous cavity and is the result of a break of a blood vessel.

Intraocular Pressure

Measurement of IOP in assessment of the eye is analogous to measurement of blood pressure in assessment of the cardiovascular system. Normal values are 8 to 21 mm Hg but may range anywhere from 0 (in cases of ruptured globe, hypotony after glaucoma surgery, and severe intraocular inflammation) to 70 or 80 mm Hg (in cases of angle-closure glaucoma). IOP may be measured by several different methods.

Applanation Tonometry. The applanation tonometer is accurate and easy to use; it can be found on most slit lamps. The Perkins tonometer is a handheld applanation model for patients unable to move into the proper position at the slit lamp (e.g., those in wheelchairs or stretchers, small children). To perform applanation tonometry, the examiner instills a drop of anesthetic (proparacaine) and a drop of fluorescein dye in the eye and sets the applanation tension at midrange, approximately 15 to 20 mm Hg. The examiner gently holds the eyelids open, taking care to not put any pressure on the globe while holding the lids. Even negligible pressure from the examiner's fingers resting on the globe can cause a significant increase in IOP. The examiner rotates the cobalt blue filter into place and turns up the light intensity. The light is directed at the tonometer tip, which also is rotated into position, and the examiner moves the tonometer directly in front of the patient's cornea. The examiner instructs the patient to open both eyes wide and slowly moves the tonometer forward until it gently touches the cornea (Fig. 1–14). Because of the prismatic effect of the tonometer tip,

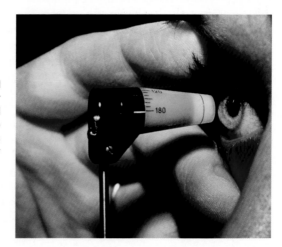

FIGURE 1–14 Applanation tonometry. The tonometer head has an area such that the surface tension force of the tear film and the elastic tension within the cornea are equal and cancel each other. The prismatic doubling head of the applanator splits the tear meniscus into two identifiable mires for measurement of the intraocular pressure when gently touched to a patient's cornea.

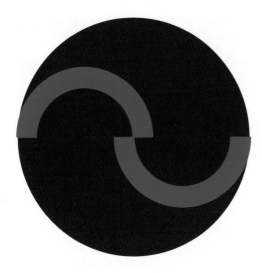

FIGURE 1–15 Tonometric mires. The fluorescein rings just overlap, producing the end point at which intraocular pressure is measured.

two green half circles are seen when the tonometer tip is fully applanated (Fig. 1–15). These shapes are known as *tonometric mires* and shift in relation to each other as the tonometer scale is rotated. The goal is to align the mires so that the inside edge of one just touches the inside edge of the other. At this point the examiner reads the IOP from the scale. The scale is marked in centimeters of mercury; for conversion to millimeters of mercury (standard notation), the scale reading is multiplied by 10.

Tonometer Pens. A tonometer pen (e.g., Tono-Pen) is an electronic device that is very easy to use and relatively accurate (Fig. 1–16). The accuracy diminishes as the pressure moves farther outside the normal range. Drawbacks include expense and fragility of the pens, but these devices are extremely effective for determining the IOP in emergency situations.

Manual Assessment. Manual assessment provides only a crude measure and is extremely inaccurate when performed by nonophthalmologists. The examiner palpates the globe through closed lids using a gentle ballotting motion and compares the eyes. The examiner's eye may be used as a control. Although providing only a gross estimate of IOP, manual assessment can be extremely useful in cases such as the evaluation of a red eye that is thought to represent angle-closure glaucoma. The involved eye will be markedly firm to palpation when compared with the fellow eye. Use of this method should be avoided in recently operated eyes or in cases of a suspected ruptured globe.

Funduscopic Evaluation

A direct ophthalmoscope is invaluable for the primary care physician. The light source is bright enough to evaluate the pupils, a cobalt blue filter often is built into the instrument for use with fluorescein staining of the cornea, and the instrument allows an excellent evaluation of the fundus. If an abnormality in the posterior pole is suspected, the eyes may be dilated.

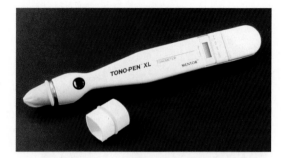

FIGURE 1–16   A handheld tonometry pen (Tono-Pen).

The physician should instill a weak mydriatic agent after vision assessment and pupillary exam. Tropicamide 0.5% or 1% and phenylephrine 2.5% are good choices; with both, effects are reversed in 4 to 6 hours. Atropine drops should not be used because they produce dilation for as long as 1 to 2 weeks. Pupillary dilation causing an attack of angle-closure glaucoma is extremely uncommon. A simple test to determine relative safety in dilation involves shining a penlight parallel to the iris at the temporal corneal limbus (see Fig. 11–5). If the anterior chamber is deep, the light reflex will be seen across the cornea to the nasal side. If the iris is bowed forward significantly, the light reflex will be obstructed by the "mound," thus blocking the transmission of light to the nasal side of the cornea. In this instance, the patient should be referred to an ophthalmologist for pupillary dilation and examination when necessary. It is imperative that whenever dilating agents are instilled in the eyes, clear documentation in the patient's record, including the agent and the time of instillation, must be performed.

Documenting the time of dilation and the agents used for dilation in the chart is an important step. Even in undilated eyes, examination with the direct ophthalmoscope can give useful information pertaining to the clarity of the ocular media and refractive error. A diminished red reflex or irregularities in the red reflex may result from cloudy media (e.g., corneal or lens opacities, vitreous blood) and unusual refractive errors. The −3 to −4 diopter lens on the ophthalmoscope (the red 3 or 4) usually generates a comfortable view of the fundus. If the examiner has difficulty seeing the fundus, different lenses may be rotated into position until a clear image appears. The direct ophthalmoscope evaluates the optic nerve head, retinal vessels, and macula. For examination of the periphery, use of an indirect ophthalmoscope, necessitating the expertise of an ophthalmologist, is indicated (Fig. 1–17).

The examiner's right eye is used to assess the patient's right eye, and the examiner's left eye assesses the patient's left eye. The optic nerve head is most easily seen by having the patient look straight ahead and approaching with the ophthalmoscope from a slightly temporal angle. The examiner looks for abnormalities in shape and color. The margins should be sharp and vessels crisp as they cross the edge of the disc. If this is not seen, the disc may be edematous. The examiner notes any hemorrhages or infarctions of the nerve fiber layer ("cotton-wool spots") near the nerve head. Pallor of the nerves (resulting from optic atrophy) may indicate an old optic neuropathy and should be evaluated by an ophthalmologist. Increased intracranial pressure

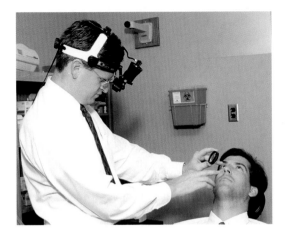

FIGURE 1-17 Indirect ophthalmoscopy. The examiner views the retina through a handheld lens that is coaxial with the headset loupes and light source. This provides an exceptional view of the entire retina.

(papilledema) is one cause of disc edema. Marked or asymmetrical cupping of the nerve is a possible sign of glaucoma.

The best view of the macula is obtained when the patient looks directly at the examining light. (The macula is examined last because of the patient's light sensitivity.) A small reflex of light seen hovering directly over the fovea (the foveal light reflex) is one indicator of normal foveal anatomy. Hemorrhage, exudates, microaneurysms, and areas of edema are findings in microvascular disease. The examiner should note whether these signs are localized to one area of the retina (as in a vascular occlusion), are diffusely scattered throughout one retina (as in ocular ischemia or radiation retinopathy), or constitute generalized findings in both eyes (as in systemic diseases such as diabetes and hypertension). The depth of hemorrhage is difficult to determine; however, deep hemorrhages tend to be small and irregular ("dot and blot" hemorrhages), whereas superficial hemorrhages follow the nerve fiber layer and are flame shaped. Retinal edema gives the retina a grayish appearance and also is present in areas of vascular occlusion. In central retinal artery occlusions and conditions in which the nerve fiber layer is thickened, a red spot (the cherry-red spot) usually is present in the central macular region. This phenomenon occurs as the normal choroidal blood flow is viewed through the fovea centralis, the only area of the retina lacking ganglion cells and a nerve fiber layer. Cherry-red spots also occur in metabolic storage diseases (e.g., Tay-Sachs disease) as a result of accumulation in the retina of the products of abnormal enzyme pathways.

Evaluation of the retinal circulation is difficult with the direct ophthalmoscope, but dilation of the pupil facilitates observation of the vessels. Venous occlusions have associated retinal hemorrhages, exudates, and retinal thickening from edema. Arteriovenous nicking is present in hypertensive retinopathy. In atherosclerotic disease (especially carotid disease), cholesterol emboli may lodge in the retinal arterioles at their bifurcations and are therefore noticeable on ophthalmoscopic examination. These small, sometimes white or refractile bodies in the lumen of the vessels are known as *Hollenhorst plaques*.

Additional Diagnostic Tests

Gonioscopy

In the anterior chamber angle of the eye, aqueous drains from the anterior chamber. This area is not accessible for viewing on routine slit lamp examination because of the optical properties of the cornea. A magnified view of the anterior chamber angle can be obtained using a slit lamp and a contact gonioscopic lens (along with a topical anesthetic such as proparacaine). Goldmann and Zeiss lenses are equipped with periscopic mirrors through which the angle is examined with reflected light (Fig. 1–18). Gonioscopy is useful in differentiating various forms of glaucoma (e.g., open angle, narrow angle, closed angle, neovascular, angle recession) and for viewing pathologic conditions in the angle (e.g., peripheral iris anomalies, tumors, foreign bodies, traumatic injury to the angle).

Tear Function Test

The Schirmer tear test performed with and without anesthesia evaluates tear adequacy and often aids in the diagnosis of dry eye syndrome. The Schirmer test performed without anesthesia measures basal tear secretion and reflex tear secretion. The Schirmer test performed with anesthesia measures basal tear secretion only by eliminating the irritation that causes reflex tearing. To perform the test, the examiner first dries the inferior cul-de-sac with a cotton swab and places one end of Whatman 41 filter paper strips (5 mm by 30 mm) over the lateral third of the lower lid (Fig. 1–19). The patient may continue blinking normally or keep the eyes closed. After 5 minutes, the examiner removes the strips and measures the length of strip wetted by tears. Without anesthesia, wetting of less than 15 mm of a Schirmer strip indicates dry eyes. With anesthesia, the interpretation is as follows: 0 to 5 mm of wetting, severe dry eyes; 5 to 10 mm of wetting, moderately dry eyes; 10 to 15 mm of wetting, mildly dry eyes; and greater than 15 mm of wetting, normal tear function.

Primary Dye Test

The primary dye test evaluates tear drainage function (e.g., patency of puncta, canaliculi, lacrimal sac, nasolacrimal duct). The examiner instills fluorescein dye into the lower cul-de-sac and places a small, cotton-tipped applicator approximately 3.5 to

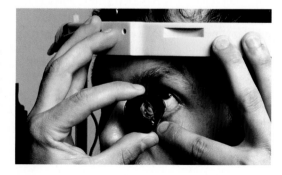

FIGURE 1–18 Gonioscopy. A Goldmann gonioscope lens being placed on the patient's eye. The indirect gonioscope lens is a solid contact lens within which a small mirror is mounted, allowing the anterior chamber angle structures to be easily viewed. The full circumference of the angle may be viewed with 360-degree rotation of the lens.

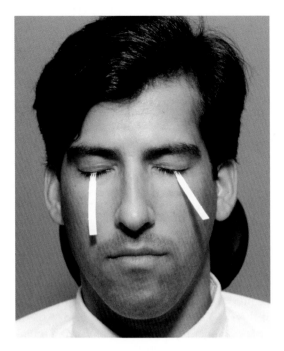

FIGURE 1–19 Schirmer tear test. Patients may keep eyes open or closed.

4 cm into the nose under the inferior meatus. After 2 minutes, the examiner removes the cotton swab. If the swab is stained with fluorescein, the system is patent. If no dye is present, either the cotton tip was in the wrong position or the system is blocked at some point.

A shortcut to this test is the "dye disappearance test," which grossly evaluates the patency of the nasolacrimal system. The examiner instills a single drop of fluorescein in each eye. If one eye retains fluorescein dye after 3 to 5 minutes while the other eye clears, asymmetry of nasolacrimal drainage is indicated.

Exophthalmometry

A Hertel exophthalmometer measures the amount of anterior protrusion of the globes (Fig. 1–20). The examiner faces the patient, palpates the patient's lateral orbital rims, places the concave sites on the side of the Hertel instrument over each rim, and records the base (or distance between these two points) from the instrument. This measurement is the baseline for accurately assessing the degree of protrusion in future examinations. For example, in Graves disease and with orbital tumors, this measurement changes with progression of the disorder. The examiner observes the mirror on the side of the patient's right eye while the patient keeps the gaze of that eye fixed on the examiner's left eye or left ear. The front of the cornea lines up with the scale, and the distance is in millimeters. The process is repeated for the left eye looking at the examiner's right eye or ear. Normal range is 12 to 20 mm, and no asymmetry greater than 2 mm should be seen.

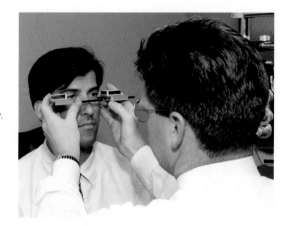

FIGURE 1–20 Hertel exophthalmometry.

Perimetry

The next step in evaluating abnormal confrontation visual field findings, perimetry provides a more accurate assessment of the extent of a patient's visual field. Kinetic testing (Goldmann perimetry) involves the examiner moving a light of varying intensity from areas outside the visual field toward fixation, with the patient responding when the light is seen. Automated or static perimetry is computerized and involves variable intensity lights that are flashed at different locations in the visual field. The patient again acknowledges each time the light is seen. A printout of this assessment of the visual field is obtained for each time the test is performed, which enables the clinician to monitor the disease state (Fig. 1–21).

Eye Patching

When the eye patch is properly applied, patching helps promote epithelial wound healing (Fig. 1–22). Usually an antibiotic ointment such as erythromycin or polymyxin B/bacitracin (e.g., Polysporin) is instilled before patching. The lids must be closed, and the patch must be snug enough to keep the lids from opening underneath the patch, thereby causing an iatrogenic corneal abrasion. Indiscriminate patching may be harmful, especially in cases of possible infection, because a warm, protected environment under a patched lid can facilitate bacterial growth (e.g., with contact lens–related corneal injury). Some researchers advocate patching in patients with extremely large abrasions only.

Eyedrops

When dilated pupils are seen in patients in the emergency room setting, pharmacologic agents often are the cause. Transdermal patches (e.g., scopolamine) and aerosolized medications (e.g., albuterol) are possible offending agents, and the patient may not realize their effects. Instillation or ingestion of ophthalmic medications belonging to other family members (e.g., Visine, Vasocon) also can result in dilated

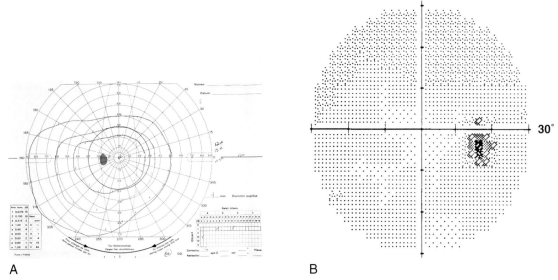

FIGURE 1–21 **Formal perimetry testing (visual fields). A,** Normal Goldmann visual field. **B,** Normal Humphrey visual field.

pupils. "Red-top" ocular medications are mydriatic and cycloplegic agents (i.e., they dilate and block accommodation).

Used chronically, gentamicin ophthalmic drops and ointments are quite toxic to the corneal epithelium. Neomycin ophthalmic drops and ointments can cause an allergic reaction in up to 10% of patients receiving these agents. Better choices for routine broad-spectrum antibiotic coverage are fluoroquinolones (e.g., ciprofloxacin [Ciloxan], ofloxacin [Ocuflox], gatifloxacin [Zymar], moxifloxacin [Vigamox]), polymyxin B/trimethoprim (Polytrim), and sulfacetamide drops or erythromycin and polymyxin B/bacitracin (e.g., Polysporin) ointments. These agents are much less damaging to the cornea and therefore more appropriate for routine coverage when epithelial regrowth is desired (e.g., in cases of corneal abrasion).

Examiners should *never* prescribe or hand a bottle of topical anesthetic drops to the patient and must always keep track of the bottle after instilling the drops into the patient's uncomfortable eye. Patients often want to keep the bottle of the "good drops" and will steal it without the examiner's knowledge. Topical anesthetic abuse can lead to more serious injury of the eye (because of the anesthesia) and also retards wound healing as a toxic effect.

Frequency of Examination

How often should patients have their eyes examined? The primary care physician must take an active role in reminding patients to schedule periodic ophthalmologic exams; this often is the only way to identify potentially serious eye disease (e.g., glaucoma, macular degeneration, diabetic retinopathy). Patients with ocular complaints should be examined and the underlying disorder treated as outlined previously. Those without

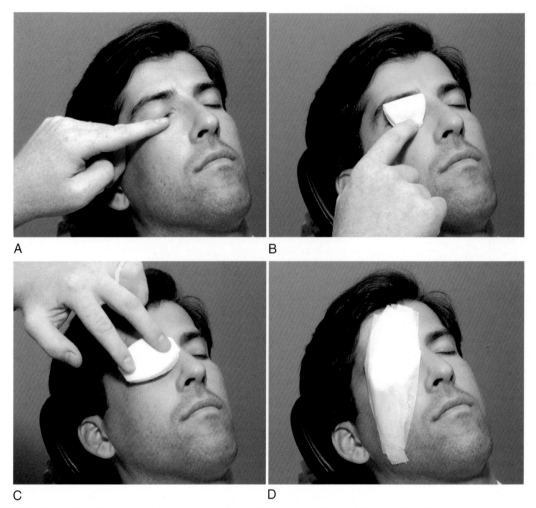

FIGURE 1–22   Application of a pressure patch. A, The patient closes both eyes; the examiner must ensure good closure of the eyelids. **B,** The examiner applies an eye pad to the closed eyelids, either lengthwise or folded in half (*shown*). **C,** The examiner places a second patch lengthwise over the first patch. **D,** Finally, the examiner secures the patches with tape placed from the center of the forehead to the angle of the jaw across the patched eye. Usually, an antibiotic ointment is applied before patching, and the patient's progress should be monitored daily.

symptoms but with risk factors for the development of eye problems (e.g., patients taking certain medications, especially corticosteroids and hydroxychloroquine [Plaquenil]; those with diabetes mellitus; those with a family history of glaucoma, cataracts, strabismus, or retinal detachments or any familial eye condition; patients older than 65 years of age) should be examined regularly, depending on their age.

Newborns. All newborns should have a general screening exam while in the nursery. High-risk characteristics for ocular disease in newborns include maternal rubella, vene-real or acquired immunodeficiency syndrome (AIDS)-related infections, and a family history of retinoblastoma, metabolic or genetic disease, or congenital eye disorders. Screening for retinopathy of prematurity is needed for newborns weighing 1500 g or less, selected infants whose birthweights are between 1500 g and 2000 g and who have an unstable clinical course, and those with a gestational age of 32 weeks or less.

Preschool Children. Every child should receive a screening ocular examination by $3\frac{1}{2}$ years of age. *Amblyopia* is the most common ocular problem among preschool children; this is the failure of the visual system to develop in one or both eyes because the brain receives a blurred or distorted image. The underlying cause often is a large asymmetry in refractive error between the two eyes, cataract formation in one eye, or strabismus (misalignment of the eyes). Diminished visual acuity in a young child warrants an ophthalmic search for these disorders.

School-Aged Children. Children who have no evidence of ocular disease or special risk factors for disease should be seen at a frequency determined by the ophthalmologist. In general, every 2 to 3 years is the preferred interval.

Adults. The frequency of significant eye disease in the adult population younger than 35 years of age is low. A routine glaucoma evaluation at age 35 is advisable for normal patients. Periodic reevaluation should be performed approximately every 2 to 5 years for normal adults. Patients at special risk for eye disease should undergo examination at intervals determined by an ophthalmologist. Patients with diabetes generally are seen at diagnosis and annually thereafter. Patients at risk for glaucoma are seen annually. Adults 65 years of age and older should be examined every 2 years.

Once the patient gains access to ophthalmologic care, regular follow-up examinations are arranged. The primary care provider can play a crucial role in helping reduce the incidence of serious eye disease by reminding patients of the need for periodic evaluations and promptly referring any patient at risk for the development of ocular problems.

CHAPTER 2

Ophthalmic Differential Diagnosis

DAVID A. PALAY

This chapter presents an overview of the common symptoms and signs associated with ocular disorders. More in-depth discussion of specific topics can be found in relevant chapters of this book. Here, clinical "pearls" are provided to quickly guide the reader to the appropriate diagnosis.

Symptoms

Visual Loss

Visual loss is a common symptom of ophthalmic conditions. The patient's subjective description of visual loss, however, often correlates poorly with the examiner's objective measurements. Some patients with profound visual loss contact the physician long after the onset of symptoms, and their subjective complaints may be relatively minor. By contrast, patients with relatively minor objective visual loss may seek medical attention immediately after the onset of symptoms and overstate complaints. Because of this disparity between reported symptoms and clinical findings, obtaining an accurate visual acuity measurement in each eye is essential. The physician should perform confrontational visual field tests, because substantial field loss can be present with normal visual acuity. Patients with hemianopic defects (blindness in one half of the visual field) often relate the disease to the eye on the side of the defect rather than the true abnormality of the right or left hemifield. Finally, the physician should evaluate color vision, because its loss is specific for central retinal or optic nerve dysfunction.

More recent visual loss requires more urgent evaluation, so the physician should determine the duration of the visual loss. Bilateral visual field loss that respects the vertical meridian is almost always associated with cerebral lesions including or posterior to the optic chiasm. Uniocular visual field loss results from direct involvement of the eye or optic nerve anterior to the optic chiasm. Patients sometimes mistake uniocular disease for binocular disease. For example, if a patient has unrecognized poor vision in one eye caused by a chronic disease and the contralateral eye is unaffected, a loss of vision in the good eye is sometimes interpreted as acute visual loss in both eyes.

Acute, Painless Loss of Vision. In cases of acute, painless loss of vision, no injection of the conjunctiva occurs. The following listing provides information on these types of disorders.

ADDITIONAL HISTORY	KEY EXAM FEATURES
Vitreous Hemorrhage	
Patients report the sensation of "spider webs" clouding the vision or the recent onset of floaters. Associated systemic diseases include diabetes, sickle cell anemia, and coagulopathy due to medical condition or anticoagulant drugs.	If the vitreous hemorrhage is extensive, decreased red reflex and poor visualization of the retina are found. Mild vitreous hemorrhages may be difficult to see with the direct ophthalmoscope.
Retinal Detachment	
Retinal detachment commonly occurs in highly myopic persons or may occur after eye surgery or trauma. The onset may be preceded by acute symptoms of flashes or floaters. Patients report a loss of visual field or describe a "curtain" covering part of their vision.	Detachment may be difficult to recognize with the direct ophthalmoscope. Indirect ophthalmoscopic evaluation is indicated.
Retinal Artery Occlusion	
Occlusion is caused by emboli and may be associated with carotid artery disease and valvular heart disease. It may be associated with previous episodes of interference with the vision by a "cloud" that eventually clears (amaurosis fugax). The visual loss is abrupt and almost complete.	With central retinal artery occlusion, vision often is limited to hand motions or light perception. Emboli may be visualized in the retinal arterioles. With central retinal artery occlusion, findings include diffuse retinal whitening and a cherry-red spot in the macula.
Retinal Vein Occlusion	
Occlusion is most commonly associated with hypertension and rarely with blood dyscrasias.	Occlusion results from a thrombosis of the retinal veins. Ophthalmoscopic findings include numerous retinal hemorrhages and occasional "cotton-wool spots." The veins are tortuous and dilated.
Exudative Macular Degeneration	
Macular degeneration usually occurs in older individuals (over the age of 60 years) and may progressively worsen over several days. It is associated with an abnormal distortion of straight lines (metamorphopsia).	Retinal hemorrhage is noted in the macular region.

ADDITIONAL HISTORY	KEY EXAM FEATURES

Ischemic Optic Neuropathy

Visual loss usually is sudden. The disorder often is associated with giant cell arteritis (arteritic anterior ischemic optic neuropathy), and patients may have symptoms of jaw claudication, scalp tenderness, neck pain, and weight loss (age usually 60 years or older). Nonarteritic anterior ischemic optic neuropathy occurs in a younger age group (40 years of age and older) and often is associated with hypertension and/or diabetes.

An afferent pupillary defect is present. The optic nerve head is swollen on ophthalmoscopic examination.

Optic Neuritis

Visual loss usually occurs over several days. Pain with eye movement may be present. The disorder usually is associated with multiple sclerosis (in patients 15 to 45 years of age).

An afferent pupillary defect is present. Two thirds of patients have a normal optic disc; one third have optic disc edema.

Cerebral Infarct

A history of previous vascular disease or strokes may be reported.

A bilateral loss of visual field usually occurs. If the infarct involves the occipital lobe, visual acuity may be reduced. Ocular examination findings are normal.

Functional Visual Loss

A history of recent stress or earlier psychologic problems is usually reported.

Examination findings are normal.

Acute, Painful Loss of Vision. The following group of disorders cause acute visual loss and are associated with severe pain. In addition, marked injection of the conjunctiva often occurs as a result of ocular inflammation.

ADDITIONAL HISTORY	KEY EXAM FEATURES

Corneal Ulcer

A history of recent trauma or contact lens wear usually is reported. Sleeping in contact lenses greatly increases the risk of developing an infectious corneal ulcer.

The penlight exam may show a corneal abrasion, but an early corneal infiltrate can be difficult to identify. As the infection progresses, a white infiltrate is seen in the cornea. With extensive infections, a layering of white cells may be seen in the anterior chamber (hypopyon).

Recurrent Erosion Syndrome

A history of sudden onset of severe eye pain, blurred vision, and redness, occurring in the middle of the night or on awakening, is typical.

Exam shows a corneal abrasion that stains with fluorescein.

Uveitis

The origin of uveitis often is idiopathic. Common systemic associations include sarcoidosis, syphilis, tuberculosis, and human leukocyte antigen HLA-B27–associated disorders (e.g., Reiter syndrome, ankylosing spondylitis, inflammatory bowel disease, psoriasis). A history of sensitivity to light also is noted.

The pupil may be small, sluggish, or nonreactive to light. A circular injection of the eye surrounding the cornea (circumlimbal flush) is seen. The red reflex may be diminished, particularly with corneal edema and vitreous inflammation. Uveitis usually is unilateral but may affect both eyes.

Acute Angle-Closure Glaucoma

Acute angle-closure glaucoma usually occurs in older persons and more commonly in those who are farsighted. It may be precipitated by an advancing cataract. A full-blown attack may be preceded by a history of blurred vision, halos around lights, and pain precipitated by dark conditions (e.g., after being in a movie theater). Markedly elevated intraocular pressure can cause a headache and nausea and vomiting. Systemic symptoms may be out of proportion to visual symptoms, so patients can be misdiagnosed.

In its acute form, it is always unilateral. The eye is red, and the pupil is mid-dilated and nonreactive. Vision usually is diminished initially because of corneal edema, but it may be subsequently diminished by optic nerve damage from prolonged elevated intraocular pressure. Intraocular pressure usually is elevated to levels above 50 mm Hg.

Endophthalmitis

Most cases of endophthalmitis are associated with recent eye surgery. Rarely, endophthalmitis (e.g., fungal endophthalmitis) may develop from another source of infection in the body.

In addition to markedly decreased vision and injection of the eye, a mucopurulent discharge may be present. A layering of white cells in the anterior chamber (hypopyon) is common. The red reflex is diminished because of vitreous inflammation. In fungal endophthalmitis, findings on the anterior segment exam may be entirely normal.

Chronic, Progressive Loss of Vision.   The following disorders may cause chronic, progressive loss of vision.

ADDITIONAL HISTORY	KEY EXAM FEATURES

Refractive Error

The patient may already wear contacts or glasses.

The visual acuity is near normal when the patient looks through a pinhole.

Cataract

Cataract is one of the most common causes of chronic, progressive visual loss and may be associated with a family history of cataracts, diabetes, or chronic corticosteroid use. Patients may complain of multiple images when looking with only one eye. As the cataract progresses, objects become blurred, and distinguishing objects up close and at a distance is difficult.

The visual acuity may be slightly improved with the pinhole. Pupil responses are normal. The normal red reflex is diminished, and visualizing the fundus with a direct ophthalmoscope can be difficult.

Open-Angle Glaucoma

Open-angle glaucoma is more common in patients with a family history of glaucoma, nearsighted patients, patients with diabetes, and African American patients. Visual acuity may remain normal until very late in the disease process, so patients with severe glaucoma may be relatively asymptomatic.

Elevated intraocular pressure of 22 mm Hg or greater and increased optic nerve cupping of 0.6 or greater are significant.

Atrophic Macular Degeneration

Atrophic macular degeneration usually is seen in patients older than age 60 years. It may be associated with a family history of macular degeneration.

With early disease, multiple hyaline nodules (drusen) are seen in the fundus. With advancing disease, retinal atrophy occurs, leaving a large scar or an atrophic area in the central macula.

Brain Tumor

Manifestations may include headache, nausea on awakening, and variable neurologic symptoms and signs.

The pattern of visual field loss varies with the location of the tumor. Tumors posterior to the optic nerve chiasm do not produce optic nerve atrophy or afferent pupillary defects. Tumors involving the chiasm or intrinsic to the optic nerve produce afferent pupillary defects and optic nerve atrophy.

Distorted Vision (Metamorphopsia)

Metamorphopsia is the perception that straight lines are distorted or bowed. This abnormality usually results from macular dysfunction and can be tested for with an Amsler grid (see Fig. 1–12). Conditions that elevate the retina (fluid under the retina), such as exudative macular degeneration, cause the lines on an Amsler grid to bow in (micropsia). By contrast, conditions that cause contraction of the retina, such as an epiretinal membrane, cause bowing out of the lines (macropsia).

Transient Visual Loss

A common patient complaint is vision that tends to fluctuate when the eyes blink. This fluctuation commonly results from a poor tear film on the ocular surface, with dry eyes as the causative factor. Blinking reestablishes the tear film momentarily and can lead to a sudden improvement in vision that deteriorates as the tear film dissipates. Excessive mucus production from dry eyes also may cloud the vision. Fluctuation in vision may be associated with new-onset diabetes. Elevations in blood glucose level cause swelling of the lens and progressive nearsightedness.

As patients pass the age of 40 years, they have more difficulty accommodating and focusing on near objects. Alterations in distance also may be difficult, such as in suddenly changing focus from close objects to far objects and vice versa. This condition is termed *presbyopia*.

Temporary interference with ocular blood flow by an embolus to the retinal circulation may cause the sensation that a curtain or cloud has come over the vision. This disturbance is termed *amaurosis fugax*. If the embolus does not clear, a central or branch retinal artery occlusion occurs. An impending thrombosis of the central retinal or a branch retinal vein can cause transient visual loss. Carotid artery or vertebrobasilar insufficiency also can cause transient visual symptoms that may be associated with movements in the neck. Papilledema caused by increased intracranial pressure may result in transient bilateral visual loss lasting a few seconds. Many systemic medications can cause transient visual symptoms, particularly those with hypotension as a possible side effect.

Night Blindness

The examiner must distinguish a patient's decreased ability to function in the dark from true night blindness. Young patients with uncorrected myopia often complain of decreased ability to function, particularly when driving at night. Commonly, they are unable to see street signs until they are close to the signs. This problem usually can be corrected with eyeglasses. Similarly, patients with cataracts may complain of difficulty driving at night because of excessive glare and visual distortion. True night blindness can occur with retinitis pigmentosa, vitamin A deficiency, and systemic medications such as phenothiazines. Patients with true night blindness have difficulty seeing any stars in the sky on a clear night and may be unable to ambulate without assistance in a dark environment such as a movie theater.

Flashes

The sudden onset of flashes in the peripheral visual field suggests traction of the vitreous on the peripheral retina. This phenomenon may occur during the evolution of a posterior vitreous detachment or as the vitreous pulls on a tear in the retina. Retinal tears and detachments are more common in highly myopic persons and patients who have undergone intraocular surgery. The flashes may be more pronounced in the dark and especially apparent with rapid eye movement. In addition, retinal flashes may be associated with the sudden onset of floaters, which can indicate debris or blood in the vitreous cavity. Because a tear in the retina can lead to a retinal detachment, urgent consultation with an ophthalmologist is required.

A second type of flashing light can occur with a migraine. These flashes have a distinctive quality and often are described as scintillations or zigzagging lights that march across the visual field. They may last a few minutes or as long as 30 minutes and can be associated with transient visual field loss. Headache may not follow the visual symptoms, and the patient may have a prior history of migraines without any visual symptoms. Often a family history of migraines or a history of carsickness as a child is reported. Hormonal changes such as with pregnancy, menopause, use of birth control pills, and the menstrual cycle may trigger an attack, as can stress and alcohol use.

Floaters

Many patients report seeing floaters, particularly when they look at a bright, white background or into the blue sky. These floaters are caused by small aggregates in the vitreous cavity, which result from a normal aging process of the vitreous (syneresis). The acute onset of vitreous floaters may be associated with uveitis affecting the vitreous cavity or the sudden onset of bleeding in the vitreous cavity. Disorders associated with vitreous hemorrhage include diabetes and sickle cell anemia. The acute onset of floaters, particularly if associated with flashing lights, may be a sign of a posterior vitreous detachment or a retinal tear with an impending retinal detachment. Therefore urgent ophthalmic referral for indirect ophthalmoscopy is essential. Detection of a retinal tear with direct ophthalmoscopy is almost impossible; most tears occur in the peripheral retina.

Photophobia

Photophobia, particularly if associated with eye pain, redness, and decreased vision, is a symptom of uveitis. The same symptoms may occur 3 or 4 days after an acute ocular injury as a result of traumatic iritis. Photophobia and increased sensitivity to loud noises can be associated with an acute migraine. Meningeal irritation also may cause photophobia.

Halos around Lights

Cataracts commonly cause patients to see halos around lights, particularly when they are driving at night. Episodic decreased vision, redness, and halos around lights may be symptoms of impending angle-closure glaucoma. Conditions that cause corneal edema also can result in halos. Halos can occur as a complication of LASIK eye surgery.

Double Vision (Diplopia)

The examiner must distinguish monocular from binocular diplopia. Binocular diplopia results from a misalignment of the eyes: When one eye fixates on a target, the other eye sees the image slightly displaced from the image in the fixating eye. For this reason, binocular diplopia disappears when either eye is covered. If the images are side by side, the disorder is termed *horizontal diplopia*. If upper and lower images are seen, it is termed *vertical diplopia*.

In monocular diplopia, the image is split within the eye and focuses poorly on the retina, resulting in a double image or ghosting of the image. Because monocular diplopia is intrinsic to the eye, it persists when the uninvolved eye is covered.

Monocular Diplopia. Common causes of monocular diplopia include (1) uncorrected refractive error, (2) dry eye with irregular corneal surface, (3) corneal scar, and (4) cataract.

Binocular Diplopia. The following disorders cause binocular diplopia:

ADDITIONAL HISTORY	KEY EXAM FEATURES
Third Nerve Palsy	
Third nerve palsy may be associated with aneurysm, microvascular infarct (particularly with diabetes or hypertension), tumor, trauma, and uncal herniation. Some patients may experience pain.	A droopy eyelid is seen on the involved side. The pupil may be fixed and dilated. If the pupil is involved, the probable cause of the disorder is an aneurysm (of the posterior communicating artery). If the pupil is not involved, microvascular ischemia usually is the cause. Because the third nerve controls superior, inferior, and medial movements, the eye is usually turned down and out.
Fourth Nerve Palsy	
The fourth nerve controls vertical eye movement, so fourth nerve palsy causes vertical diplopia. Some patients report difficulty reading but may have no symptoms otherwise. This palsy may occur with trauma, microvascular infarct (particularly with diabetes or hypertension), tumor, and aneurysm.	The involved eye is higher than the uninvolved eye. The deviation may be so slight that detecting the difference on gross examination is difficult. Patients may demonstrate a head tilt that eliminates the double vision.
Sixth Nerve Palsy	
The sixth nerve controls lateral eye movements. Patients therefore complain of horizontal diplopia. Sixth nerve palsy may be associated with trauma, microvascular infarct (from diabetes or hypertension), increased intracranial pressure, temporal arteritis, cavernous sinus tumor, and aneurysm.	An inability to move the eye outward with the involved eye turned in (esotropia) is significant.
Decompensated Strabismus	
The patient may report a history of strabismus or previous eye muscle surgery.	Horizontal (esotropia/exotropia) or vertical deviation may be present depending on the muscles involved.

ADDITIONAL HISTORY	KEY EXAM FEATURES

Myasthenia Gravis

Patients may have the typical symptoms of myasthenia gravis, including fatigue, weakness, and difficulty swallowing, chewing, and breathing; these symptoms may fluctuate during the day. The double vision also tends to fluctuate during the day and worsens with fatigue.

Droopiness of eyelids that worsens toward the end of the day or when the affected person is fatigued is significant. With sustained upgaze, the drooping may worsen. Systemic edrophonium chloride (Tensilon) often helps reverse the eyelid droop and/or correct the double vision. Weakness of the facial muscles and limb muscles may be noted, but no pupil abnormalities are present.

Thyroid Eye Disease

Eye disease usually is associated with hyperthyroidism; however, patients may have a normal functioning thyroid gland. The eye disease may be present even when the systemic disease is under good control.

Unilateral or bilateral proptosis may be present, and the conjunctiva can be injected or filled with fluid (chemosis). Eye movement may be limited, particularly up and out. When the patient looks down slowly, the upper eyelids may lag behind the eye movement such that the superior sclera is visible (lid lag). The proptosis may lead to an inability to fully close the lids, causing dry eye signs and symptoms.

Orbital Pseudotumor

Patients report severe pain and redness, usually in one eye.

The conjunctiva is usually injected, and swelling of the conjunctiva (chemosis) may occur. The eyelids often are red and swollen. Other findings are proptosis and restriction of movement in one eye, and a palpable orbital mass may be present. The vision in the involved eye may be decreased.

Blow-out Fracture

Blow-out fracture is associated with a history of blunt trauma to the orbit.

Restricted eye movement, particularly in upgaze and/or lateral gaze, is significant. Subcutaneous air (crepitus) and numbness in the distribution of the infraorbital nerve, which involves the cheek and upper lip, are possible.

Itching and Burning

Itching and burning are nonspecific complaints that can be associated with many diseases of the lids and conjunctiva. Any acute conjunctivitis can be associated with itching and burning. Chronic itching and burning are most commonly associated with allergic conjunctivitis, blepharitis, and dry eyes.

Foreign Body Sensation

Foreign body sensation, or the feeling that a grain of sand is in the eye, is a common ocular complaint. The most common cause is dry eyes. In severe cases, superficial punctate staining of the corneal epithelium is possible. Lashes rubbing on the eye from an entropion or misdirected lashes (trichiasis) can cause a foreign body sensation. Most corneal abrasions cause severe pain, but minor abrasions may be associated with a foreign body sensation. An arc welder burn causes a punctate corneal keratopathy, and foreign body sensation may be a prominent symptom. Conjunctival and corneal foreign bodies also produce this symptom.

Severe Eye Pain

As stated, corneal ulcer, uveitis, acute angle-closure glaucoma, and endophthalmitis are disorders that cause severe eye pain and are associated with acute loss of vision. Injection of the conjunctiva and sclera with severe ocular pain but with otherwise normal findings on the eye exam usually results from scleritis. Episcleritis has a similar clinical presentation but is associated with only a mild degree of pain. Any defect in the corneal epithelium caused by contact lens wear, trauma, or recurrent erosion syndrome is associated with a severe burning pain in the eye. The instillation of a topical anesthetic agent eliminates the pain and can be a useful diagnostic test for the physician to establish whether the pain is caused by one of these entities. Orbital pseudotumor is an inflammatory disease of the orbit associated with severe orbital pain. Important signs include proptosis, restriction of ocular motility, injection and edema of the conjunctiva and lids, optic nerve swelling, and in some cases, visual loss.

Excessive Tearing

An overflow of tears from the eye onto the cheek is termed *epiphora*. Impairment of tear drainage can occur with lid malposition. Ectropion is an outward turning of the lid that results in an inability of the tears to enter the puncta. Obstructions of the nasolacrimal drainage system distal to this area also can result in excessive tearing in both adults and children. External ocular irritation can cause reflex tearing and an overflow of tears from the eye. Two common examples include turning in of the lids (entropion) and presence of abnormal lashes rubbing on the cornea (trichiasis), stimulating tear production. Dry eyes produce less tear volume, which results in drying of the cornea and conjunctiva. This can cause pain and inflammation, stimulating lacrimal gland production of tears, resulting in paradoxical tearing despite a dry eye. In the neonate, excessive tearing can be the earliest sign of congenital glaucoma, necessitating urgent ophthalmologic examination.

Eyelid Twitching

Any irritation of the conjunctiva or cornea can cause eyelid twitching. Occasional twitching of the lids usually is associated with stress. Caffeine or other stimulants can cause a similar reaction. Severe spasm of the lids with a functional impairment is termed *benign essential blepharospasm*. Rarely, multiple sclerosis is associated with lid spasm.

Signs

Conjunctivitis

Any type of ocular inflammation can be associated with a secondary conjunctivitis. Corneal ulcers, angle-closure glaucoma, endophthalmitis, and uveitis are associated with conjunctival inflammation. Conjunctivitis, as opposed to scleritis and episcleritis, usually involves the entire conjunctiva (not just a section), is associated with a discharge, and is not associated with pain. (Table 2–1 outlines common ophthalmic disorders that manifest primarily as a conjunctivitis.)

Eyelid Swelling and Erythema

Patients with blepharitis often complain of fullness or swelling in the eyelids, although the lids may not appear thick on clinical evaluation. Examination of the lid margin often shows inflammation and crusting along the lashes. A chalazion is an acute inflammation of the meibomian glands and can cause diffuse erythema and inflammation of one eyelid. The examiner often can palpate a nodule in the center of the area of inflammation. In patients with preseptal and orbital cellulitis, erythema and swelling of the eyelids are frequently seen. In contrast with an acute chalazion, both lids are involved, and the inflammation extends to the skin beyond the lids. In addition, patients usually have a fever and an elevated white blood cell count. Contact dermatitis with secondary lid swelling may develop after prolonged use of a topical medication. Clinically, erythema and an eczematous reaction of the skin are present. Symptoms include itching and irritation.

Ptosis (Droopy Eyelid)

Table 2–2 details disorders that result in ptosis.

Small Pupil

When one pupil is smaller than the other, the size disparity between pupils is greater in darkness than in well-lit conditions. It can occur in Horner syndrome and is associated with ptosis on the same side. Tertiary syphilis is associated with Argyll Robertson pupils. These bilaterally small pupils react poorly to light. When the eyes fixate on a near target, the pupils constrict normally (light-near dissociation). The use of miotic drops (e.g., pilocarpine), traumatic iritis, uveitis, and recent eye surgery may be associated with a small pupil.

Table 2–1   Ophthalmic Disorders Associated with Conjunctivitis

Acute or Chronic	Unilateral or Bilateral	Key Symptoms	Degree of Injection	Discharge Type	Other Features
Viral Conjunctivitis					
Acute	Bilateral, possibly asymmetric	Itching, burning, soreness	4+	Watery	Preauricular lymphadenopathy
Bacterial Conjunctivitis					
Acute	Unilateral or bilateral	Burning, general irritation	3+	Heavy, mucopurulent	Lids possibly adherent
Herpes Simplex Conjunctivitis					
Acute	Unilateral	Photophobia, mild irritation	1-2+	None	Dendritic ulcer on the cornea or vesicles on the lid possible
Adult Chlamydial Conjunctivitis					
Subacute/ chronic	Usually unilateral	Burning, general irritation	2+	Scant, mucopurulent	Usual occurrence in young, sexually active adults
Allergic Conjunctivitis					
Chronic	Bilateral	Itching	2+	Stringy, mucoid	Usual occurrence in atopic persons, possible seasonal symptoms
Blepharitis					
Chronic	Bilateral	Itching, burning, foreign body sensation	1-2+	Usually none	Inflammation and crusting of lid margins
Dry Eye					
Chronic	Bilateral	Foreign body sensation	1+	Mucoid in severe cases	Punctate fluorescein staining of the cornea
Cavernous Sinus AV Fistula					
Chronic	Unilateral	Double vision, audible bruits	1-4+	None	Elevated intraocular pressure, proptosis, possible vision loss

AV, arteriovenous.

Large Pupil

With an abnormally large pupil, the size disparity between pupils is greater in light than in darkness. Inadvertent deposition of any alpha-adrenergic or anticholinergic agent into the eye can cause a large pupil. The unilateral use of dilating drops is a common cause of an abnormally large pupil. Scopolamine patches for the control of seasickness can result in a fixed, dilated pupil if the patient rubs the eye after touching the patch. With eye trauma, the iris sphincter muscle can be damaged, and an abnormally large pupil can result. Tears in the iris sphincter can sometimes be appreciated on slit lamp examination. Third nerve palsy may cause a dilated pupil and is associated with ptosis, decreased elevation, decreased depression, and decreased

Table 2–2   Disorders Causing Ptosis

History	Degree of Ptosis	Motility	Pupil
Third Nerve Palsy			
Double vision, possible severe pain	Moderate to severe	Decreased elevation, depression, and medial movement	Dilated and unreactive or normal
Horner Syndrome			
Asymptomatic	Mild	Normal	Small
Myasthenia Gravis			
Fatigue, difficulty swallowing or breathing, double vision	Variable, possible worsening on sustained upgaze	Any abnormality or no abnormality	Normal
Senile Ptosis			
Possible history of recent eye surgery	Variable	Normal	Normal

Table 2–3   Disorders Resulting in Proptosis

Acute or Chronic	Unilateral or Bilateral	Conjunctival Injection (Redness)	Pain	Fever	Other Features
Thyroid Eye Disease					
Subacute	Bilateral but possibly asymmetric	0-4+, variable depending on extent of disease	None	No	Possible association with systemic thyroid abnormalities
Orbital Pseudotumor					
Acute	Usually unilateral	3-4+	Severe, particularly with eye movement	No	Possible decreased vision and diplopia
Optic Nerve Tumor					
Chronic	Unilateral	0	None	No	Slow-onset visual field loss
Cavernous Sinus AV Fistula					
Acute onset, chronic course	Unilateral	1-4+, variable depending on flow rate	Variable	No	Elevated intraocular pressure, double vision, possible visual loss, audible bruit or pulsating exophthalmos
Cellulitis					
Acute	Unilateral	4+	Moderate to severe	Yes	Most common association with sinusitis, elevated white blood cell count

AV, arteriovenous.

medial movement of the eye. Adie's pupil is an idiopathic abnormality of the pupil that results in unilateral dilation. The pupil is hypersensitive to weak cholinergic drops such as pilocarpine 0.125%. Traumatic iritis, uveitis, angle-closure glaucoma, and recent eye surgery may be associated with a large pupil.

Proptosis

Proptosis is an abnormal protrusion of the eye (Table 2–3).

CHAPTER 3

The Red Eye

JAY H. KRACHMER

This chapter presents an overview of conditions causing a red eye. Most of these topics are treated in more depth elsewhere in this book.

An awareness of the broad spectrum of potential causes for this finding is extremely helpful, because appropriate management depends on a correct diagnosis. Some disorders that may be associated with a red eye (e.g., angle-closure glaucoma, intra-ocular foreign body) may result in loss of vision and require prompt referral for ophthalmologic management. Other causative disorders and conditions (e.g., stye, conjunctivitis) either are self-limiting or can be simply managed without referral. Accordingly, the following discussion is divided into (1) vision-threatening disorders that may be the cause of a red eye and (2) disorders that pose no inherent threat to vision.

Vision-Threatening Causes of Red Eye

Hyphema

A hyphema usually is caused by trauma (Fig. 3–1). After a visual acuity measurement is obtained, the eye should be protected by a shield or glasses, and the patient should be referred to an ophthalmologist for further evaluation and management. Serious cornea, lens, glaucoma, and retina problems can result without proper treatment.

Angle-Closure Glaucoma

Angle-closure glaucoma occurs when the iris is positioned against the trabecular mesh-work, blocking the flow of aqueous out of the eye and raising the intraocular pressure. When this occurs acutely, the pressure can be very high. The patient has pain and often nausea and vomiting. Light directed across the pupil demonstrates the iris up against the cornea. The pupil is irregular in contour and usually mid-dilated and does

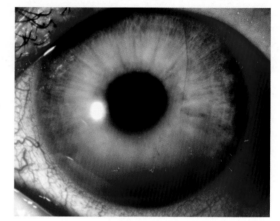

FIGURE 3–1 Traumatic hyphema. Blood is present in the anterior chamber after an injury.

not react properly to light (Fig. 3–2A). Slit lamp examination discloses the flat or nearly flat anterior chamber (Fig. 3–2B). The patient must be sent immediately to an ophthalmologist for evaluation and management.

Severe Dry Eye

The most common setting for the occurrence of severe dry eye is in Sjögren syndrome associated with rheumatoid arthritis. The cornea demonstrates a poor light reflex, and mucus often is seen adherent to the surface (Fig. 3–3). A tear production test (Schirmer test) reveals 0, 1, or 2 mm of tear production after 5 minutes. Corneal thinning, ulceration, infection, and perforation can lead to loss of vision or even loss of the eye (Fig. 3–4). Another, less common severe dry eye condition is ocular cicatricial pemphigoid. Scarring of the bulbar conjunctiva with adhesion to the palpebral conjunctiva is seen in this condition (Fig. 3–5).

Corneal Lesions

A variety of corneal conditions threaten vision. Contact lens–induced corneal stromal scarring can occur (Fig. 3–6). A small *Pseudomonas* infiltrate (Fig. 3–7) in a contact lens wearer can turn overnight into a large ulcer with severe intraocular inflammation. The cornea can be infected with a variety of organisms. Examples are bacteria (Fig. 3–8), fungi (Fig. 3–9), *Acanthamoeba* (Fig. 3–10), and viruses, such as herpes simplex virus (Fig. 3–11). A herpes ulcer typically, but not always, demonstrates a dendritic or branching pattern on fluorescein staining. Herpetic iritis can be part of the clinical picture (Fig. 3–12).

Iritis and Scleritis

Iritis, episcleritis, and scleritis are conditions in which the eye is red and usually painful, but without discharge. The injection causing the red eye in iritis typically is concentrated around the cornea—a clinical entity termed *circumlimbal flush* (Fig. 3–13). White blood cells and fibrin from the aqueous humor precipitate on the back of the

FIGURE 3–2 **A,** A mid-dilated pupil in a patient with acute angle-closure glaucoma. **B,** In the same patient, note the lack of depth in the anterior chamber demonstrated by the iris beam against the corneal beam (1).

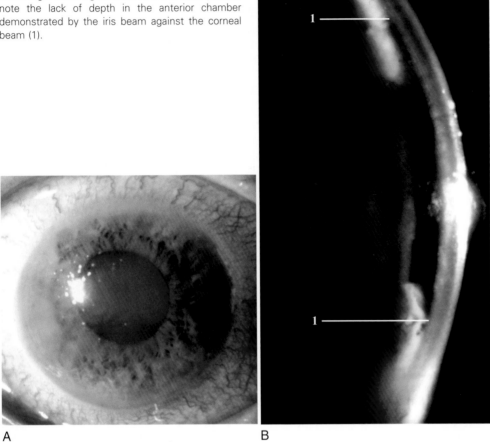

A   B

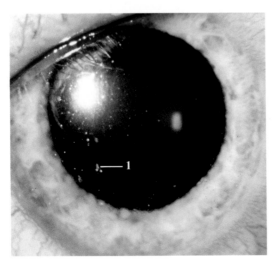

FIGURE 3–3 Dry eye (keratoconjunctivitis sicca) in a patient with Sjögren syndrome associated with rheumatoid arthritis. Mucus can be seen stuck to the corneal surface (1).

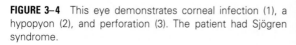
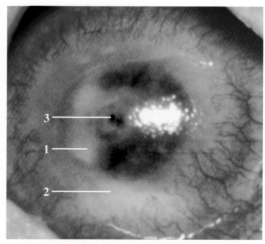

FIGURE 3–4 This eye demonstrates corneal infection (1), a hypopyon (2), and perforation (3). The patient had Sjögren syndrome.

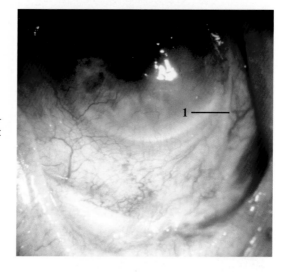

FIGURE 3–5 Scarring (1) of the bulbar conjunctiva with adherence to the palpebral conjunctiva (symblepharon) in a patient with ocular cicatricial pemphigoid.

cornea (Fig. 3–14). If the pupil is not dilated, adhesions (synechiae) may form between the iris and cornea or the iris and lens (Fig. 3–15). Iritis can lead to glaucoma, cataracts, and even retinal and optical nerve disorders.

Episcleritis itself is not a serious condition (Fig. 3–16). Because it is very difficult to differentiate from scleritis, however, the patient should be referred to an ophthalmologist.

Scleritis is a more serious condition (Figs. 3–17 and 3–18). It can be associated with systemic vasculitis. Choroidal effusions, macular edema, and optic neuritis can threaten vision.

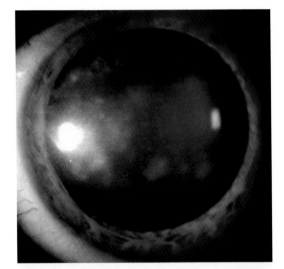

FIGURE 3–6   Contact lens–induced corneal scarring.

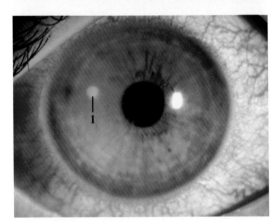

FIGURE 3–7   A tiny bacterial infiltrate (1) in a soft contact lens wearer.

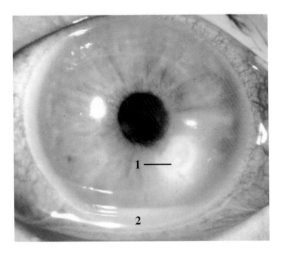

FIGURE 3–8   Staphylococcal ulcer (1) with white blood cells and fibrin (a hypopyon) in the anterior chamber (2).

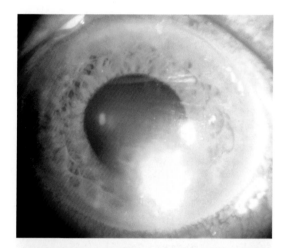

FIGURE 3–9 A fungal corneal ulcer.

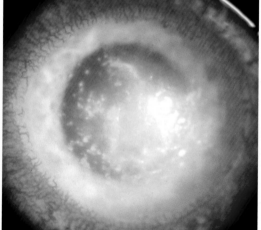

FIGURE 3–10 This eye exhibits the early phase of *Acanthamoeba* keratitis.

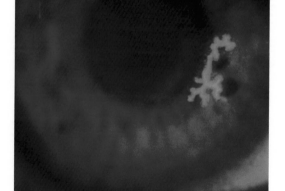

FIGURE 3–11 A herpes simplex dendritic corneal ulcer.

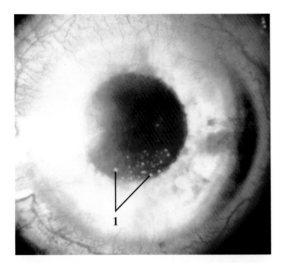

FIGURE 3–12 Herpetic iritis. Note the white blood cell and fibrin precipitates on the posterior cornea (1), termed *keratic precipitates*.

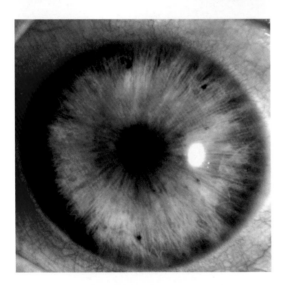

FIGURE 3–13 Iritis. Note the violaceous hue (*between lines*). The eye was red and painful without discharge.

Intraocular Foreign Bodies

Intraocular foreign bodies can cause serious ocular problems, such as endophthalmitis (Fig. 3–19). Most important is a history of the patient's working with metal on metal, such as hammering, and then feeling a strike to the eye. Entrance sites can be microscopic.

Orbital Disease

Orbital disease from inflammation (Fig. 3–20), infection (Fig. 3–21), and tumor is characterized by proptosis or protrusion of the eye, reduction in extraocular movements, and often compression of the optic nerve.

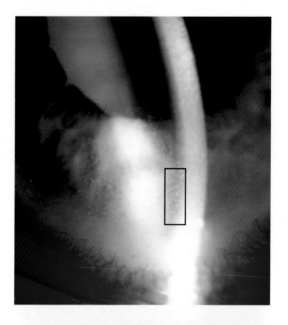

FIGURE 3–14 In iritis, cells (especially white blood cells) and flare (produced by fibrin in the anterior chamber)—referred to as "cells and flare"—can precipitate on the posterior cornea (*box*). These deposits are keratic precipitates (see Fig. 3–12).

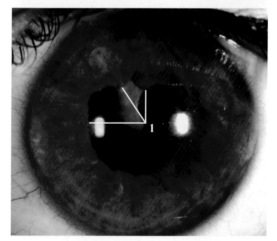

FIGURE 3–15 This eye, in a patient with inactive iritis, demostrates an adhesion between the iris and lens—posterior synechiae (1).

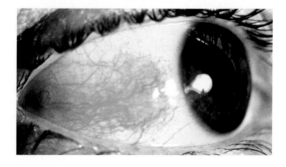

FIGURE 3–16 Eye of a patient with episcleritis.

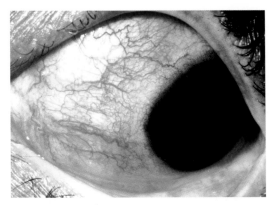

FIGURE 3–17   Note the deeper vessels in this eye of a patient with diffuse scleritis.

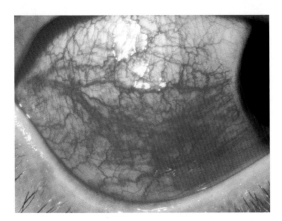

FIGURE 3–18   The patient had nodular scleritis. An elevated, more localized patch of inflammation is present.

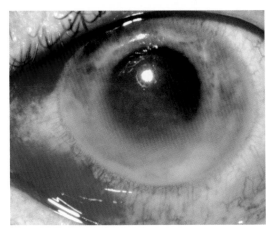

FIGURE 3–19   A history of hammering metal on metal with the finding of subconjunctival hemorrhage should alert the examiner to the presence of an intraocular foreign body. In this example, the eye has become infected (endophthalmitis).

FIGURE 3–20   The patient had thyroid eye disease with orbital inflammation resulting in proptosis.

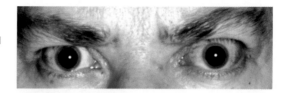

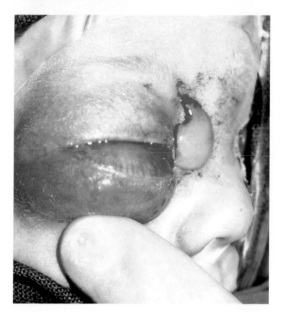

FIGURE 3–21   Orbital cellulitis arising from infectious sinusitis.

Usually conjunctivitis is either self-limiting or easily treated without permanent sequelae. An exception is bacterial conjunctivitis caused by *Neisseria gonorrhoeae* (Fig. 3–22). The gonococcal organism can penetrate an intact corneal epithelium, quickly leading to massive corneal ulceration and loss of the eye. In gonococcal conjunctivitis, a copious purulent discharge is present. Gram-negative intracellular cocci are easily seen on microscopic examination of scrapings and grown on culture. The patient should be immediately referred to an ophthalmologist. When gonococcal infections occur in newborns, the signs are seen a few days after birth.

Non–Vision-Threatening Causes of Red Eye

Although the following conditions ordinarily do not pose a threat to vision, certain etiologic factors or cases of unusual severity may place the patient at risk. In such instances, however, the nature of the condition generally is obvious, and the patient is then promptly referred for ophthalmologic care.

Nasolacrimal Duct Blockage

Blockage of the nasolacrimal duct can be seen in infants and adults. In infants, opening of the nasolacrimal duct is delayed. Massaging the nasal corner of the eye in and down

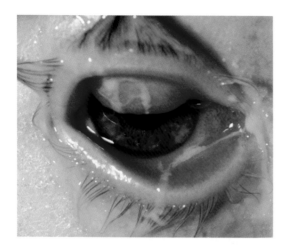

FIGURE 3–22   Gonococcal conjunctivitis. Note the copious purulent material.

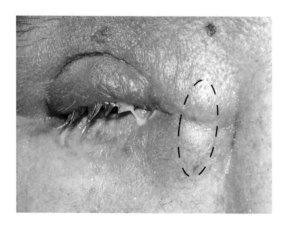

FIGURE 3–23   Dacryocystitis in an adult patient. The enlarged nasolacrimal sac is outlined.

toward the nose, and waiting several months, results in resolution in 75% to 80% of cases. In infants, use of topical and systemic antibiotics plus a little bit of time usually is sufficient. Lacrimal probing may be required in some cases, however. In adults, the nasolacrimal duct can become obstructed from a variety of causes (Fig. 3–23). Infection of the lacrimal sac, or dacryocystitis, necessitates referral for ophthalmologic management.

Preseptal Cellulitis

Cellulitis anterior to the orbital septum—preseptal cellulitis—is seen in a variety of disorders (Fig. 3–24). Causes include inflammation of the lacrimal gland (dacryoadenitis), styes, chalazia, and insect bites. If the cause of the preseptal cellulitis is known and if it is certain that the patient does not have orbital cellulitis, the primary care practitioner can treat the condition as appropriate for the cause.

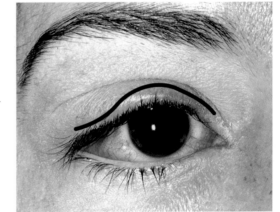

FIGURE 3–24 Preseptal cellulitis from lacrimal gland inflammation. Note the S-shaped configuration of the upper lid.

FIGURE 3–25 A lower lid stye (1).

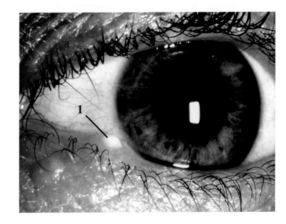

Stye (Hordeolum)

A stye or hordeolum is the result of staphylococcal infection and blockage of glands along the lid margin (Fig. 3–25). Hot compresses with slight pressure and topical antibiotics usually are enough to successfully treat the condition. Use of a sterile needle to open the lesion followed by hot compresses and topical antibiotics also is appropriate if it does not spontaneously open.

Chalazion

A chalazion results from blockage of the glands deeper in the eyelid, the meibomian glands (Fig. 3–26). In a majority of cases, the chalazion will absorb, or drain and absorb, following days and sometimes weeks of hot compresses. If absorption fails to occur, it would be appropriate to refer the patient to an ophthalmologist for surgical excision.

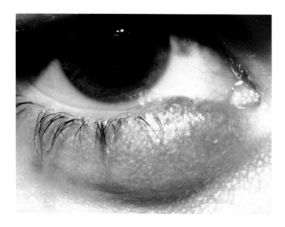

FIGURE 3–26 A large chalazion of the lower lid.

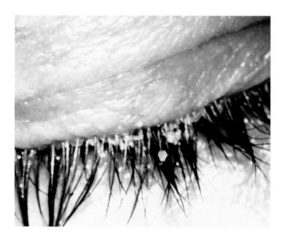

FIGURE 3–27 Seborrheic blepharitis. Note the dandruff flakes on the eyelashes.

Blepharitis

Blepharitis, or inflammation of the eyelids, is a very common disorder. Hot compresses and careful lid hygiene constitute the mainstay of treatment for blepharitis. The three most common types are seborrheic blepharitis (Fig. 3–27), staphylococcal blepharitis (Fig. 3–28), and blepharitis due to meibomian gland dysfunction (Fig. 3–29). Magnification often is required to make the correct diagnosis. In seborrheic blepharitis, in addition to hot compresses, dandruff shampoo should be used on the scalp and eyebrows but not on the eyelids.

In staphylococcal blepharitis, infection of the lid margins results in red, pitted, and even ulcerated margins, with loss of lashes and misdirected lashes. In addition to hot compresses, antibiotic ointment should be used twice a day to the lid margins.

Meibomian Gland Dysfunction

Meibomian gland dysfunction involves the posterior lid margins. It can be an isolated finding or associated with rosacea of the face. In addition to hot compresses, in patients

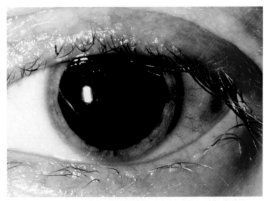

FIGURE 3–28   Staphylococcal blepharitis. The lid margins are very red and under high magnification demonstrate tiny ulcerations.

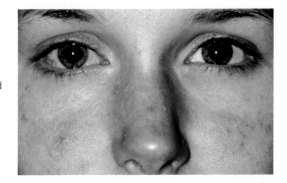

FIGURE 3–29   The patient had blepharitis and associated rosacea due to sebaceous gland dysfunction.

able to take tetracyclines, treatment includes a 4 to 6 week course of doxycycline (50 to 200 mg/day). Doxycycline is contraindicated in children, pregnant women, and breastfeeding mothers.

Pediculosis

A far less common cause of blepharitis is pediculosis, or lice infestation (Fig. 3–30A and B). It is easily treated by manually removing some of the lice and then suffocating remaining lice with a bland ointment.

Structural Abnormalities of the Eyelids

Three structural abnormalities of the eyelids that can produce red eyes are *entropion*, turning in of the eyelid (Fig. 3–31); *ectropion* (Fig. 3–32), turning out of the eyelid; and *trichiasis* (Fig. 3–33), with misdirected lashes that rub the globe. If the lashes are few enough in number, the primary care practitioner or even the patient can pull them out. In more extensive cases, the patient should be referred for surgical management.

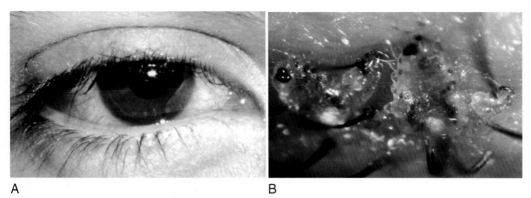

A   B

FIGURE 3–30   Blepharitis due to pediculosis. A, At first glance, this appears to be a routine case of blepharoconjunctivitis. **B,** Under high magnification, lice can be seen.

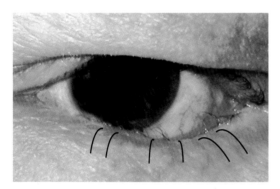

FIGURE 3–31   Involutional entropion. Turning in of the lid is part of the aging process.

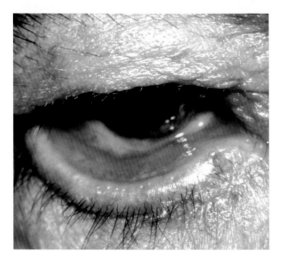

FIGURE 3–32   Ectropion. In this patient, ectropion of the lower lid was due to lid laxity with aging.

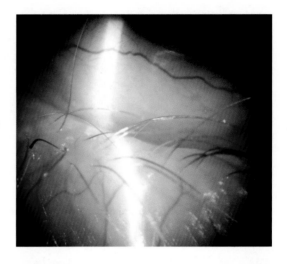

FIGURE 3–33 Trichiasis. In this condition, lashes from the eyelid rub against the globe.

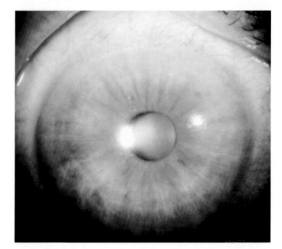

FIGURE 3–34 Mild dry eye with resultant minimal degradation of the light reflex.

Dry Eyes

Dry eyes may be classified as mild, moderate, or severe. Patients with severe dry eyes and those requiring artificial tears more than 4 or 5 times a day should be referred for ophthalmologic management. The condition of mild dry eyes is an extremely common disorder (Fig. 3–34). The patient complains of red, irritated eyes that feel dry, burn, and sometimes have reflex tearing. Typically, the drying worsens during the day. A clue that the surface is dry is the lack of a sharp light reflex secondary to a poor tear film. A positive response to the use of preservative-free artificial tears usually is diagnostic.

Conjunctivitis

Conjunctivitis is an inflammation of the conjunctiva. If the classic signs of inflammation—hyperemia, edema, discharge—are not present, the condition probably is not conjunctivitis.

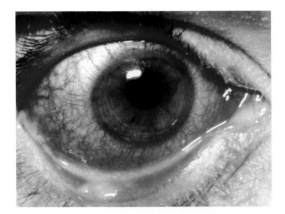

FIGURE 3–35 Bacterial conjunctivitis with purulent discharge.

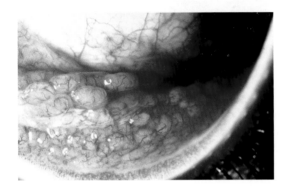

FIGURE 3–36 **Follicular conjunctivitis.** The smooth, rounded follicles with vascularization can be seen.

Major pathogenic agents of conjunctivitis are bacteria, viruses, *Chlamydia*, allergy, foreign bodies, and toxins, including medications. Each of these categories has characteristic features. Because conjunctivitis usually is self-limiting, laboratory workup typically is not warranted.

Bacterial conjunctivitis is characterized by a purulent discharge and probably is more common in children (Fig. 3–35). Simple bacterial conjunctivitis should be treated with broad-spectrum topical antibiotics. A common dosing schedule is every 2 hours while the patient is awake for the first day and then four times a day until a week of therapy is completed.

Viral conjunctivitis can be seen as an isolated condition or in combination with or following a viral upper respiratory tract infection. Discharge is mixed but mainly watery. With adequate magnification, the examiner may be able to see tiny rounded subepithelial follicular lesions (Fig. 3–36). Preauricular adenopathy also is a common finding.

Viral conjunctivitis can be extremely contagious. The patient should be considered contagious for 7 to 10 days after the onset of clinical signs. Children should be kept out of school and workers away from the work place where others might become infected. The examiner should use gloves and make certain that any furnishings or equipment exposed to the patient is cleaned.

FIGURE 3–37 The patient had epidemic keratoconjunctivitis and demonstrates the very common findings of ecchymosis of the lids and subconjunctival hemorrhages.

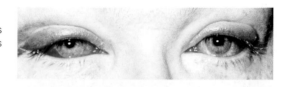

FIGURE 3–38 Subepithelial infiltrates in epidemic keratoconjunctivitis, which are best seen using a broad oblique slit lamp beam.

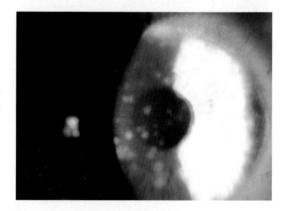

Many different viruses can cause infection, but adenovirus is frequently implicated. Some types of adenovirus cause a combination of conjunctivitis, sore throat, and fever known as *pharyngeal conjunctival fever.* Other types cause an extremely contagious condition known as *epidemic keratoconjunctivitis* (EKC) (Fig. 3–37). At times, epidemics of this disorder have closed schools and physicians' offices.

In most cases of EKC, subepithelial infiltrates may be observed by the end of the second week. These infiltrates can be seen only with the high magnification of the slit lamp (Fig. 3–38). Photophobia can be extreme and last for several weeks or longer.

Treatment of viral conjunctivitis should include careful cleansing of the eyes with a warm washcloth. The examiner cannot always be certain whether the conjunctivitis is viral or bacterial without expensive cultures. It is therefore reasonable to use topical broad-spectrum antibiotics, four times a day for a week. Artificial tears also can be soothing.

Conjunctivitis in the newborn is seen in four common settings. Toxic conjunctivitis is seen within the first 48 hours after the use of perinatal prophylactic antibiotics. Bacterial conjunctivitis usually manifests 2, 3, or 4 days after birth. Chlamydial conjunctivitis usually is seen 5 to 10 days after birth (Fig. 3–39A and B). Herpes simplex conjunctivitis manifests 6 to 14 days after birth.

In addition to inclusion conjunctivitis in the newborn, the chlamydial organism causes inclusion conjunctivitis in the adult (Fig. 3–40). Because chlamydial conjunctivitis is a sexually transmitted disease, transmission from the genitourinary tract of the patient and any sexual partner should be considered. Other serotypes of *Chlamydia* cause trachoma, a leading cause of blindness in underdeveloped countries.

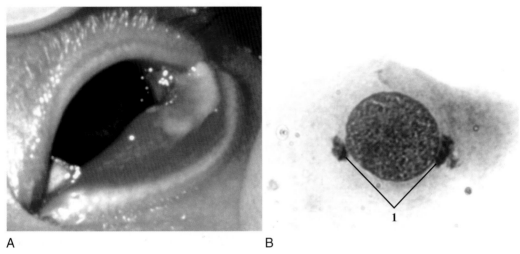

A   B

FIGURE 3–39   A, The patient was a newborn with chlamydial conjunctivitis. **B,** Intracytoplasmic inclusion bodies (1) were found after scraping the palpebral (lid) conjunctiva followed by Giemsa staining.

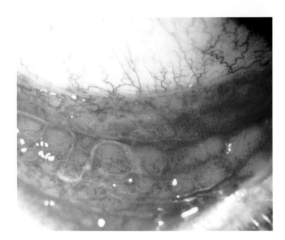

FIGURE 3–40   Follicular conjunctivitis in an adult patient with chlamydial conjunctivitis.

The discharge in chlamydial conjunctivitis is mucopurulent. In the acute infection, it is very copious. Chlamydial conjunctivitis if not treated adequately becomes chronic, at which time the discharge is less profuse.

In acute infections, especially in the newborn, gram-positive inclusion bodies can be seen in the cytoplasm of conjunctival epithelial cells. If inclusion conjunctivitis is considered in the adult, a DNA Genprobe for *Chlamydia* laboratory test can be performed.

In the newborn, because chlamydial pneumonitis can occur along with the conjunctivitis, systemic erythromycin, 50 mg/kg per day in two to four divided doses is given for 2 weeks. In adult inclusion conjunctivitis, doxycycline, 100 mg two times a day for 3 weeks is used. If the patient is unable to take tetracyclines, erythromycin,

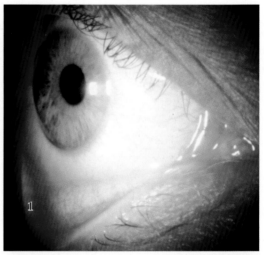

FIGURE 3–41   Chemosis (edematous swelling of the conjunctiva) is seen in a patient with marked allergic conjunctivitis (1).

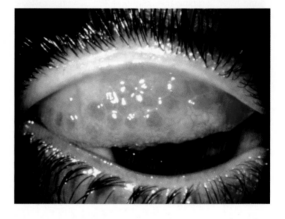

FIGURE 3–42   Vernal conjunctivitis. The characteristic vascular vegetative papillary lesions are evident.

250 mg four times a day is used instead. Infected sexual partners should receive treatment as well.

Allergic conjunctivitis is most common during the spring and fall allergy seasons (Fig. 3–41). It usually is associated with other mucous membrane reactions. Intense itching and a watery mucoid discharge are typical. In markedly acute cases, the conjunctiva can become extremely edematous.

Vernal conjunctivitis is an unusual form of allergic conjunctivitis. Flipping the upper lid reveals very large tufts of reactive tissue (Fig. 3–42). Vernal conjunctivitis requires referral of the patient to an ophthalmologist for management, because corneal complications are frequent (Fig. 3–43).

Another setting in which allergic conjunctivitis can be seen is that of topical drug allergy (Fig. 3–44). As in other allergic settings, itching is the key symptom. It is difficult to make the diagnosis of allergy without a complaint of itching. Because the drops also contact the lids and skin, reaction in the lids as well as conjunctiva is obvious.

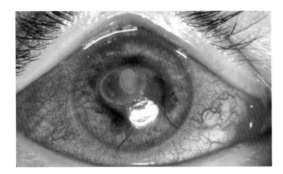

FIGURE 3–43 Severe corneal scarring due to vernal blepharo-keratoconjunctivitis.

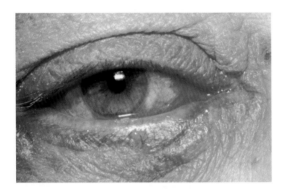

FIGURE 3–44 Drug allergy resulted in the inflammation of the lids and conjunctiva seen in this eye.

Treatment of allergic conjunctivitis will depend on the particular setting in which it is seen. Cold compresses bring quick relief. In the case of seasonal allergic conjunctivitis, treatment with systemic antihistamines is important. Topical antihistamines are effective. Topical nonsteroidal anti-inflammatory agents are helpful because they bring rapid reduction of inflammation and relief of itching. Topical mast cell stabilizers can require days before benefit is realized, but when they are effective, they are safe drugs with great benefit. Because patients vary in their response to these anti-inflammatory medications, trial of various combinations often is needed. In patients without systemic manifestations, topical medications alone are sufficient.

Another expression of conjunctivitis is that due to foreign material irritating the conjunctiva. A bicycle ride on a windy, dusty day can produce this form. On eversion of the upper lid (Fig. 3–45A and B), if no objects are found in the eye, topical anesthetic followed by irrigation with an eyewash will usually remove microscopic foreign bodies previously not visible.

Conjunctivitis also can be produced by eye rubbing. A previously normal, healthy eye can exhibit pathologic changes from eye rubbing that range from mild irritation to lid and corneal disease (Fig. 3–46). Chronic irritation from a contact lens against the palpebral conjunctiva, the conjunctiva on the back of the lid, can cause conjunctivitis. Mucous discharge deposits on the lens reduce vision and further irritate the eye.

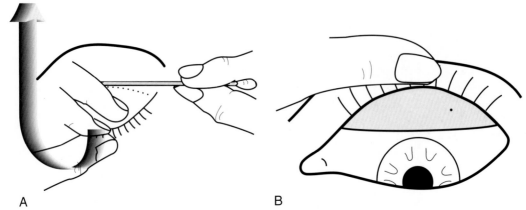

A   B

FIGURE 3–45　To evert the upper lid, ask the patient to look down and to continue looking down until completion of examination of the upper lid. Looking up will flip the lid back. Place the wooden end of a cotton-tipped applicator at the upper lid fold (**A**); then grasp the eyelashes and pull the lid down and out and over the applicator (**B**).

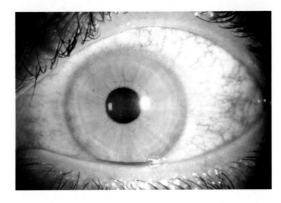

FIGURE 3–46　This eye is red from irritation caused by rubbing.

Environmental toxins can irritate the conjunctiva, producing a watery and often mucoid discharge. Toxins from a molluscum contagiosum lesion produce a chronic follicular conjunctivitis (Fig. 3–47).

Subconjunctival Hemorrhage

A subconjunctival hemorrhage usually is a spontaneous event (Fig. 3–48). It can be seen associated with trauma, Valsalva maneuver, systemic anticoagulation, and high blood pressure. In patients who experience repeated episodes of subconjunctival hemorrhages without an obvious cause, a further workup should be done to rule out the rare occurrence of a hematologic disorder.

Pinguecula

A pinguecula is a small, fleshy, pink to yellow benign growth located a few millimeters from the 3 o'clock to 9 o'clock limbus (Fig. 3–49). It probably represents

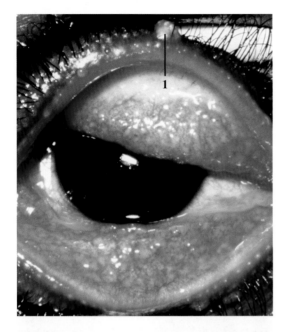

FIGURE 3–47 Molluscum contagiosum conjunctivitis caused by toxins from the lesion at the upper lid margin (1).

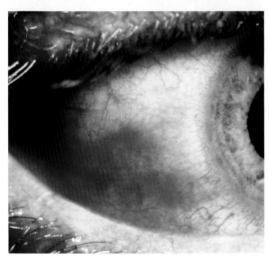

FIGURE 3–48 Subconjunctival hemorrhage. The blood takes approximately 1 week to clear completely, and may become yellow in the process.

a reaction to environmental exposure. An inflamed pinguecula constitutes a red eye condition that is treated with a short course of vasoconstrictive and antihistamine drops.

Pterygium

A pterygium is a fibrovascular growth extending from the conjunctiva onto the cornea, usually nasally but rarely temporally (Fig. 3–50). This lesion also is caused by environmental exposure. Indications for excision are reduced vision and sometimes cosme-

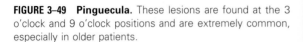

FIGURE 3–49   Pinguecula. These lesions are found at the 3 o'clock and 9 o'clock positions and are extremely common, especially in older patients.

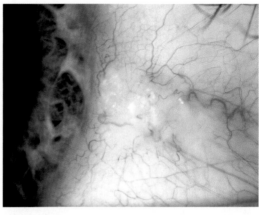

FIGURE 3–50   Pterygium. These lesions are found in the horizontal meridian, most commonly nasally.

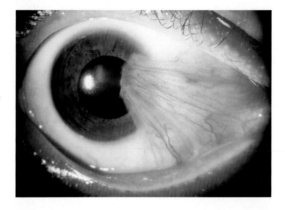

sis. If its appearance or location is unusual, the patient should be referred for ophthalmologic management.

Corneal Epithelial Injury

A scratch to the corneal epithelium produces a corneal abrasion with severe pain (Fig. 3–51). A fluorescein drop used with a cobalt blue light shows the green-staining lesion. Instillation of antibiotic ointment and application of a patch worn until the next day for comfort usually constitute adequate treatment. Instillation of antibiotic drops without patching also is acceptable and is supported by recent studies. A cold compress can be used to relieve discomfort, with addition of an oral analgesic if pain is extreme. Use of broad-spectrum antibiotic drops should be continued until the lesion has healed. With persistent pain, the patient should be referred for evaluation to determine whether infection, iritis, or some other reason for the continued discomfort is present. After healing, the corneal epithelium can later break down; the resultant lesion is termed a *recurrent erosion* (Fig. 3–52).

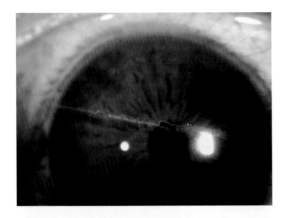

FIGURE 3–51 The patient suffered a "paper cut" of the cornea. Such lesions are extremely painful because of the highly innervated tissue.

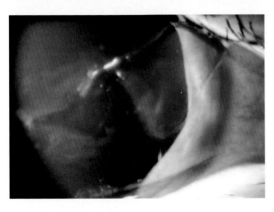

FIGURE 3–52 Sometimes after the corneal epithelium heals from an abrasion, an erosion of the epithelium (recurrent erosion) may occur. The most common time for this to happen is during the night or especially on awakening.

Simple abrasions in contact lens wearers should be treated with antibiotics but without patching. These patients are more prone to the development of secondary infection.

Tiny surface corneal foreign bodies, from low-velocity injuries, can result in conjunctivitis (Fig. 3–53). Rust rings can form around and under an iron foreign body; these can be carefully removed under slit lamp exmination (Fig. 3–54). It is essential to remember that high-velocity injuries, especially those resulting from metal on metal as in hammering, may result in intraocular foreign bodies.

Eye Rubbing

A common cause of a chronic red eye is eye rubbing. Possible mechanisms include excessive use of tissues and accidentally rubbing the eye into the pillow during sleep. Treatment consists of awareness and avoidance of eye rubbing. Use of artificial tears can be helpful during the healing process.

Eyestrain

Eyestrain is a very common cause of red eyes (Fig. 3–55). Strain can be caused by wearing eyeglasses of improper prescription or by the need for glasses, or may result

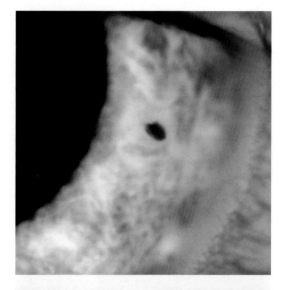

FIGURE 3–53 A small superficial corneal foreign body.

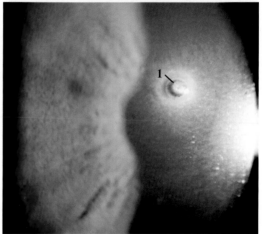

FIGURE 3–54 A rust ring (1) that developed following implantation of an iron corneal foreign body.

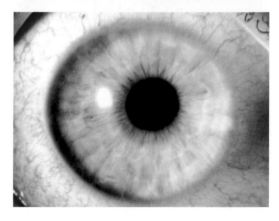

FIGURE 3–55 Eyestrain is a very common cause of a mildly red eye.

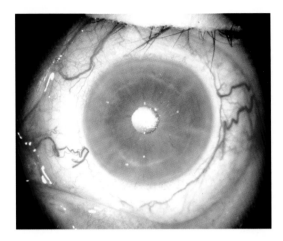

FIGURE 3–56 Marked conjunctival vascular dilatation in a patient with a carotid artery–cavernous sinus fistula.

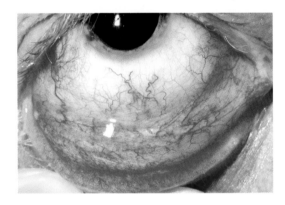

FIGURE 3–57 Dilated palpebral and bulbar conjunctival vessels in a patient with polycythemia vera.

from long periods of reading, driving, or using the computer, which frequently are accompanied by decreased blinking. In these situations, the eyes often are dry and can be helped with artificial tears. Some patients may find relief with the use of a cool or warm damp washcloth placed over the eyes.

Uncommon Conditions

Two very uncommon red eye–producing conditions, both characterized by very dilated conjunctival vessels but no discharge, are carotid artery–cavernous sinus fistula (Fig. 3–56) and polycythemia vera (Fig. 3–57). These conditions are mentioned to remind the examiner to keep an open mind concerning the etiology of the red eye.

CHAPTER 4

Eyelid Abnormalities

TED H. WOJNO

Related Anatomy

In adults, the upper lid usually rests at a point between the upper limbus (corneoscleral junction) and upper pupillary border. The lower lid margin usually rests along the inferior limbus. A small amount of scleral "show" (visibility of the sclera between lid and limbus) is not abnormal in the lower lid but is abnormal in the upper lid. In most people, the upper lid has a distinct crease where fibers from the levator muscle insert; this is covered by a small fold of skin. A lower lid crease sometimes is present and is less well defined than that in the upper lid. The upper and the lower lids join at the medial and the lateral canthi (Fig. 4–1).

The tarsal plates are composed of dense, collagenous tissue that forms the "skeleton" of the lids. Vertically oriented meibomian oil glands within the tarsi have orifices visible just posterior to the lashes (Fig. 4–2). The tarsal plates are attached to the orbital rims by the medial and lateral canthal tendons.

Elevation of the upper lid is primarily the work of the levator muscle (innervated by the third cranial nerve) and is assisted by Müller's muscle (through sympathetic innervation). Third nerve palsy results in moderate drooping of the lid (at least 3 mm lower than usual), a condition known as *ptosis*, whereas sympathetic palsy results in mild lid drooping (1 to 2 mm lower than usual).

The orbicularis muscle, innervated by the seventh cranial nerve, is responsible for involuntary blinking and forceful lid closure. The lids are separated from the orbit by the orbital septum, a fibrous membrane that functions to prevent the spread of superficial infections into the orbit. Thinning of the septum with age allows the orbital fat to prolapse anteriorly, causing characteristic bulges, or "bags," in the lids.

Ectropion

Symptoms

- Irritation, burning, and foreign body sensation occur.
- Tearing results from punctal malposition.

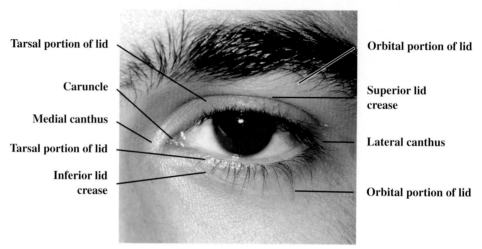

Tarsal portion of lid

Caruncle

Medial canthus

Tarsal portion of lid

Inferior lid crease

Orbital portion of lid

Superior lid crease

Lateral canthus

Orbital portion of lid

FIGURE 4–1   Eyelid structures.

Signs

- An out-turned lower lid margin is evident, often with a visible space between the globe and the lid (Fig. 4–3).

Etiology

- *Involutional*: The disorder is caused by lower lid laxity, which occurs with aging.
- *Cicatricial*: The disorder is caused by a scar on the lower lid skin.
- *Paralytic*: The disorder is caused by a seventh nerve palsy.
- *Mechanical*: The disorder is caused by a mass on the lower lid or cheek.
- *Congenital*: The disorder rarely has a congenital origin.

Treatment

- Surgery is performed to correct any causative abnormality.

Entropion

Symptoms

- Irritation, burning, and foreign body sensation occur.
- Tearing results from lashes abrading the globe.

Signs

- An in-turned lower lid margin is evident (Fig. 4–4).

Etiology

- *Involutional*: The disorder is caused by lower lid laxity, which occurs with aging.
- *Cicatricial*: The disorder is caused by a scar on the conjunctival surface such as from a chemical burn.
- *Congenital*: The disorder rarely has a congenital origin.

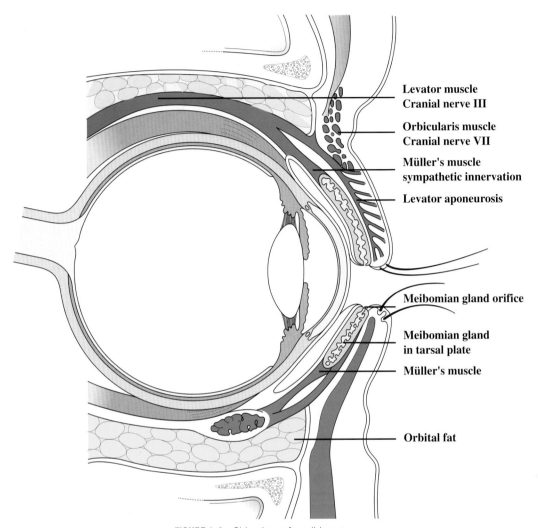

Levator muscle
Cranial nerve III

Orbicularis muscle
Cranial nerve VII

Müller's muscle
sympathetic innervation

Levator aponeurosis

Meibomian gland orifice

Meibomian gland
in tarsal plate

Müller's muscle

Orbital fat

FIGURE 4–2 Side view of eyelid anatomy.

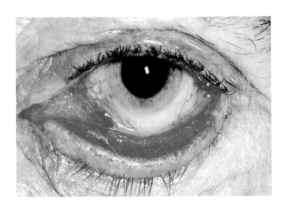

FIGURE 4–3 Involutional ectropion.

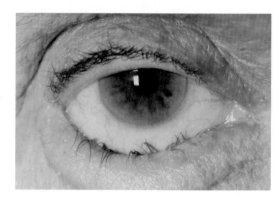

FIGURE 4–4   Involutional entropion.

Treatment

• Surgery is performed to correct any causative abnormality.

Trichiasis

Symptoms

• Irritation, burning, and foreign body sensation are reported by the patient.
• Tearing results from lashes abrading the globe.

Signs

• Lashes on a normally positioned lid margin are posteriorly misdirected (Fig. 4–5).

Etiology

• *Spontaneous*: The disorder usually affects an isolated lash or two and often occurs at the site of a previous stye.
• *Previous injury*: An inflammatory process of the conjunctiva results from injuries such as a chemical burn or a disease such as ocular cicatricial pemphigoid.

Associated Diseases

• The disorder may coexist with cicatricial entropion.

Treatment

• Isolated lashes are removed with forceps.
• Extensive lash abnormalities are corrected with surgery.

Lagophthalmos

Symptoms

• Irritation, burning, and foreign body sensation are reported by the patient.
• Tearing is caused by failure of the "lacrimal pump."

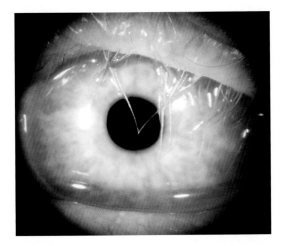

FIGURE 4–5 Trichiasis. The lashes are rubbing on the cornea.

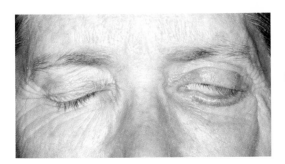

FIGURE 4–6 Lagophthalmos of the left eye due to seventh nerve palsy.

Signs

• The patient cannot completely close the eye (Fig. 4–6).

Etiology

Possible causes include the following:
• Severe lower lid laxity
• Seventh nerve palsy
• Proptosis
• Overcorrected ptosis repair or blepharoplasty
• Scarring changes in upper or lower lid

Treatment

• The following applies to seventh nerve palsy:
  ○ *Mild*: Artificial tears or tear ointments are used. The eye is taped shut at night.
  ○ *Moderate to severe*: Lid margins are sutured together (tarsorrhaphy).
  ○ *Permanent*: A gold weight is surgically inserted into the upper lid.
• For other causes, the primary problem is treated.

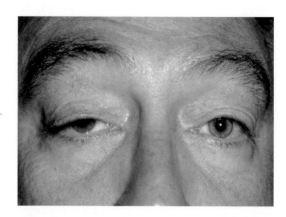

FIGURE 4–7 Ptosis of the right upper lid.

Ptosis

Symptoms

- Obstruction of the superior visual field occurs.
- Reading is difficult, with acquired ptosis usually worse in downgaze.
- The patient is concerned about the cosmetic appearance of the lid.
- If the ptosis is congenital or acquired in early childhood, amblyopia often is present.

Signs

- The upper lid margin is in an abnormally low position (Fig. 4–7).

Etiology

- *Congenital*: The disorder usually results from a malformed levator muscle.
- *Acquired*: A thinning or detachment of the levator aponeurosis is present.
- *Horner syndrome*: The disorder involves 1 to 2 mm of ptosis with a small pupil on the same side (see Chapter 12).
- *Third nerve palsy*: With ophthalmoplegia, more than 3 mm of ptosis is present (see Chapter 12).
- *Myasthenia gravis*: Ptosis varies in severity and may worsen with sustained upgaze (see Chapter 12).

Treatment

- For congenital or acquired lesions, surgery is performed to tighten the levator aponeurosis or resect the levator muscle.
- For other causes, the primary problem is treated.

Floppy Eyelid Syndrome

Symptoms

- Irritation, burning, foreign body sensation, and discharge are reported by the patient.

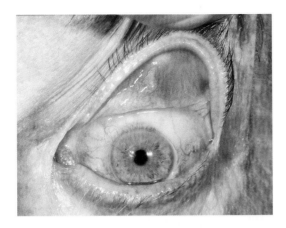

FIGURE 4–8 Floppy eyelid syndrome demonstrating ease with which upper lid is everted.

Signs

- The disorder is usually unilateral or asymmetrical.
- Chronic conjunctivitis that is nonresponsive to topical antibiotics is present.
- A giant papillary reaction (papillae greater than 1 mm in size) of the tarsal conjunctiva occurs, giving the surface a red cobblestone or velvety appearance.
- A characteristic finding is the ability to evert the patient's upper lid by simply pulling upward from the lateral brow area (Fig. 4–8).

Etiology

- An abnormal laxity of the lateral canthal tendon and tarsal plate is present in affected persons.
- The upper lid everts during sleep and rubs against the pillow, leading to severe irritation of the conjunctiva and mucus secretion.

Treatment

- A Fox shield (plastic or metal shield usually worn after cataract surgery) is taped over the eye at night to prevent the lid from rubbing on the pillow.
- Surgery is necessary to tighten the upper and lower lids horizontally; the procedure may need to be repeated after several years.

Seborrheic Keratosis

Symptoms

- Patients usually are symptom free.
- Occasional itchiness is reported.

Signs

- The lesion usually is well demarcated with variable pigmentation, a "stuck-on" appearance, and a cerebriform surface (Fig. 4–9).
- A lobulated papillary or pedunculated frond sometimes is present at the lid margin.

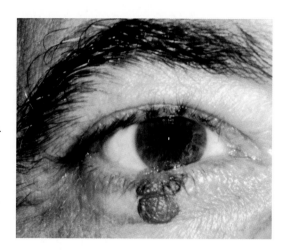

FIGURE 4–9 Seborrheic keratosis.

Differential Diagnosis

Considerations in the differential diagnosis include the following:
- Nevus
- Basal cell carcinoma
- Melanoma

Treatment

- Seborrheic keratoses are benign lesions, usually requiring no treatment.
- A superficial shave biopsy or an excision can be performed if lesions are cosmetically undesirable.

Actinic Keratosis

Symptoms

- Patients usually are symptom free.
- Occasional itchiness is reported.

Signs

- The disorder varies in morphologic appearance, ranging from a flat, scaly lesion to a papilloma to a cutaneous horn (Fig. 4–10).

Etiology

- The disorder results from overexposure to actinic radiation.

Differential Diagnosis

Considerations in the differential diagnosis include the following:
- Squamous cell carcinoma
- Verruca
- Seborrheic keratosis

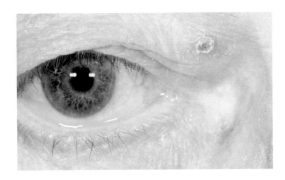

FIGURE 4–10 Actinic keratosis.

Associated Factors and Diseases

- The disorder is more common in fair-skinned persons.
- A lesion may develop into squamous cell carcinoma.

Treatment

The three treatment options are as follows:
- Surgical excision is performed.
- Patients undergo cryotherapy.
- Topical 5-fluorouracil (e.g., Efudex) is prescribed.

Xanthelasma

Symptoms

- Patients usually are symptom free.
- The disorder is a cosmetic deformity.

Signs

- A bilateral, plaquelike yellow lesion usually is present (Fig. 4–11).
- The lesion is found in the medial upper and lower lids.

Etiology

- The origin usually is idiopathic.

Associated Factors and Diseases

- The disorder affects middle-aged to elderly persons, predominantly women.
- The disorder occasionally is associated with hyperlipidemia or diabetes.

Treatment

- Surgical excision of the involved skin is performed.
- A skin graft often is necessary following removal of a large lesion.

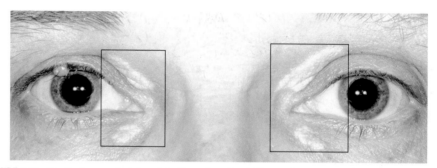

FIGURE 4–11 Xanthelasma of all four lids (*boxed outlines*). The patient also has an intradermal nevus on the right upper lid margin.

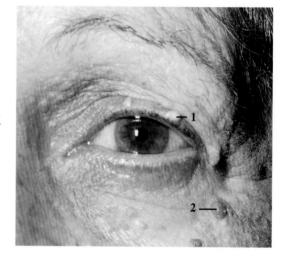

FIGURE 4–12 Epithelial inclusion cyst (1) of the left upper lid. The patient also has a seborrheic keratosis (2) of the lower lid and lateral canthus.

Epithelial Inclusion Cyst

Symptoms

• Patients usually are symptom free.

Signs

• The cyst is slow-growing, white, round, and firm (Fig. 4–12).
• The diameter of the cyst usually is less than 1 cm.

Etiology

• Formation of the cyst follows traumatic implantation of epidermis into the dermis.

Differential Diagnosis

Considerations in the differential diagnosis include the following:

- Milium (small retention cyst of a hair follicle)
- Syringoma (adenoma of an eccrine sweat gland)
- Hydrocystoma (cyst of an eccrine sweat gland)
- Trichoepithelioma (squamous cell cyst of a hair follicle)
- Basal cell carcinoma

Associated Diseases

- The disorder is rarely associated with Gardner syndrome.

Treatment

- Excision or marsupialization of the cyst is performed.

Basal Cell Carcinoma

Symptoms

- Patients usually are symptom free.

Signs

- *Nodular*: Most commonly, a solid, pearly lesion is covered with telangiectatic vessels and a central ulceration (Fig. 4–13).
- *Infiltrative*: Rarely, a superficial, erythematous patch is present.
- The most common locations are the lower lid and the medial canthus.

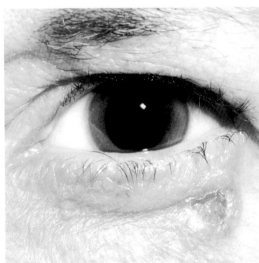

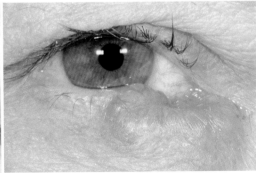

B

A

FIGURE 4–13   A, A relatively flat basal cell carcinoma.
B, A typical nodular basal cell carcinoma.

Etiology

• The disorder results from overexposure to actinic radiation.

Differential Diagnosis

Considerations in the differential diagnosis include the following:
• Milium (small retention cyst of a hair follicle)
• Syringoma (adenoma of an eccrine sweat gland)
• Hydrocystoma (cyst of an eccrine sweat gland)
• Trichoepithelioma (squamous cell cyst of a hair follicle)

Associated Factors and Diseases

• It is the most common primary eyelid malignancy, occurring in 80% to 90% of cases.
• The disorder is more common in basal cell nevus syndrome and xeroderma pigmentosum.
• The carcinoma rarely metastasizes but is locally destructive.

Treatment

• The preferred approach is surgical removal by Mohs' technique followed by reconstruction; use of this technique results in a high cure rate (98%) and spares as much normal tissue as possible. Surgical excision with frozen section control is an acceptable alternative with a high cure rate (95%).
• Radiation therapy (80% to 90% cure rate) usually is reserved for patients unable or unwilling to have surgery.

Follow-up

• The site is examined for recurrence.
• Sun-exposed body parts are inspected for additional lesions.

Squamous Cell Carcinoma

Symptoms

• Patients usually are symptom free.

Signs

• An infiltrative, erythematous patch, often with ulceration, is a common sign of squamous cell carcinoma (Fig. 4–14).
• A nodular, erythematous lesion, often with ulceration, is an uncommon finding.

Etiology

• The disorder results from overexposure to actinic radiation.

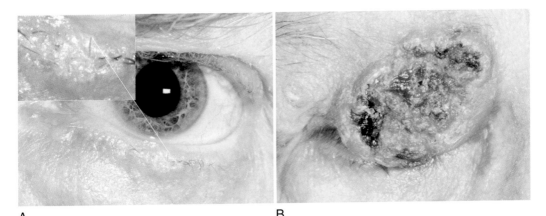

FIGURE 4–14 **A,** A typical small squamous cell carcinoma (*inset*). **B,** A large nodular squamous cell carcinoma.

Differential Diagnosis

Considerations in the differential diagnosis include the following:
- Basal cell carcinoma
- Actinic keratosis
- Verruca

Associated Factors and Diseases

- It is the second most common primary eyelid malignancy (5% to 10% of cases).
- It is more common in fair-skinned persons.
- It is more common in patients with xeroderma pigmentosum, those who have undergone radiation therapy, and immunosuppressed patients, such as those with human immunodeficiency virus (HIV) infection.
- The carcinoma may metastasize.

Treatment

- Surgery as for basal cell carcinoma is performed.
- Radiation usually is ineffective.

Follow-up

- Follow-up involves the same procedures as for basal cell carcinoma.

Blepharitis

Symptoms

- Irritation, burning, and foreign body sensation are reported by the patient.
- Excessive tearing (epiphora), photophobia, and intermittent blurred vision are other complaints.

Signs

- Erythema of the lid margin occurs.
- Dandruff-like deposits (scurf) are found on the lashes.
- Fibrinous scales surrounding individual lashes (collarettes) are seen.
- Lash loss occurs.
- Recurrent, mild conjunctivitis is present.
- Thick, cloudy secretions from the meibomian orifices result with digital pressure on the lid.

Etiology

Three distinct types of blepharitis may occur:
- Seborrhea (Fig. 4–15A) often is associated with dandruff of the brows and scalp.
- Staphylococcal infection (Fig. 4–15B) often is associated with styes (hordeola).

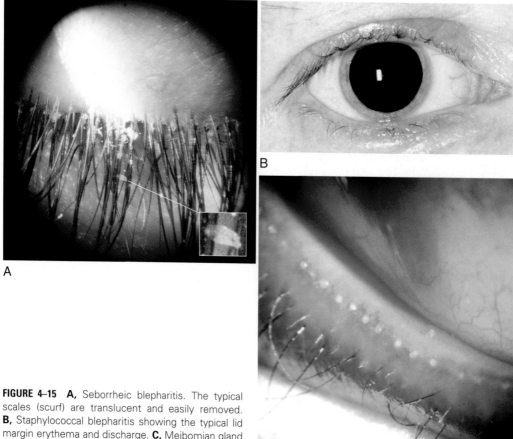

A

B

C

FIGURE 4–15 A, Seborrheic blepharitis. The typical scales (scurf) are translucent and easily removed. **B,** Staphylococcal blepharitis showing the typical lid margin erythema and discharge. **C,** Meibomian gland dysfunction showing thick secretions.

- Meibomian gland dysfunction (posterior lid margin disease and meibomianitis) (Fig. 4–15C) often is associated with chalazia.
- A combination of any of the three types can cause the disorder.

Differential Diagnosis

Considerations in the differential diagnosis include the following:
- Infiltrative lid neoplasm (e.g., squamous cell carcinoma, sebaceous cell carcinoma)
- Discoid lupus erythematosus

Treatment

- The lid margins are scrubbed daily with a cotton-tipped applicator dipped in dilute baby shampoo to remove scurf, collarettes, and bacteria. Massage of the lid margins may help express the abnormal meibomian secretions.
- Antibiotic treatment consists of the following:
  - A topical antibiotic ointment such as erythromycin or polymyxin B/bacitracin (e.g., Polysporin) is applied to the lid margins at night if lid scrubs are ineffective.
  - A 4 to 6 week course of doxycycline (50 to 200 mg/day) is added to improve meibomian gland function. Doxycycline is contraindicated in children, pregnant women, and breastfeeding mothers.

Follow-up

- The disorder frequently recurs and sometimes is recalcitrant to treatment.

Stye (Hordeolum)

Symptoms

- The subacute onset of a painful nodule or pustule of the eyelid is reported by the patient.

Signs

- A painful, erythematous, often pointed nodule is present on the skin surface (external stye) (Fig. 4–16) or conjunctival surface (internal stye).

Etiology

- Usually the disorder is caused by a staphylococcal infection of a sebaceous gland of the lid.

Differential Diagnosis

Considerations in the differential diagnosis include the following:
- Chalazion
- Inclusion cyst
- Lid tumor

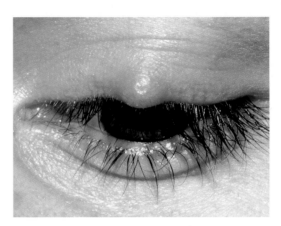

FIGURE 4–16 External stye.

Treatment

- Warm compresses and topical antibiotic drops such as fluoroquinolones (e.g., Vigamox, Zymar) or polymyxin B/trimethoprim (Polytrim) are applied three to four times a day.
- Incision and drainage are performed if improvement is not obtained with use of compresses and antibiotics or if the patient wants rapid relief of symptoms.

Follow-up

- The focus of follow-up evaluation is to ensure that preseptal cellulitis does not occur.

Chalazion

Symptoms

- Patients usually are symptom free or report a minimally tender nodule of the lid.

Signs

- A firm, well-demarcated nodule is present just below the lid margin (Fig. 4–17A).
- Usually a grayish discoloration is visible on the conjunctival surface (Fig. 4–17B).

Etiology

- A chronic, lipogranulomatous inflammation of a meibomian gland is present.
- The disorder is more common with meibomian gland dysfunction.

Differential Diagnosis

Considerations in the differential diagnosis include the following:
- Hordeolum
- Inclusion cyst
- Lid tumor

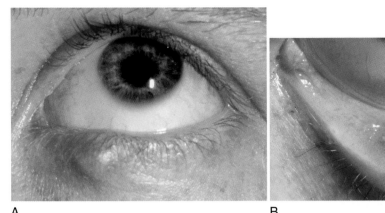

A   B

FIGURE 4–17 **A,** A typical chalazion appearing as a pea-sized nodule. **B,** The conjunctival appearance of the same chalazion.

Treatment

- Early treatment (during the first 5 days) consists of application of frequent, warm compresses to open the inflamed gland.
- Intermediate treatment (for first 2 to 3 weeks) consists of injection of triamcinolone. Steroid injections can result in depigmentation and are contraindicated in darkly pigmented individuals.
- Late treatment (after 1 month) entails marsupialization of the encysted meibomian gland using a conjunctival approach.

Molluscum Contagiosum

Symptoms

- Irritated skin, conjunctivitis, and keratitis secondary to viral shedding into the tear film are typical ophthalmic symptoms.

Signs

- Round, umbilicated, pearly-white lesions of the skin are present (Fig. 4–18).
- Lesions usually are multiple.

Etiology

- The disorder is caused by a poxvirus.

Differential Diagnosis

Considerations in the differential diagnosis include the following:
- Verruca
- Herpes zoster
- Herpes simplex

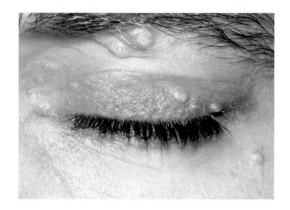

FIGURE 4–18   Multiple lesions of molluscum contagiosum.

Associated Factors and Diseases

- It is more common in children, sexually active adults, and patients with HIV infection.

Treatment

- The lesion is destroyed using excision, curettage, electrocautery, or cryotherapy.

Herpes Simplex Dermatitis

Symptoms

- Mild to moderately painful blepharitis occurs.

Signs

- Vesicular eruption on the skin of the lids or lid margin is present (Fig. 4–19).
- The eruption progresses to an ulcerative lesion with escharification.

Etiology

- The disorder commonly is caused by infection with herpes simplex virus 1 (human herpesvirus 1).
- Infection with herpes simplex virus 2 is uncommon.

Differential Diagnosis

Considerations in the differential diagnosis include the following:
- Molluscum
- Verruca
- Herpes zoster

Workup

- A viral culture is performed if necessary.

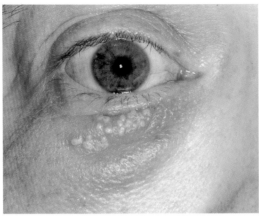

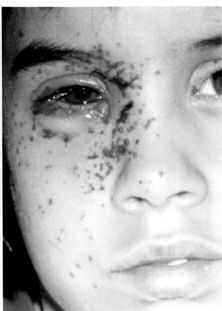

FIGURE 4–19 Herpes simplex dermatitis. A, Involvement of the eyelids. B, In this patient, the dermatitis affects the face and eyelids.

Treatment

- In mild cases, good hygiene is encouraged to prevent secondary bacterial infection.
- In moderate to severe cases, the following regimen is recommended:
  - Topical polymyxin B/bacitricin (e.g., Polysporin) ointment to prevent secondary bacterial infection
  - Trifluridine (Viroptic) drops to prevent secondary herpetic keratitis
  - Oral acyclovir (Zovirax) or famciclovir (Famvir) or valacyclovir (Valtrex)

Follow-up

- The patient is referred to an ophthalmologist, who monitors for subtle signs of herpetic keratitis.

Contact Dermatitis

Symptoms

- Generalized pruritic or painful eyelid occurs.

Signs

- In acute cases, erythema and edema of the eyelid occur (Fig. 4–20).
- In chronic cases, manifestations of the acute disorder as well as scaling and lichenification are present.
- Generally, the inflammation has a well-demarcated border.

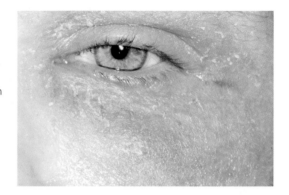

FIGURE 4–20   Contact dermatitis from tape used to secure an eye patch.

Etiology

• Pollen, dust, chemicals, and cosmetics are causative agents.

Differential Diagnosis

Considerations in the differential diagnosis include the following:
• Atopic dermatitis
• Seborrheic dermatitis
• Psoriasis
• Preseptal cellulitis

Workup

• A thorough history of the exposure is obtained.
• The possibility of infection is excluded.
• Patch testing may be necessary.

Treatment

• Patients are advised to avoid contact with the suspected cause.
• A topical corticosteroid such as fluorometholone 0.1% ophthalmic ointment is applied to the lids. Prolonged use of such agents can be associated with glaucoma and cataracts.

Essential Blepharospasm

Symptoms

• Irritation, burning, and foreign body sensation are reported by the patient.
• An inability to keep the eyes open, frequent blinking, and photophobia are other complaints.

Signs

• Obvious, frequent blinking, and an inability to open the eyes are evident (Fig. 4–21).

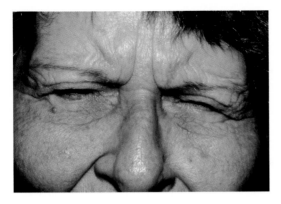

FIGURE 4–21   The patient had essential blepharospasm.

Etiology

- The disorder probably results from an abnormality of the basal ganglia or midbrain.

Differential Diagnosis

- Any secondary cause of blepharospasm such as iritis, corneal foreign body, or keratitis is identified.

Associated Factors and Diseases

- The disorder often is associated with other dystonic movements of the face and neck (Meige syndrome).
- The disorder sometimes is associated with peripheral dystonias of the legs, arms, and back and Parkinson's disease.
- A family history of the disorder occasionally is reported.

Treatment

- Botox (botulinum toxin) injections into the eyelids and other affected facial muscles are administered. Botox produces a positive response in approximately 90% of patients.
- Oral medication with clonazepam (Klonopin) can be tried if Botox is ineffective or not maximally effective.
- Surgery (orbicularis myectomy or differential section of the seventh cranial nerve) is performed if administration of Botox and oral medication fail.

Follow-up

- Botox injections usually need to be repeated every 2 to 3 months.

CHAPTER 5

Conjunctival Abnormalities

DAVID A. PALAY

Related Anatomy

The conjunctiva is a thin, transparent mucous membrane that lines the inner surface of the lids and outer surface of the eye. The portion of the conjunctiva on the eye is the bulbar conjunctiva, and the portion of the conjunctiva on the lid is the palpebral conjunctiva. The point of transition between these two zones is the fornix. An inferior and a superior fornix normally are present (Fig. 5–1). Glands in the conjunctiva produce the components of the tear film; a healthy conjunctiva is therefore essential for maintaining a healthy corneal surface. The conjunctiva also serves as a barrier against infection. Medially, the two important conjunctival structures are the plica semilunaris and the caruncle (Fig. 5–2).

Viral Conjunctivitis

Symptoms

- The onset of the disorder is acute.
- Redness, watering, soreness, and general discomfort are typical complaints.
- The second eye usually is involved 3 to 7 days after the first, and the symptoms are less severe in most cases.

Signs

- Diffuse injection of the conjunctiva with a watery discharge is present (Fig. 5–3).
- In severe cases, erythema and edema often are found in the lids (Fig. 5–4).

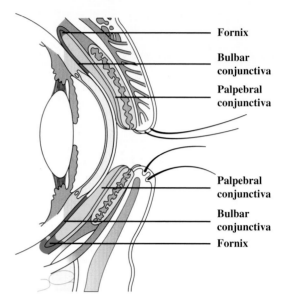

FIGURE 5–1   The region of the conjunctiva.

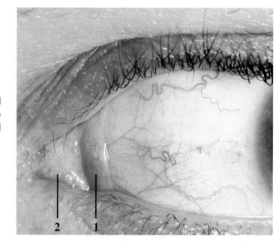

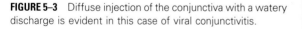

FIGURE 5–2   Conjunctiva, normal anatomy. The medial fold in the conjunctiva is the plica semilunaris (1). The caruncle (2) is an elevated mass that has features of both skin and conjunctiva.

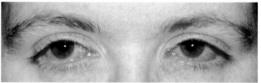

FIGURE 5–3   Diffuse injection of the conjunctiva with a watery discharge is evident in this case of viral conjunctivitis.

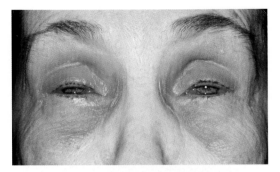

FIGURE 5–4 In this severe case of viral conjunctivitis, erythema and swelling of the lids and periocular skin are noted in addition to the diffuse injection of the conjunctiva.

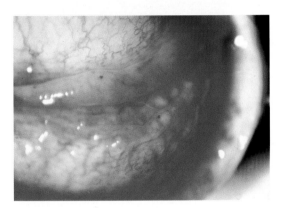

FIGURE 5–5 Small, elevated, cystic-appearing lesions termed *follicles* commonly occur on the palpebral conjunctiva in viral conjunctivitis.

- A follicular response in the conjunctiva is evident in most cases (Fig. 5–5).
- Preauricular adenopathy is common; patients may report tenderness in this region. Bacterial conjunctivitis is almost never associated with preauricular adenopathy, which can be a differentiating feature.
- Subepithelial infiltrates can develop in the cornea 2 to 3 weeks after the acute infection (Fig. 5–6). They result from the body's immune response to viral antigens and can cause decreased vision and photosensitivity.

Etiology

- Adenovirus infection (epidemic keratoconjunctivitis) usually is the cause.

Treatment

- The disease is self-limiting.
- Symptoms are treated, usually with cold compresses, artificial tears, and a vasoconstrictor-antihistamine combination (e.g., naphazoline plus pheniramine maleate [Naphcon-A], naphazoline plus antazoline phosphate [Vasocon-A]) four times a day if the itching is severe.
- Patients are counseled about the highly contagious nature of this viral infection. Infected persons involved in patient care should be excused from work until the acute signs and symptoms have resolved (usually in 5 to 14 days).

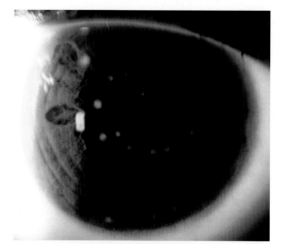

FIGURE 5–6 Subepithelial infiltrates may be noted in the cornea 2 to 3 weeks after the acute viral infection.

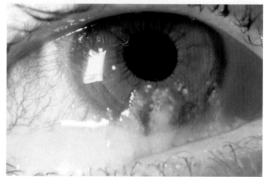

FIGURE 5–7 Diffuse injection of the conjunctiva with a thick, purulent discharge is evident in this case of bacterial conjunctivitis.

Bacterial Conjunctivitis

Symptoms

- Redness, irritation, and adhesion of the lids (especially in the morning) are typical complaints.

Signs

- A mucopurulent exudate is found in the fornix and on the lid margin (Figs. 5–7 and 5–8).
- In cases of diffuse conjunctivitis, erythema and edema of the lids sometimes are observed.
- *Neisseria gonorrhoeae* and *Neisseria meningitidis* cause a "hyperacute" conjunctivitis characterized by an exuberant mucopurulent discharge (Fig. 5–9). Because the organism can rapidly invade the cornea, causing tissue destruction and ocular perforation, infection with *Neisseria* species results in a potentially serious form of conjunctivitis (Fig. 5–10).

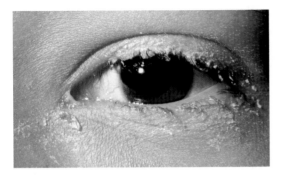

FIGURE 5–8 In this case of bacterial conjunctivitis, the purulent material has dried, creating a thick crust of material on the lid and lid margin.

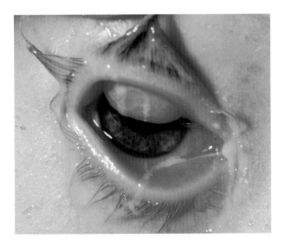

FIGURE 5–9 Bacterial conjunctivitis resulting from infection with *Neisseria gonorrhoeae*. A thick, mucopurulent discharge can be seen on the conjunctiva and lids.

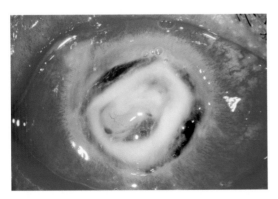

FIGURE 5–10 In this case of bacterial conjunctivitis resulting from infection with *Neisseria gonorrhoeae*, a central corneal perforation is evident, and retina plugs the perforation site.

Etiology

- Any of several bacterial species can cause conjunctivitis; *Staphylococcus aureus*, *Haemophilus* species, *Streptococcus pneumoniae*, and *Moraxella* species are the most common agents. *N. gonorrhoeae* and *N. meningitidis* are rarely the cause.

Workup

- Gram stain and conjunctival culture are performed in any cases suggestive of conjunctivitis caused by *Neisseria* species.
- Most cases do not require extensive workup, because broad-spectrum antibiotics eradicate the infection.

Treatment

- A broad-spectrum antibiotic, such as a fluoroquinolone (e.g., ciprofloxacin [Ciloxan], ofloxacin [Ocuflox], moxifloxacin [Vigamox], gatifloxacin [Zymar]), or polymyxin B/trimethoprim (Polytrim), or sulfacetamide drops, is administered four to six times a day.
- Drops are preferred over ointments because the latter can cause blurring of the patient's vision.
- For conjunctivitis caused by *Neisseria* species, the following apply:
  - Urgent referral to an ophthalmologist is necessary.
  - The eyes are irrigated with saline solution and the lids are cleansed four to six times a day.
  - Topical antibiotics (e.g., bacitracin, erythromycin ointment) are applied four to six times a day.
  - A single dose (1 g) of ceftriaxone (Rocephin) is injected intramuscularly in adults. In patients with severe penicillin allergy, medication with an oral fluoroquinolone (e.g., ciprofloxacin) for 7 days may be effective.
  - A twice-a-day oral dose of doxycycline (100 mg) is administered for 3 weeks to treat a concomitant chlamydial infection that may be present. Tetracycline and doxycycline are contraindicated in children, pregnant women, and breastfeeding mothers.
  - Sexual partners are counseled and treated.

Adult Chlamydial Conjunctivitis

Symptoms

- The onset of the disorder is acute or subacute.
- Redness, foreign body sensation, tearing, and photosensitivity are typical complaints.

Signs

- The conjunctivitis is more often unilateral than bilateral.

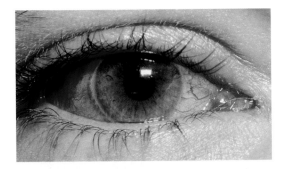

FIGURE 5–11 Diffuse injection of the conjunctiva is evident in this case of adult chlamydial conjunctivitis.

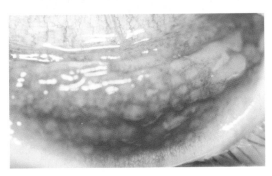

FIGURE 5–12 The inferior palpebral conjunctiva demonstrates multiple cystic-appearing lesions (follicles) in adult chlamydial conjunctivitis.

Etiology

- Ocular inoculation usually results from chlamydial infection of the genitalia.
- Diffuse injection of the conjunctiva with a scant mucopurulent discharge is present (Fig. 5–11).
- A follicular response in the conjunctiva usually is present (Fig. 5–12).
- Preauricular adenopathy is possible.

Workup

- Giemsa stain of a conjunctival scraping may show basophilic inclusion bodies (Fig. 5–13).
- Direct fluorescent antibody staining of conjunctival scrapings can be useful; however, a high incidence of false-negative results has been reported.

Treatment

- Medication entails oral tetracycline (250 mg) four times a day for 3 weeks or oral doxycycline (100 mg) twice a day for 3 weeks. Tetracycline and doxycycline are contraindicated in children, pregnant women, and breastfeeding mothers. If tetracyclines are contraindicated or not tolerated, oral erythromycin (250 mg) four times a day for 3 weeks is an effective alternative.
- Topical treatment consists of application of erythromycin ointment two to four times a day for 3 weeks.
- Sexual partners also are given appropriate treatment.

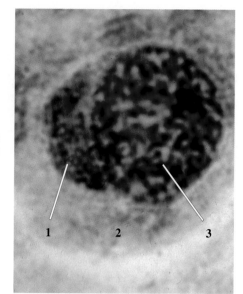

FIGURE 5–13   An epithelial cell from a conjunctival scraping obtained from a patient with adult chlamydial conjunctivitis shows basophilic inclusion bodies (1), the cell cytoplasm (2), and the cell nucleus (3).

Allergic Conjunctivitis

Symptoms

- The most predominant symptom is intense itching.

Signs

- The conjunctivitis is almost always bilateral.
- Mild conjunctival injection is present.
- A stringy mucoid discharge is evident.

Associated Factors and Diseases

- The disorder is usually seasonal, often occurring in persons with a history of atopic disease.
- Some airborne allergies (e.g., animal dander, dust, plant pollens, ragweed, mold spores) can incite a type I hypersensitivity reaction with acute swelling of the conjunctiva (chemosis) (Fig. 5–14).

Treatment

- Systemic allergy evaluation is performed with consideration of desensitization treatment and removal of allergens from the patient's environment.
- Systemic antihistamines are administered.
- Several topical preparations may be useful:
  - Topical vasoconstrictor-antihistamine combinations (e.g., naphazoline plus pheniramine maleate [Naphcon-A], naphazoline plus antazoline phosphate

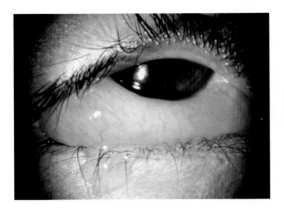

FIGURE 5–14 Acute allergic conjunctivitis caused by an airborne allergen. A diffuse conjunctivitis with swelling of the conjunctiva (chemosis) is present.

[Vasocon-A]) can be used four times a day for several days, but their chronic use can be associated with a worsening of the conjunctivitis from rebound vasodilation after discontinuation of the vasoconstrictor.
- Topical antihistamines (e.g., levocabastine [Livostin]) are applied four times a day as the symptoms warrant.
- Mast cell stabilizers (e.g., cromolyn sodium [Crolom], lodoxamide tromethamine [Alomide], pemirolast potassium [Alamast]) are applied three or four times a day. These agents require 10 to 14 days of use to reach their maximal effectiveness.
- Topical nonsteroidal agents (e.g., ketorolac tromethamine [Acular]) are applied four times a day as symptoms warrant.
- If these treatments fail, patients should be referred to an ophthalmologist for further treatment and consideration of topical corticosteroid therapy.

Conjunctivitis Associated with Blepharitis

Symptoms

- Burning, itching, and foreign body sensation are typical complaints.
- Unlike dry eyes, in which symptoms worsen as the day progresses, symptoms in this disorder usually are worse in the morning. Blepharitis, however, often is associated with dry eyes; therefore, this distinction may not be useful in patients with severe dry eyes associated with blepharitis.

Signs

- Diffuse injection and inflammation of the lid margin involving the meibomian glands are present (Fig. 5–15).
- Moderate conjunctival injection is found.
- In rare cases, vascularization of the cornea occurs (Fig. 5–16).
- The disorder usually is bilateral but may be asymmetrical.

Etiology

Three distinct types of blepharitis may occur and cause conjunctivitis:

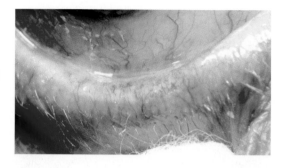

FIGURE 5-15 In blepharitis, the lid margin is thickened, and vascularization of the lid margin is evident.

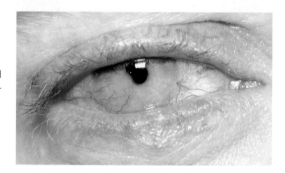

FIGURE 5-16 In severe blepharitis with rosacea, the lid margins and conjunctiva are inflamed, and corneal vascularization and scarring are present.

- Seborrhea often is associated with dandruff of the brows and scalp.
- Staphylococcal infection often is associated with styes (hordeola).
- Meibomian gland dysfunction (posterior lid margin disease and meibomianitis) often is associated with chalazia.
- Any combination of these causes is possible.

Associated Factors and Diseases

- Blepharitis is one of the most common causes of chronic conjunctivitis.
- Meibomian gland dysfunction is a disorder of the sebaceous glands frequently associated with rosacea, which is a sebaceous gland dysfunction of the skin (Fig. 5–17).

Treatment

- The underlying blepharitis is treated (see Chapter 4).

Pinguecula

Symptoms

- Patients are symptom free.

Signs

- An elevated, fleshy conjunctival mass is located on the sclera adjacent to the cornea (Fig. 5–18).

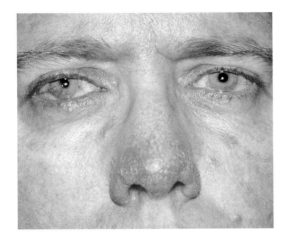

FIGURE 5–17 Occurring with greater frequency in females, rosacea often manifests with erythema, telangiectasia, and acne.

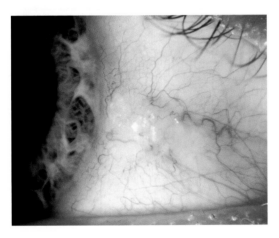

FIGURE 5–18 Pinguecula. Pingueculae are elevated, fleshy conjunctival masses located in the interpalpebral region, most commonly on the nasal side. These lesions are yellow or light brown.

- The pinguecula is yellow or light brown.
- Rarely, the pinguecula can become acutely inflamed.

Etiology

- The disorder usually is associated with chronic actinic exposure, repeated trauma, and dry and windy conditions.

Treatment

- No treatment usually is necessary; in rare cases in which the pinguecula is chronically irritated or cosmetically undesirable, resection is performed.

Conjunctival Intraepithelial Neoplasia

Symptoms

- Patients are symptom free.

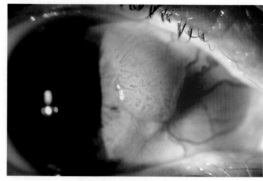

FIGURE 5–19 Conjunctival intraepithelial neoplasia. This raised, gelatinous lesion demonstrates hairpin-shaped vascular loops.

Signs

- An elevated, gelatinous mass, usually arising at the junction of the conjunctiva and cornea (Fig. 5–19), is present.
- Distinctive hairpin-shaped vascular loops are seen within the lesion.

Etiology

- The disorder usually is associated with chronic sun exposure in older white patients.

Treatment

- Surgical resection is indicated, because these lesions are dysplastic and can progress to invasive squamous cell carcinoma.

Nevi

Symptoms

- Patients are symptom free.

Signs

- Benign pigmented lesions of the conjunctiva are found (Fig. 5–20).
- The nevi usually occur on the conjunctiva covering the globe.
- The lesions are freely mobile over the sclera.
- In rare cases, a nevus may progress to a malignant melanoma (Fig. 5–21).

Workup

- A biopsy of nevi that show documented growth or change in appearance is done.

Treatment

- Resection of suspicious lesions is performed.

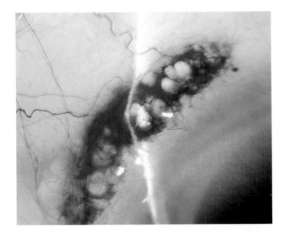

FIGURE 5–20 Nevi are benign pigmented lesions of the conjunctiva. Occasionally, clear cystic spaces develop within the lesion.

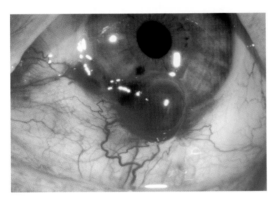

FIGURE 5–21 In this case of malignant melanoma of the conjunctiva, the tumor is elevated, pigmented, and highly vascular.

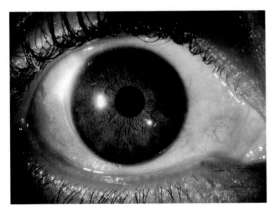

FIGURE 5–22 In racial melanosis, a flat, deeply pigmented lesion of the conjunctiva commonly is found near the limbus.

Racial Melanosis

Symptoms

- Patients are symptom free.

Signs

- This lesion of the conjunctiva is flat and deeply pigmented (Fig. 5–22).
- The lesion usually is found on the conjunctiva overlying the globe.
- The disorder occurs primarily in darkly pigmented patients and has no malignant potential.

Treatment

If the lesion is cosmetically undesirable, resection is performed.

CHAPTER 6

Corneal Abnormalities

DAVID A. PALAY

Related Anatomy

The cornea is the primary refractive element of the eye, and any disturbance in corneal clarity results in visual impairment. The cornea has five layers: the epithelium, Bowman's layer, the stroma, Descemet's membrane, and the endothelium (Fig. 6–1). The epithelium is four to six layers thick and composed of nonkeratinized, stratified squamous epithelium. Bowman's layer is a thin, acellular area composed of collagen fibers. The stroma constitutes 90% of the corneal thickness and is composed primarily of keratocytes, collagen, and proteoglycans. Descemet's membrane is a thin, collagenous layer produced by the endothelium. The endothelium is one cell layer thick and is responsible for removing fluid from the cornea, thereby preventing corneal edema. The cornea is approximately 12 mm in diameter and has a central thickness of 0.5 mm. The peripheral cornea is 0.65 mm thick (Fig. 6–2).

Dry Eye

Symptoms

- Foreign body sensation, irritation, dryness, and mild redness are characteristic.
- Patients may report symptoms out of proportion to the signs present.
- Symptoms worsen as the day progresses and may be exacerbated by smoke, cold, low humidity, wind, prolonged use of the eye without blinking, and contact lens wear.

Signs

- The disorder usually is bilateral.
- Mild conjunctival injection is present primarily medially and laterally.
- Excessive mucus production is evident (Fig. 6–3).
- Punctate staining of the cornea is found with fluorescein dye (Fig. 6–4).

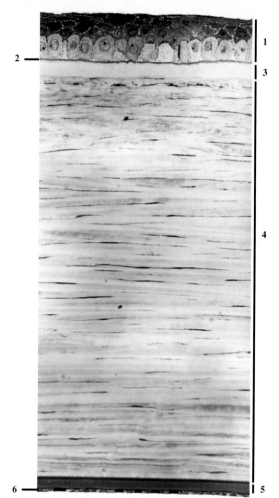

FIGURE 6–1 The normal cornea. The epithelium (1), epithelial basement membrane (2), Bowman's membrane (3), stroma (4), Descemet's membrane (5), and endothelium (6).

Associated Factors and Diseases

- Most cases of dry eye are idiopathic and occur in older persons. In younger persons, contact lens wear may precipitate dry eye signs and symptoms.
- Any eyelid abnormality resulting in poor lid closure, such as seventh nerve palsy and ectropion, can lead to exposure and drying of the cornea (Fig. 6–5).
- Graft-versus-host disease can cause severe dry eyes.
- Collagen-vascular diseases such as rheumatoid arthritis and systemic lupus erythematosus often are associated with dry eyes. The combination of dry eyes and dry mouth is termed *primary Sjögren syndrome*. The combination of dry eyes, dry mouth, and collagen-vascular disease, most commonly rheumatoid arthritis, is termed *secondary Sjögren syndrome*.
- The disorder often is associated with blepharitis.

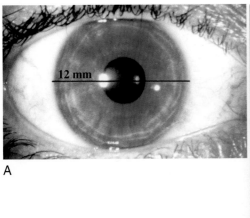

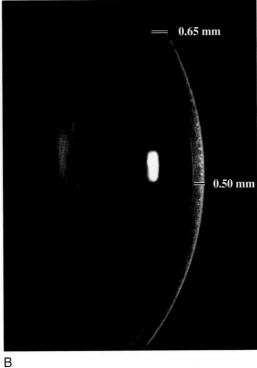

FIGURE 6–2   A, The normal cornea is 12 mm in diameter. **B,** The central thickness is 0.5 mm, and the peripheral thickness is 0.65 mm.

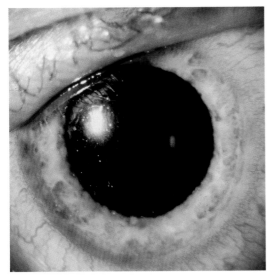

FIGURE 6–3   In this case of dry eye, the corneal surface is dry, and mucus is evident on the surface.

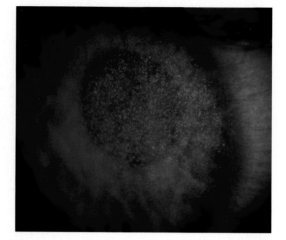

FIGURE 6–4   Punctate staining of the cornea with fluorescein dye in dry eye. The areas of abnormal epithelium stain green.

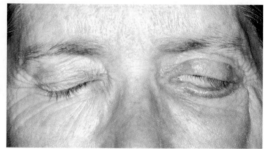

FIGURE 6–5   In seventh nerve palsy, the inability to close the lids and the out-turning of the lower lid (ectropion) can cause dry eye.

- Sarcoidosis can cause infiltration of the lacrimal gland and is associated with dry eyes.
- Many systemic medications are associated with dry eyes. Drugs with anticholinergic properties often are implicated.

Workup: Schirmer Test

- The Schirmer tear test can be performed with or without the instillation of anesthetic drops. (The procedure is described in Chapter 1.)
  - With anesthesia, this test provides an indication of the basal tear secretion—that is, the amount of tears being produced without any noxious stimuli to the eye, which probably is a more accurate measure of tear production.
  - Without anesthesia, this test measures the ability of the lacrimal gland to produce tears in response to a noxious stimulus; a false-negative result can occur, particularly in patients in whom the diagnosis is not clear.

Treatment

- For mild cases, artificial tear preparations (e.g., polyvinyl alcohol [HypoTears], hydroxypropyl methylcellulose [Tears Naturale II]), which typically contain a

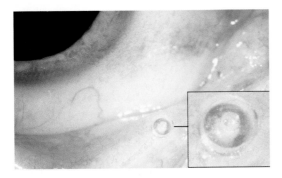

FIGURE 6–6 A silicone punctal plug *(inset)* has been placed in the right inferior punctum. The plug increases the volume of the tear film by decreasing tear outflow.

preservative, are used as symptoms warrant. Excessive use of these preparations (e.g., every 1 to 2 hours) can result in toxic effects from the preservatives.

- For more severe cases, use of a preservative-free artificial tear preparation (e.g., hydroxypropyl methylcellulose [Bion Tears], polyvinyl alcohol [Refresh, Hypo-Tears PF]) is recommended. These preparations can be used as frequently as necessary and do not cause toxic effects to the eye from preservatives.
- Artificial tear ointments (e.g., white petrolatum–mineral oil–lanolin [Refresh P.M., Lacri-Lube], white petrolatum–mineral oil [HypoTears ointment]) are used at bedtime and during the day if necessary. Ointments provide a longer-lasting effect than drops; however, a side effect is blurring of the vision.
- Insertion of punctal plugs decreases the outflow of tears through the nasolacrimal system (Fig. 6–6).

Herpes Simplex Keratitis

Symptoms

- Irritation, light sensitivity, and redness are typical.
- Pain is mild or does not occur.

Signs

- In 98% of cases the disorder is unilateral.
- Mild conjunctival injection is present.
- Epithelial dendrites are observed with fluorescein staining (Fig. 6–7).
- With advanced disease, stromal scarring and vascularization are possible (Fig. 6–8), and patients may have decreased corneal sensation.

Treatment

- Urgent referral to an ophthalmologist is necessary for confirmation and treatment.
- Topical antiviral medications usually are applied.
- **Note:** Indiscriminate use of topical corticosteroids to treat herpes simplex keratitis can result in tissue loss and ocular perforation. Therefore, it is important in the primary care setting to exclude herpes simplex keratitis prior to the treatment of a

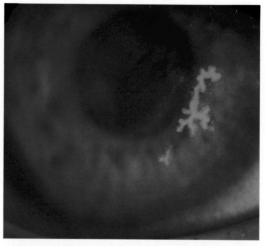

FIGURE 6–7 In this case of herpes simplex keratitis, an epithelial dendrite stains green with fluorescein dye.

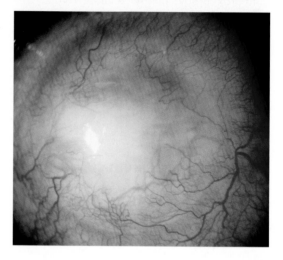

FIGURE 6–8 The corneal scarring and corneal vascularization present in this eye are due to herpes simplex keratitis.

"red eye" with a topical corticosteroid or a topical antibiotic/corticosteroid combination. Patients with herpes simplex keratitis should be referred for management to an ophthalmologist familiar with the diagnosis and treatment of this disorder.

Herpes Zoster Ophthalmicus

Symptoms

• Pain, headache, and photophobia are symptoms of this disorder.

Signs

• A vesicular rash is seen in the distribution of the first division of the fifth cranial nerve. If the tip of the nose is involved (Hutchinson's sign), ocular involvement is

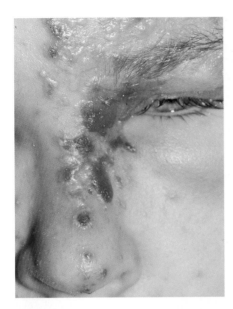

FIGURE 6–9 A vesicular rash and Hutchinson's sign are present in herpes zoster ophthalmicus.

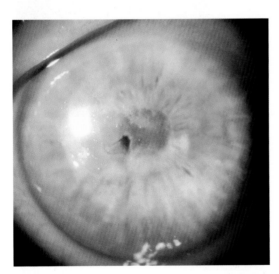

FIGURE 6–10 Severe scarring in the cornea has resulted from repeated corneal inflammation from herpes zoster ophthalmicus.

likely, because both regions are supplied by the nasociliary branch of the first division of the fifth cranial nerve (Fig. 6–9).

- Ocular findings include conjunctivitis, corneal involvement (Fig. 6–10), uveitis (Fig. 6–11), glaucoma, and scleritis (Fig. 6–12).
- Corneal involvement, uveitis, and glaucoma can develop into a chronic disorder possibly refractory to treatment.
- Rare ocular complications include optic neuritis with resultant visual loss and cranial nerve palsies with resultant diplopia.

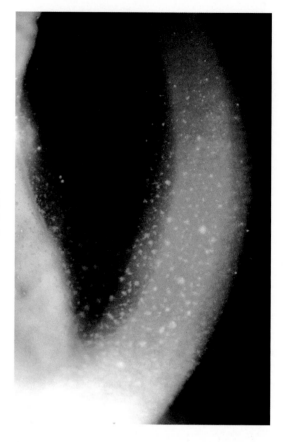

FIGURE 6–11 Uveitis has resulted from herpes zoster ophthalmicus. Multiple white keratic precipitates have formed on the posterior cornea from repeated inflammation. Many patients with this disorder also have elevated intraocular pressure, which can lead to severe glaucoma.

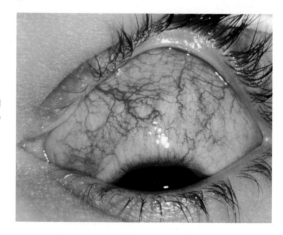

FIGURE 6–12 Injection of the conjunctiva and deep episcleral blood vessels with severe pain are present in this example of herpes zoster ophthalmicus with scleritis.

Differential Diagnosis

- The vesicular rash of herpes simplex virus does not follow a dermatomal distribution, although characteristics of the disorder may be otherwise identical to those of herpes simplex infection.

Treatment

- Oral acyclovir (800 mg) is administered five times a day for 7 to 10 days. Immunocompromised patients may require intravenous therapy. Treatment alternatives include famciclovir (Famvir), with an oral dosage of 500 mg three times a day for 7 days, and valacyclovir (Valtrex), with an oral dosage of 1 g three times a day for 7 days. The use of valacyclovir is contraindicated in immunocompromised patients. Thrombotic thrombocytopenic purpura or hemolytic-uremic syndrome has developed in some immunocompromised patients on this regimen. Bioavailability of these new agents is greater than that of oral acyclovir.
- Patients with ocular involvement should be referred to an ophthalmologist within 24 hours. Treatment usually involves administration of topical corticosteroids. Some patients have a protracted clinical course, with keratitis, uveitis, and glaucoma.

Infectious Corneal Ulcer

Symptoms

- Pain, redness, decreased vision, and photophobia are characteristic.

Signs

- A dense corneal infiltrate with an overlying defect in the epithelium is observed (Fig. 6–13).
- A layering of white cells in the anterior chamber (hypopyon) may be evident (Fig. 6–14).
- Severe corneal ulcers, particularly those resulting from gram-negative pathogens, can lead to rapid corneal destruction and ocular perforation (Fig. 6–15).
- Fungal ulcers may have a feathery border (Fig. 6–16).

Associated Factors and Diseases

- The disorder usually is associated with a history of trauma, poor lid apposition, or contact lens wear.
- Fungal ulcers usually are associated with a history of trauma involving vegetable matter or chronic topical corticosteroid use.

Treatment

- Immediate referral to an ophthalmologist is necessary for corneal scraping for Gram stain and culture.
- Bacterial ulcers often are treated with fortified antibiotics (e.g., gentamicin, cefazolin).

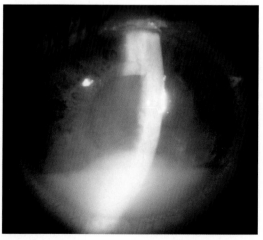

FIGURE 6–13 A dense corneal infiltrate (1) with an overlying defect in the epithelium (2) has resulted from a bacterial corneal ulcer.

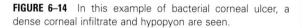

FIGURE 6–14 In this example of bacterial corneal ulcer, a dense corneal infiltrate and hypopyon are seen.

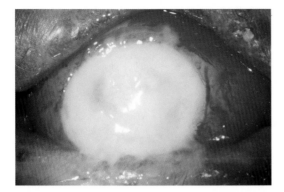

FIGURE 6–15 Severe bacterial corneal ulcer has resulted from *Pseudomonas* infection. The entire cornea is white and necrotic. Corneal perforation is imminent.

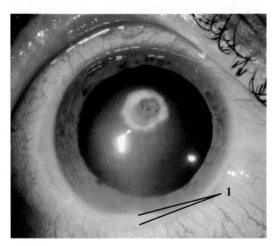

FIGURE 6–16 In this fungal corneal ulcer, the infiltrate has feathery margins. Hypopyon (1) also is evident.

Pterygium

Symptoms

- Patients usually are symptom free.
- Intermittent irritation, redness, and a mild disturbance in visual acuity may be noted.

Signs

- Fibrovascular growth extending from the conjunctiva onto the cornea is present (Fig. 6–17).

Treatment

- Surgical resection is performed for pterygia that interfere with vision or are actively growing.

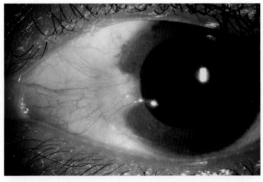

FIGURE 6–17   Fibrovascular growth extending from the conjunctiva onto the cornea is evident in this case of pterygium.

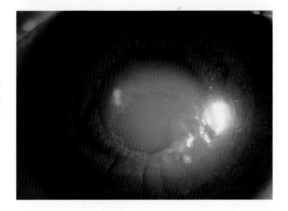

FIGURE 6–18   In this example of recurrent corneal erosion, a defect in the epithelium is evident. The adjacent epithelium is irregular and loose, and the entire area stains lightly with fluorescein dye.

Recurrent Erosion Syndrome

Symptoms

- Patients report sudden onset of severe eye pain, blurred vision, and redness in the middle of the night or on awakening.

Signs

- In the acute stage of the disorder, the epithelial defect stains with fluorescein (Fig. 6–18).
- After the epithelial defect heals, there is diffuse irregularity of the epithelial surface.

Etiology

- Poor epithelial adhesion to Bowman's membrane and the underlying corneal stroma causes the disorder.

Associated Factors and Diseases

- The disorder usually is associated with a previous episode of trauma that resulted in a corneal abrasion.

Treatment

- In the acute stage, the patient is referred to an ophthalmologist within 24 hours for confirmation and treatment.
- In chronic cases, hypertonic saline ointment (e.g., Muro #128 ointment) is used at night. The hypertonicity of the ointment promotes dehydration of the epithelium, preventing loosening during sleep with sudden shearing of the epithelium on opening the lids. The ointment also provides a lubricating function that prevents the lid from adhering to the epithelium. Therapy may be needed for many months.
- In advanced cases, surgical treatment with stromal puncture or laser treatment to the underlying stroma may be required.

Calcific Band Keratopathy

Symptoms

- A mild foreign body sensation or severe pain resulting from calcium accumulation on the cornea may be reported by the patient.

Signs

- A white accumulation of calcium is seen on the central cornea (Fig. 6–19).
- "Swiss cheese" holes usually are present in calcium deposits.

Associated Factors and Diseases

- The disorder usually is associated with chronic ocular inflammation.
- The disorder may be associated with systemic diseases causing hypercalcemia (e.g., renal failure, sarcoidosis, primary hyperparathyroidism).

Treatment

- For calcium deposits that cause discomfort or limit vision, a superficial scraping of the cornea using disodium EDTA is performed.

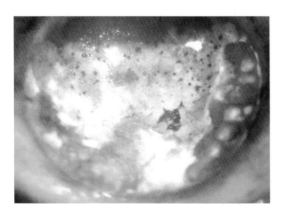

FIGURE 6–19 A white, chalky material is deposited across the cornea in this eye affected with band keratopathy. Small "Swiss cheese" holes also are seen.

Corneal Surgery

Corneal Transplantation

Corneal transplantation (penetrating keratoplasty) is performed to restore vision in patients with corneal scarring, corneal edema, or abnormal corneal shape. Donor corneas are harvested post mortem and kept in storage media for up to a week. The central area of corneal malformation is replaced with a circular piece of donor tissue and sutured into place with fine nylon sutures (Fig. 6–20).

Refractive Surgery

Laser in situ keratomileusis (LASIK) is the most common procedure used to correct refractive errors of the eye. In LASIK, a corneal flap is dissected with a microkeratome. The flap is retracted, and an excimer laser is used to reshape the stromal bed. The flap is replaced; subsequently, it heals around the peripheral cut edge (Fig. 6–21). This procedure does not cause central corneal scarring, is relatively painless, and usually results in rapid visual recovery.

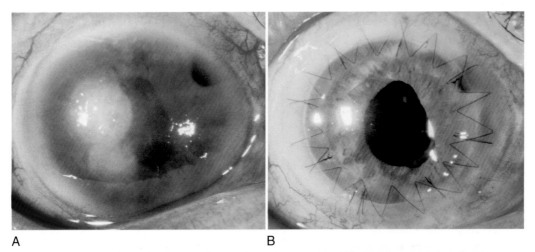

A   B

FIGURE 6–20   A, Preoperative view of a central corneal scar from a resolved bacterial corneal ulcer. **B,** The same eye 3 weeks after corneal transplantation. Fine nylon sutures hold the transplant in place. The visual axis is clear.

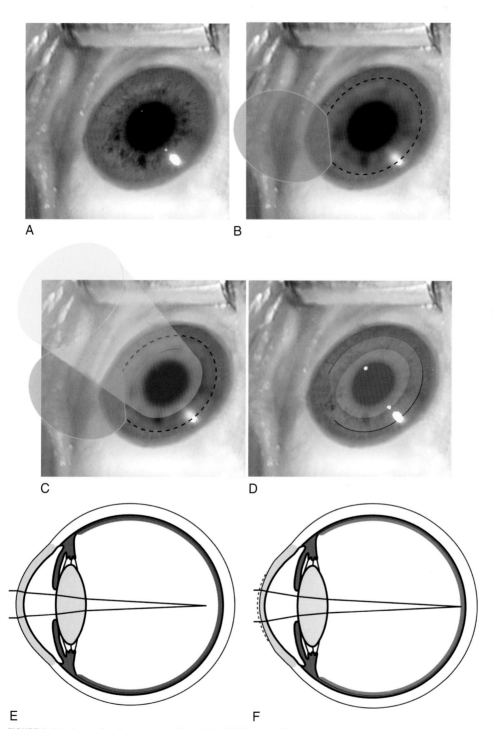

FIGURE 6–21 Laser in situ keratomileusis (LASIK) procedure. A, A lid speculum is used to retract the lids. **B,** A microkeratome *(not shown)* creates a thin corneal flap that remains attached to the underlying cornea with a small hinge. **C,** The excimer laser reshapes the stromal bed. **D,** The corneal flap is replaced; it will heal around the peripheral cut edge. **E,** In this example of the near-sighted (myopic) eye, the light is focused in front of the retina. **F,** After LASIK, the cornea has been reshaped so that light focuses directly on the retina. The cornea is less convex than the preoperative surface *(dotted line).*

117

CHAPTER 7

Scleritis

MICHAEL C. DIESENHOUSE

Related Anatomy

The episclera and sclera are composed of connective tissue, and together they provide a protective coat for the eye (Fig. 7–1). The episclera is a fascial sheath that encases the eye. It has a superficial layer, Tenon's capsule, which acts as a synovial membrane to allow smooth movements of the eye. A deeper layer of the episclera contains a network of vessels. The episclera overlies the primarily avascular sclera and is partly responsible for scleral nutrition. The sclera is composed of collagen and elastic fibers arranged randomly. Its rigid structure is necessary for vision to remain stable during eye movements. The thickness of the sclera varies, ranging from approximately 0.3 mm behind the insertion of the rectus muscles to 1.2 mm posteriorly.

Inflammatory Conditions

Inflammation of the episclera and sclera is not commonly seen in clinical practice. Confusion with more common causes of a red eye, however, may lead to a delay in diagnosis. Conjunctivitis usually involves the entire conjunctiva (not just a section), usually is not associated with pain, and generally is accompanied by a discharge. Episcleritis and scleritis usually involve a section of the eye (although sometimes the entire eye is involved), are associated with mild pain (episcleritis) or severe pain (scleritis), and are not associated with a discharge. On the patient's initial visit, distinguishing between episcleral and scleral inflammation is essential, because the management of these two diseases differs considerably. In addition, scleritis is more likely to be associated with exacerbation of a potentially serious systemic disease. A useful classification is presented in Box 7–1.

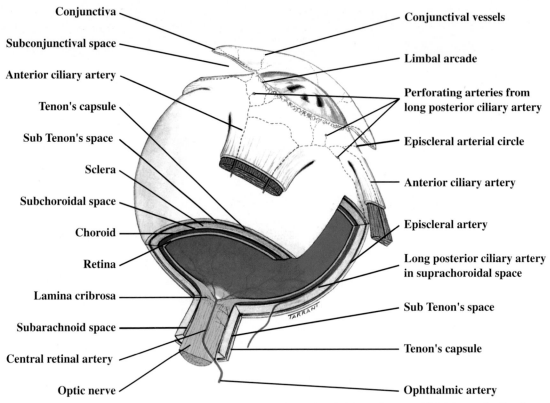

FIGURE 7–1 Anteriorly, the episclera lies between the conjunctiva and underlying sclera, to which it is attached by fibrous bands. Posteriorly, it is continuous with the muscular sheath, extends backward to cover the whole of the globe, and merges with the optic nerve sheath behind the eye. It is perforated by the ciliary vessels and nerves and the vortex veins.

Episcleritis

Symptoms

- Redness of acute onset is noted by the patient.
- If pain is present, it often is described as a dull ache localized to the eye.
- Visual acuity usually is normal.
- The patient may report a history of recurrent episodes.

Signs

- Sectoral or diffuse redness of one or both eyes is evident.
- Episcleral vessels are engorged, but the vascular pattern is not disturbed.
- If a nodule is present, it is mobile over the underlying sclera.
- Neither discharge nor corneal involvement is present.

BOX **7–1** **Classification of Episcleritis and Scleritis**

Episcleritis
- Simple
- Nodular (Fig. 7–2)

Scleritis

Diffuse Anterior
- Diffuse anterior scleritis is the most common but least destructive type (Fig. 7–3).
- Widespread involvement of the sclera is characteristic, but localized changes also are seen.

Nodular Anterior
- This form is distinguished by a painful localized elevation of the sclera, which may develop into a nodule (Fig. 7–4).
- Nodular anterior scleritis differs from nodular episcleritis in that the nodule is immobile.
- In approximately 20% of the patients, the condition progresses to necrotizing scleritis.

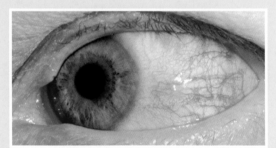

FIGURE 7–2 Nodular episcleritis in a patient with gout.

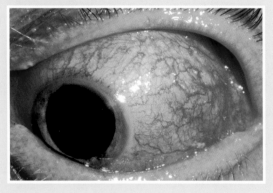

FIGURE 7–3 In diffuse anterior scleritis, widespread injection of the conjunctival and deep episcleral vessels is characteristic.

BOX **7–1**   **Classification of Episcleritis and Scleritis** (Continued)

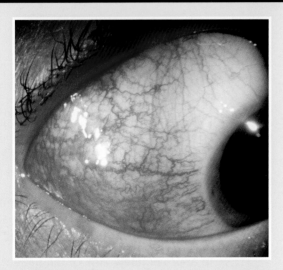

FIGURE 7–4   An elevated mass within the area of inflammation is seen in nodular anterior scleritis. Unlike the nodule in episcleritis, this nodule is immobile.

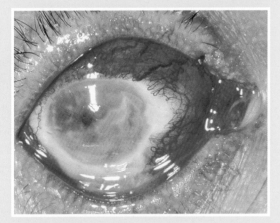

FIGURE 7–5   In this eye of a patient with rheumatoid arthritis and necrotizing scleritis, avascular areas with tissue loss are adjacent to areas of active inflammation. Prompt and aggressive immunosuppressive treatment is necessary.

Necrotizing

- Necrotizing scleritis is the least common but most destructive form (Fig. 7–5).
- Ocular and systemic complications are seen in 60% of patients.
- Progressive scleral necrosis can lead to scleral thinning and perforation of the globe.
- The disorder usually is associated with a potentially serious systemic disease.

Scleromalacia Perforans

- Scleromalacia perforans is the only form of scleritis without pain (Fig. 7–6).
- A lack of symptoms is characteristic. Some patients may note decreased vision or a change in the color of the sclera.

BOX **7–1** **Classification of Episcleritis and Scleritis** (Continued)

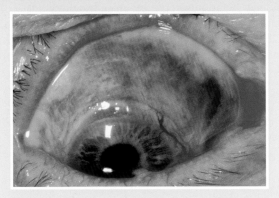

FIGURE 7–6 Marked scleral thinning, a characteristic of scleromalacia perforans, allows exposure of the underlying choroid. This gives the sclera a bluish hue, a discoloration best seen in daylight.

- Scleral necrosis and thinning are observed in the absence of inflammation.
- Perforation of the globe may occur with minor trauma.
- The disorder is predominantly bilateral and seen almost exclusively in patients with rheumatoid arthritis.

Associated Factors and Diseases

- In 75% of cases, the origin is idiopathic.
- Other causes include the following:
  - Collagen-vascular diseases
  - Atopy
  - Rosacea
  - Gout
  - Herpes zoster
  - Lyme disease
  - Syphilis
  - Bisphosphonates
- The disorder is more prevalent in young adults.

Workup

- The phenylephrine test involves instillation of a drop of phenylephrine 2.5% in the eye, which helps distinguish between dilated episcleral and scleral vessels. Unlike the deeper scleral vessels, episcleral vessels blanch when topical phenylephrine is applied.

Treatment

- Referral to an ophthalmologist is necessary for confirmation and treatment. A careful review of systems should be performed.

- Most cases are self-limited and resolve without treatment.
- Initially, cold compresses, artificial tears, and/or a topical vasconstrictor are used. Topical corticosteroids may be administered by an ophthalmologist. Topical non-steroidal anti-inflammatory drugs (NSAIDs) are of questionable value in treatment.
- If topical medications do not provide relief, a course of an oral NSAID is instituted.
- Resistance to treatment may signify the presence of an associated systemic disease.

Scleritis

Several types of scleritis exist (see Box 7–1). Although each type has distinct characteristics, these entities have many of the same symptoms and signs.

Symptoms

- The onset of the disorder is gradual.
- The hallmark symptom is severe pain that may radiate to the temple or jaw. Often the pain awakens the patient at night.
- Photophobia is present.
- Tearing occurs.
- Vision is normal or mildly decreased.
- Episodes may recur.

Signs

- The globe is tender to palpation.
- Sectoral or diffuse edema of the sclera occurs, with engorgement of the overlying episcleral vessels.
- Nodules and scleral necrosis may be present.
- Corneal and intraocular inflammation may coexist.

Associated Factors and Diseases

- The origin usually is idiopathic, but almost half of the patients have an associated systemic disease. The inflammation of the eye may serve as a clue to an underlying disease or warn of increased severity in a known condition.
- Disorders and medications for which an association with scleritis has been documented include the following:
  - Rheumatoid arthritis
  - Systemic lupus erythematosus
  - Polyarteritis nodosa
  - Wegener's granulomatosis
  - Relapsing polychondritis
  - Ankylosing spondylitis
  - Giant cell arteritis
  - Gout
  - Herpes zoster
  - Lyme disease

- ○ Syphilis
- ○ Tuberculosis
- ○ Bisphosphonates

Workup

- In the phenylephrine test, deep episcleral and scleral vessels do not blanch when topical 2.5% phenylephrine is applied.
- The patient's eye is viewed with normal lighting. An eye with scleritis may have a bluish hue when seen in daylight, which can signify thinning of the sclera. This discoloration can be easily overlooked in a darkened room.

Treatment

- Referral to an ophthalmologist is necessary for confirmation and treatment.
- Because scleritis may be the presenting sign of a systemic disease, a thorough systemic evaluation is warranted. The management of scleritis necessitates the use of systemic medications. If an associated systemic disease is identified, therapy is appropriately modified.
- Initial treatment involves administration of oral NSAIDs or systemic corticosteroids.
- In advanced cases, cytotoxic agents may be prescribed. Because of the side effects and contraindications of these medications, the treatment protocol must be individualized for each patient.
- Treatment guidelines are based on the persistence of inflammation, with the degree of resolution of pain used to gauge disease control.
- For management of patients with scleritis, a team approach involving the ophthalmologist and the primary care physician is essential.

CHAPTER 8

Lens Abnormalities

JONATHAN H. ENGMAN • ANDREW R. HARRISON •
JAY H. KRACHMER

Related Anatomy

The lens is a biconvex and grossly transparent structure located directly behind the iris. In adults, it is approximately 9 mm in diameter and 4 mm thick. The lens consists of 65% water and 35% protein (which is the highest protein content of any body tissue). No pain fibers, blood vessels, or nerves are present in the lens.

The lens has three layers: the capsule, cortex, and nucleus (Fig. 8–1). The lens capsule is a thin, semipermeable membrane that envelops the entire lens. The posterior capsule is markedly thinner than the anterior capsule. The lens cortex is composed of lens cells, or fibers, that are produced continuously throughout life. The old lens fibers migrate centrally as new fibers are produced. The oldest lens fibers, which are those that have lost their nuclei, make up the nucleus.

The lens is held in place by ligaments known as *zonules*, which are composed of numerous fibrils that arise in the ciliary body and insert into the lens capsule. Contraction of the ciliary body causes relaxation of zonules with resultant thickening of the lens, thereby allowing the eye to focus on near objects. This phenomenon is known as *accommodation*.

Presbyopia

Symptoms

- Reading is difficult.
- Reading material is held farther from the eyes.
- Distance vision is blurry after the patient reads.

Signs

- Only near vision decreases; the ability (or inability) to see distant objects remains the same.

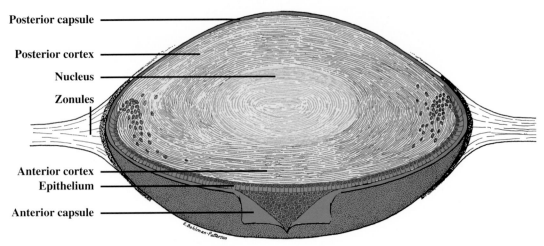

Posterior capsule

Posterior cortex

Nucleus

Zonules

Anterior cortex
Epithelium

Anterior capsule

FIGURE 8–1 Normal lens anatomy.

Etiology

- With age, the lens becomes increasingly inelastic and can no longer "thicken" to focus on near objects (Fig. 8–2). This disorder, also called "old sight," usually becomes clinically significant at the age of 40 to 45 years.

Treatment

- For patients with normal distance vision, simple reading glasses may be purchased over the counter, without a prescription, at pharmacies.
- For patients with distance vision requiring correction, the following apply:
  - ○ Spectacle correction with bifocal (distance and near) or trifocal (distance, intermediate, and near) lenses
  - ○ Monovision contact lenses in which one eye is corrected for distance vision and the other eye for near vision
  - ○ Contact lens correction of distance vision and simple reading glasses for near vision

Senile Cataract

A cataract is any opacity in the crystalline lens. Senile cataract is an age-related disorder, and four types occur: nuclear, cortical, posterior subcapsular, and dense white (Box 8–1).

Symptoms

- A slowly progressing visual loss or blurring occurs over months to years.
- Glare is a problem, particularly from oncoming headlights during night driving.
- Double vision in one eye (monocular diplopia) may be noted.
- Fixed spots in the visual field are present.

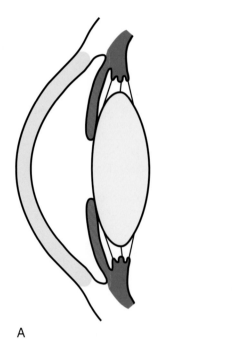 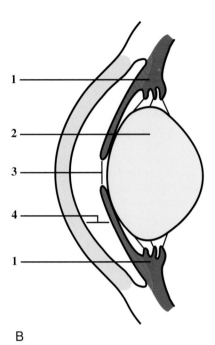

A   B

FIGURE 8–2 A, Cross section of the eye in the nonaccommodative state. **B,** During accommodation to focus on a near object, the ciliary body (1) moves forward, relaxing the zonules, which allows the lens (2) to thicken in the anteroposterior axis. The iris (3) constricts, and the space between the cornea and iris—the anterior chamber (4)—decreases.

- Color perception is reduced.
- With a nuclear cataract, near vision may improve ("second sight").
- With a posterior subcapsular cataract, near visual acuity decreases.

Signs

- Opacification of the lens is evident.

Workup

- Cataracts are best seen after dilation of the pupil. The examiner looks through the +5 lens of a direct ophthalmoscope held about 6 inches from the patient's eye.

Treatment

- For early nuclear cataracts, a change in the spectacle prescription may improve vision.
- For small central opacities, pupillary dilation may improve vision.
- Surgical removal of the lens with placement of an intraocular lens implant is performed.
- Cataract surgery is not performed with lasers. A laser may be used, however, if an after-cataract is present (see page 136).

BOX **8–1**   **Types of Senile Cataract**

Nuclear

- A yellow-brown discoloration of the central part of the lens is observed (Fig. 8–3).
- The nuclear type of cataract usually becomes evident at the age of 50 years and progresses slowly until the entire nucleus is opaque.

Cortical

- Radial or spokelike opacities in the periphery of the lens extend to involve the anterior or posterior lens (Fig. 8–4).
- Patients often are asymptomatic until the lens changes involve the central lens.

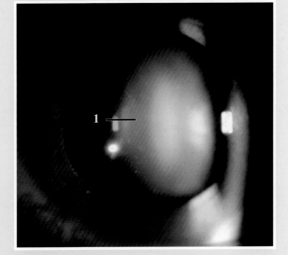

FIGURE 8–3   In cases of nuclear cataract, the yellow-brown color of the central nucleus (1) is evident.

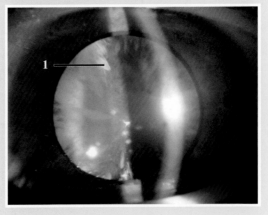

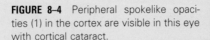

FIGURE 8–4   Peripheral spokelike opacities (1) in the cortex are visible in this eye with cortical cataract.

BOX 8–1   Types of Senile Cataract (Continued)

Posterior subcapsular

- Opacities appear in the most posterior portion of the lens adjacent to the posterior capsule, often forming a plaque (Fig. 8–5).
- Posterior subcapsular cataract most commonly is associated with systemic or topical corticosteroid use.
- Because the visual axis is involved, this type causes a disproportionate number of symptoms for its size.

Dense white

- A white discoloration of the central part of the lens is observed.
- A dense white cataract often is seen in combination with cortical and nuclear cataracts in older patients (Fig. 8–6).
- This type may be severely disabling because of the marked visual loss it produces.

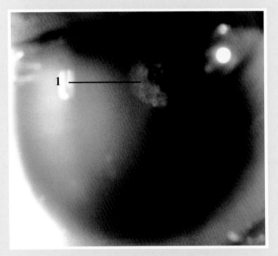

FIGURE 8–5   The central location of a posterior subcapsular cataract (1).

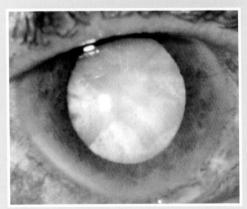

FIGURE 8–6   Advanced central (nuclear) and peripheral (cortical) opacification is seen in this eye with a dense white cataract.

Cataract Surgery

Cataract surgery is one of the most frequently performed surgical operations. Greater than 1.5 million cataract surgery procedures are performed annually in the United States. An estimated 5 to 10 million persons in the United States become visually disabled each year because of cataracts.

Indications

Cataract surgery is indicated in the following instances:
- To improve quality of life, which depends on the affected person's visual needs
- To prevent a secondary glaucoma or uveitis
- To permit visualization of the fundus to monitor patients with diseases of the optic nerve (e.g., glaucoma) or retina (e.g., diabetic retinopathy)
- To permit visualization of the fundus before retinal surgery or laser treatment

Preoperative Considerations

Every patient undergoing cataract surgery needs a complete ophthalmologic examination to rule out an underlying ophthalmic pathologic condition that may contribute to the patient's visual symptoms. Evaluation of the retina is especially important in patients with diabetes, because diabetic retinopathy can be exacerbated after cataract surgery.

Before cataract surgery, a preoperative exam is required. In many instances the patient is referred back to the primary care provider for a complete history, physical examination, and appropriate laboratory testing. Such testing may include an electrocardiogram, chest radiography, and determinations of hematocrit and potassium level, depending on the patient's medical status. With newer surgical techniques, however, minimal or no sedation is necessary, and the need for a complete medical evaluation is in question.

Advances in surgical technique also have changed anticoagulation management in the perioperative period. With small incisions, which allow for a "closed system" inside the eye, and the use of topical anesthesia, the risk of bleeding during cataract surgery is minimal, and the great majority of ophthalmologic surgeons do not recommend discontinuing anticoagulation therapy before cataract surgery. In certain procedures that may be performed in conjunction with a cataract extraction, discontinuation of anticoagulants may be warranted. Consultation with the ophthalmologic surgeon performing the operation is recommended before the primary care physician changes a patient's anticoagulation regimen.

Prognosis and Risks

The prognosis following cataract surgery using current techniques is excellent. Approximately 95% of patients obtain improved vision after cataract surgery.

Potential complications of cataract surgery, as with any ocular surgery, include infection and bleeding that can lead to blindness. The risk of infection is approximately 0.02%. The risk of retrobulbar hemorrhage is 0.1% with retrobulbar anesthesia. The risk of intraocular hemorrhage during cataract surgery is 0.06%. Possible late sequelae include retinal detachment and the development of glaucoma.

Anesthesia

In most cases, cataract surgery is performed using topical anesthesia with monitored anesthesia care. Topical anesthetic is placed on the surface of the eye, and a small amount of anesthetic is injected into the anterior chamber after the corneal incision is performed. With this technique, there is no need for retrobulbar anesthesia and therefore no risk of retrobulbar hemorrhage. Some patients require akinesia of the eyelids and eye because of an inability to cooperate or communicate during surgery, which necessitates the use of retrobulbar or peribulbar injections of anesthetic. Some surgeons utilize short-acting intravenous sedatives before performing the injections. General anesthesia is relatively rare in cataract surgery today. It may still be used for patients who are unable to lie still or who have language or hearing problems that may impair communication, potentially compromising the surgeon's ability to perform the operation safely.

Procedure

Cataract surgery is performed as an outpatient procedure. The procedure takes approximately 10 to 15 minutes to perform. Phacoemulsification is the technique used in nearly all patients undergoing cataract surgery today. Phacoemulsification is the preferred procedure because of the smaller incision size and faster visual rehabilitation. An older technique, extracapsular cataract extraction, is used in rare circumstances.

Phacoemulsification. In phacoemulsification, the surgeon makes a 2- to 4-mm incision (Fig. 8–7) and removes a circular portion of the anterior lens capsule (Fig. 8–8). A phacoemulsification instrument emits ultrasonic vibrations and provides suction for breakup and extraction of the hard nuclear lens material (Fig. 8–9). The surgeon uses

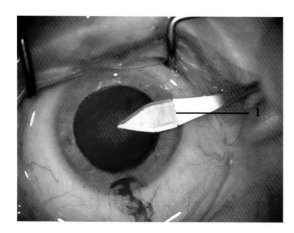

FIGURE 8–7 Phacoemulsification: A small incision is created in the cornea with a blade (1).

FIGURE 8–8 Phacoemulsification: Forceps (1) is used to tear a continuous capsulorrhexis in the anterior capsule (2).

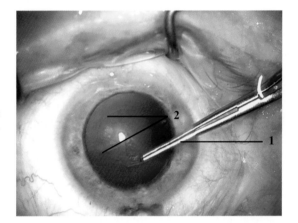

FIGURE 8–9 Phacoemulsification: The nucleus (1) is removed with the phacoemulsification handpiece (2). A second instrument (3) is used to assist in the procedure.

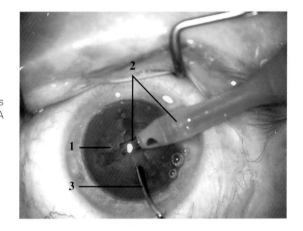

a mechanical irrigation and suction instrument to remove the lens cortex (Fig. 8–10) and then places the lens implant in the remaining capsular bag.

Flexible lens implants are now available that can be folded and introduced through a small incision into the eye, where they unfold (Fig. 8–11) and are held in place within the remaining capsular bag (Fig. 8–12). The smaller wounds may be self-sealing or require only a few sutures. This small incision technique can be performed with topical anesthesia.

Extracapsular Cataract Extraction. In extracapsular cataract extraction, the surgeon makes a 10- to 11-mm superior sclerocorneal incision and removes the anterior portion of the lens capsule. The entire nucleus is extracted through the incision. The surgeon uses a mechanical irrigation and suction instrument to remove the lens cortex, places the implant in the remaining capsular bag, and sutures the incision. The extracapsular technique is utilized only for very dense cataracts that cannot be removed with the phacoemulsification technique. Retrobulbar or peribulbar anesthesia is required for the extracapsular method.

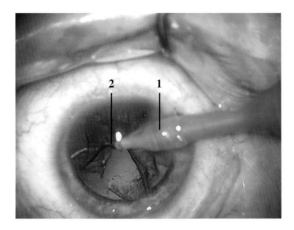

FIGURE 8–10 Phacoemulsification: A mechanical irrigation and suction instrument (1) is used to remove the lens cortex (2).

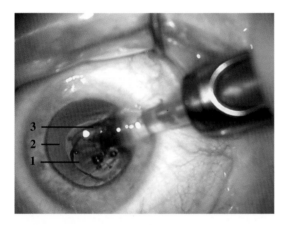

FIGURE 8–11 Phacoemulsification: The lens (1) is inserted under the anterior capsular surface (2) using a lens inserter (3).

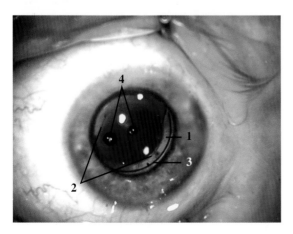

FIGURE 8–12 Phacoemulsification: New intraocular lens (1) in proper position in the remaining capsular bag. Note the edge of the anterior capsule (2) and the edge of the intraocular lens (3). Two air bubbles (4) are visible beneath the cornea.

Postoperative Care

If cataract removal is performed using local or topical anesthesia, the patient can go home shortly after the surgery. The patient usually is ambulatory on the day of the procedure. The patient is seen in the ophthalmologist's office for evaluation the following day and often is able to return to work within a day or two. The patient typically is given antibiotic and steroid drops for the first few weeks after surgery. The postoperative course usually is painless; therefore, prescription painkillers are not necessary. An updated spectacle prescription usually is given 3 to 8 weeks after surgery.

After-Cataract (Secondary Membrane/Posterior Capsular Opacity)

In 10% to 30% of patients who have undergone cataract surgery, the posterior capsule subsequently opacifies (Fig. 8–13), producing significant visual distortion. The opacity usually is noted several months to years after cataract surgery. Treatment involves a noninvasive technique (posterior capsulotomy) using the neodymium:YAG laser to

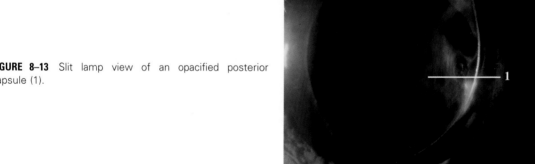

FIGURE 8–13 Slit lamp view of an opacified posterior capsule (1).

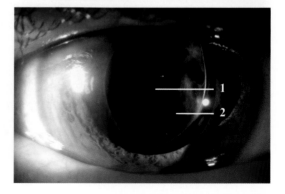

FIGURE 8–14 After-cataract treatment with laser: View of open posterior capsule (1) after the laser procedure. Note the peripheral opacified posterior capsule (2).

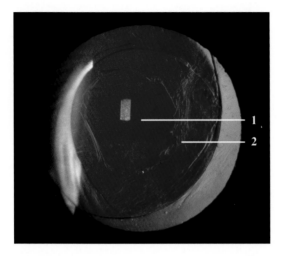

FIGURE 8–15 After-cataract treatment with laser: Open central posterior capsule (1) viewed using retroillumination. Again, note the peripheral opacified posterior capsule (2).

create a small opening in the center of the opacified posterior capsule (Figs. 8–14 and 8–15). A complication of this procedure is a transient rise in intraocular pressure, which may require medical treatment. The most serious complication is retinal detachment, which may occur weeks to months after the procedure in up to 1% of patients.

CHAPTER 9

Uveitis

TERRY KIM • DOUGLAS M. BLACKMON

Related Anatomy

The uveal tract is a heavily pigmented and highly vascular structure composed of three distinct anatomic components: the iris, ciliary body, and choroid (Fig. 9–1). The iris represents the most anterior portion of the uveal tract and is the only portion that is directly visible by external or slit lamp examination. It is located behind the cornea (with the space between the cornea and iris known as the *anterior chamber*) and is responsible for giving the eye its color. The central opening of the iris is the pupil, which constricts or dilates, depending on the amount of light entering the eye. The ciliary body is contiguous with the iris and has numerous functions, including aqueous humor production and accommodation. The choroid has a posterior location and lies between the retina and the sclera. Its main role is to provide a blood supply to the outer retina. These three components together form a continuous uveal lining that can be affected by inflammatory conditions within the eye.

Uveitis is a general term used to describe any inflammatory condition involving the uveal tract. Different classifications and terminology are used to denote the specific sites of the uveal tract primarily involved. For the anterior segment of the eye the terms *iritis* and *iridocyclitis* describe inflammation of the iris and of the iris–ciliary body complex, respectively. The terms *vitritis*, *retinitis*, and *choroiditis* designate inflammation in the relevant parts of the posterior segment of the eye. In this book, the term *anterior uveitis* means any inflammation of the iris and/or ciliary body, and the term *posterior uveitis* denotes any inflammation of the vitreous, retina, and/or choroid.

Identification of the segment of the eye primarily affected by uveitis guides formulation of a differential diagnosis, workup, and treatment. Some disorders appear exclusively as an anterior or a posterior uveitis, although in a few such disorders (e.g., sarcoidosis, Behçet syndrome, syphilis, tuberculosis), the inflammation can be either anterior or posterior. Because of the close anatomic and functional relationships of the vitreous, retina, and choroid, pinpointing the principal site of involvement, especially

Iris + Ciliary body + Choroid = Uveal tract

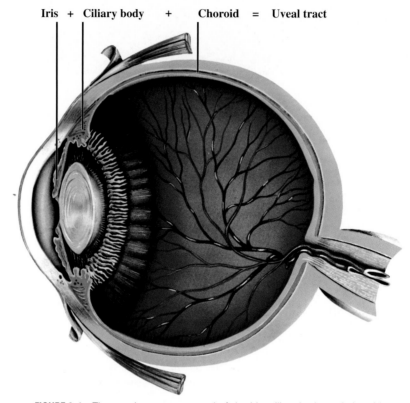

FIGURE 9–1 The uveal tract, composed of the iris, ciliary body, and choroid.

in the posterior segment, often is difficult. Classification of a uveitis as anterior or posterior may be difficult, because both segments may be involved. A severe anterior uveitis may result in anterior vitreous changes, whereas a vitritis may manifest with signs in the anterior chamber. When both segments of the uveal tract are definitely involved, the condition is called *panuveitis*. The term *endophthalmitis* is reserved for cases in which the inflammation is predominantly centered within the vitreous—a special type of posterior uveitis remarkable for its severity, necessitating prompt diagnostic workup and treatment (see Chapter 10).

Anterior Uveitis

Symptoms

- Redness, photophobia, and pain are characteristic.
- Vision is normal or decreased.
- The onset of symptoms is acute or insidious.
- Possible nonocular symptoms (e.g., back pain, joint stiffness, dysuria) are caused by various systemic disorders associated with uveitis.

Signs

- The disorder is unilateral or bilateral.
- Conjunctival injection is seen, primarily surrounding the cornea (ciliary injection) (Fig. 9–2).
- Deposits on the posterior surface of the cornea (keratic precipitates) vary in size and appearance (fine and whitish precipitates in nongranulomatous uveitis and large, grayish, "mutton-fat" precipitates in granulomatous uveitis) (Figs. 9–3 and 9–4).
- Floating inflammatory cells and protein (seen as "flare") in the anterior chamber are detectable only with the aid of a slit lamp biomicroscope. If severe enough, these inflammatory cells can layer in the anterior chamber (hypopyon) (Fig. 9–5).
- Adhesions of the iris to the front surface of the lens (posterior synechiae) may form, which may result in a small or irregularly shaped pupil (Fig. 9–6A). A 360-degree distribution of posterior synechiae may inhibit normal aqueous flow to create iris bombé and angle-closure glaucoma (Fig. 9–6B).
- A constricted pupil is evident, even without posterior synechiae.

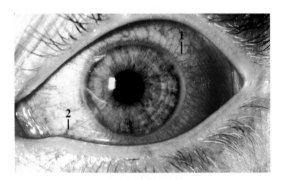

FIGURE 9–2 Marked ciliary injection (1) in addition to generalized conjunctival injection (2) in this eye of a patient with ankylosing spondylitis.

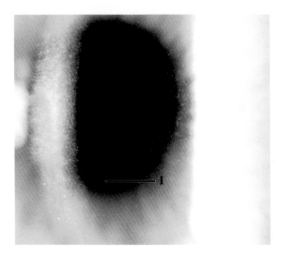

FIGURE 9–3 Fine keratic precipitates (1) with a nongranulomatous anterior uveitis.

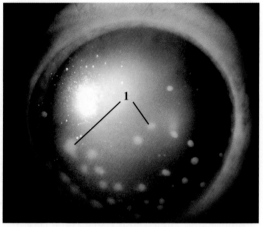

FIGURE 9–4   "Mutton-fat" keratic precipitates (1) are diffusely scattered on the posterior surface of the cornea.

FIGURE 9–5   Accumulation of inflammatory cells forming a hypopyon in the anterior chamber.

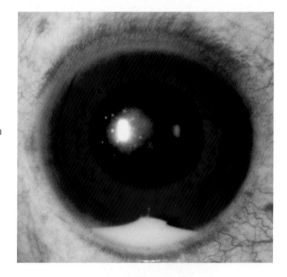

- Nodules of inflammatory cells are found on the iris surface. These lesions are termed *Koeppe nodules* if they are located at the pupillary margin and *Busacca nodules* if located on the remainder of the iris surface (Fig. 9–7).

Etiology

- Most cases have an idiopathic origin.
- Many local and systemic associations have been identified, as outlined in Box 9–1.

Associated Factors and Diseases

- Cataract and glaucoma are associated with anterior uveitis.
- Low intraocular pressure (hypotony) may be present.

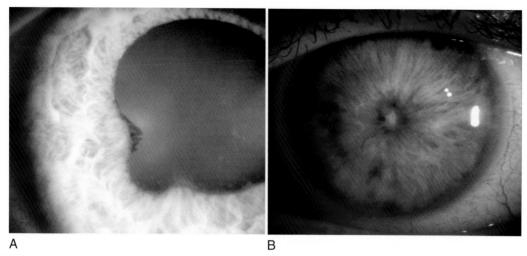

A   B

FIGURE 9–6   A, Posterior synechiae causing iris pigment deposition on the anterior lens surface and an irregularly shaped pupil. **B,** Posterior synechiae in a 360-degree distribution inducing miosis and iris bombé, which may lead to pupillary block glaucoma.

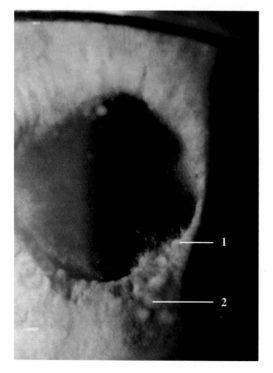

FIGURE 9–7   Koeppe (1) and Busacca (2) nodules of sarcoid uveitis.

BOX **9–1**   **Classification of Anterior Uveitis**

Autoimmune disorders
- HLA-B27 positive anterior uveitis
- Ankylosing spondylitis
- Reiter syndrome
- Inflammatory bowel disease (ulcerative colitis and Crohn's disease)
- Psoriatic arthritis
- Juvenile rheumatoid arthritis

Infections
- Syphilis
- Tuberculosis
- Lyme disease
- Herpes simplex
- Herpes zoster

Malignancies*
- Lymphoma
- Leukemia

Other conditions
- Idiopathic disease
- Trauma
- Postoperative complication
- Sarcoidosis
- Behçet syndrome

---

*Noninflammatory conditions in which the clinical findings can mimic those with an anterior uveitis.

- Elevated intraocular pressure may be associated with pupillary block glaucoma, toxoplasmosis, and infections due to herpes simplex virus and herpes zoster virus.

Differential Diagnosis

Considerations in the differential diagnosis include the following:
- Conjunctivitis (injected conjunctiva but *no* cells or flare in the anterior chamber)
- Sclerouveitis (uveitis secondary to an inflammation of the sclera)
- Intraocular malignancy (e.g., leukemia)

Workup

- A careful history and complete ocular examination are necessary. A history of ocular trauma incurred 2 to 3 days before presentation may facilitate the diagnosis of traumatic iritis.

- The general physical examination is directed at possible systemic findings with the various conditions associated with an anterior uveitis.
- For patients with unilateral, nongranulomatous, first-episode disease and unremarkable history and physical findings, no systemic workup is needed.
- For patients with bilateral, granulomatous, recurrent disease and unremarkable history and physical findings, the followings steps are taken:
  - A nonspecific diagnostic workup is initiated, including complete blood count (CBC), erythrocyte sedimentation rate (ESR) (preferably using the Westergren method), antinuclear antibody (ANA) titer, rapid plasma reagin (RPR) or Venereal Disease Research Laboratory (VDRL) testing, fluorescent treponemal antibody absorption (FTA-ABS) test or microhemagglutination assay for *Treponema pallidum* (MHA-TP), purified protein derivative (PPD) testing with anergy panel, chest radiograph, and Lyme titer (for cases occurring in an endemic area and as indicated).
  - The diagnostic workup is supplemented with other tests and subspecialty consultations if the need for any of these measures is strongly indicated by symptoms, history, or physical findings (e.g., determination of angiotensin-converting enzyme level for ruling out sarcoidosis, sacroiliac spine x-ray examination for ruling out ankylosing spondylitis, consultation with a rheumatologist for ruling out psoriatic arthritis).

Treatment

- Patients should be referred to an ophthalmologist within 24 hours.
- A topical cycloplegic agent (e.g., homatropine hydrobromide 5%, atropine sulfate 1%) is administered two or three times a day to stabilize the blood-aqueous barrier, decrease pain, and prevent formation of posterior synechiae.
- A topical corticosteroid (e.g., Pred-Forte 1%, Flarex 0.1%) is administered 4 to 6 times a day. An ophthalmologist initiates this prescription.

Prognosis

- Overall, the prognosis is excellent for patients with a first-time, nongranulomatous anterior uveitis and less favorable for patients with a recurrent, granulomatous type.

Posterior Uveitis

Symptoms

- Vision is commonly decreased or blurred.
- Floaters are seen.
- Redness, pain, and photophobia are occasional symptoms.
- The onset is acute or insidious.

Signs

- The disease can be unilateral or bilateral.
- Inflammatory cells within the vitreous cause a hazy view of the fundus of the eye (Fig. 9–8).

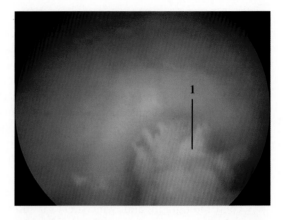

FIGURE 9–8 Inflammatory vitreous cells causing a hazy view of the fundus in this case of lens-induced posterior uveitis. Note the large lens fragment (1).

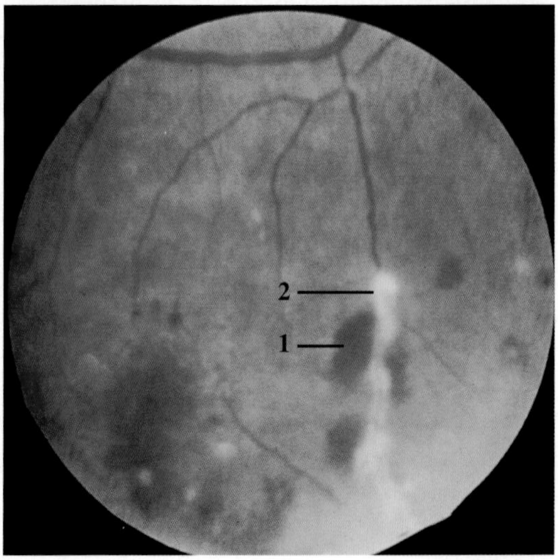

FIGURE 9–9 Sarcoid posterior uveitis showing retinal hemorrhage (1) and vascular sheathing (2).

- Optic disc swelling and edema are observed.
- Retinal and choroidal hemorrhages, exudates, infiltrates, and vascular sheathing are seen (Fig. 9–9). These abnormalities can be difficult to discern without indirect ophthalmoscopy; the view also may be lessened by a constricted pupil and interference from overlying inflammatory cells.

Etiology

- Toxoplasmosis is the most common cause of posterior uveitis (Fig. 9–10).
- In patients with acquired immunodeficiency syndrome (AIDS) who have symptoms of a posterior uveitis, cytomegalovirus retinitis and syphilis should be ruled out or confirmed (see Chapter 10).
- Many local and systemic associations have been noted, as outlined in Box 9–2.

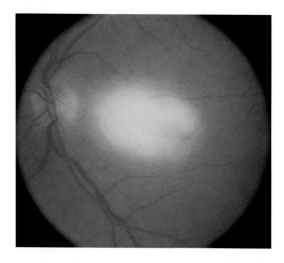

FIGURE 9–10 Toxoplasmosis lesion located near the optic disc.

Associated Factors and Diseases

Associated disorders include the following:
- Chorioretinal scars
- Exudative retinal detachment
- Macular edema
- Epiretinal membrane

Differential Diagnosis

Considerations in the differential diagnosis include the following:
- Retinal detachment
- Intraocular malignancy (e.g., retinoblastoma)
- Intraocular foreign body

Workup

- A careful history and complete ocular examination are essential.
- The general physical examination is directed at possible systemic findings with the conditions associated with a posterior uveitis.
- A nonspecific diagnostic workup and other tests and subspecialty consultations may be initiated if the need for any of these measures is strongly indicated by symptoms, history, or physical findings.

Treatment

- Patients should be referred to an ophthalmologist within 24 hours.
- Topical cycloplegic and topical corticosteroid agents are administered by an ophthalmologist if anterior inflammation is present.

BOX 9–2   **Classification of Posterior Uveitis**

Autoimmune disorders
- Vogt-Koyanagi-Harada syndrome (uveoencephalitis)
- Polyarteritis nodosa
- Lens-induced posterior uveitis

Infections
- Toxoplasmosis
- Toxocariasis
- Ocular candidiasis
- Ocular histoplasmosis
- Cytomegalovirus
- Acute retinal necrosis (herpes zoster)
- Tuberculosis
- Syphilis

Malignancies*
- Retinoblastoma
- Malignant melanoma
- Lymphoma
- Leukemia

Other conditions
- Idiopathic disease
- Sarcoidosis
- Behçet's syndrome

---

*Noninflammatory conditions in which the clinical findings can mimic those with a posterior uveitis.

- Decisions regarding further treatment (e.g., periocular corticosteroid injections, intravitreal antibiotic injections, systemic medications, potential intraocular surgery) need to be made by an ophthalmologist.

Prognosis

- The prognosis varies greatly depending on the etiology, severity of inflammation, and promptness of appropriate therapy.

CHAPTER 10

Retina

TIMOTHY W. OLSEN

The retina is a highly specialized, neurosensory tissue that forms from an extension of the central nervous system during embryogenesis. Retinal tissue translates focused light energy into a complex series of electrical impulses transmitted through the optic nerve, optic chiasm, and visual tracts to the occipital cortex, resulting in the perception of vision. The examining physician has a unique opportunity, owing to the transparency and clarity of the ocular tissues, to directly examine living, functional neurologic tissue and the accompanying vasculature.

The retinal vasculature may be viewed directly, photographed, or imaged with angiographic dyes such as fluorescein or indocyanine green. The vascular changes seen in the retina often are representative of the systemic vasculature. A skilled clinician will take advantage of this unique window to the human body and incorporate the knowledge gained from ophthalmoscopy into the overall assessment of a patient.

This chapter discusses retinal findings that can serve as a guide for primary care physicians in diagnosing systemic disease and common retinal disorders.

Related Anatomy

The optic nerve is a key landmark that is important for the examining physician to identify during ophthalmoscopy. The optic nerve lies just nasal to the fovea and is best visualized as the examiner approaches the patient's eye from a slightly temporal approach. As the clinician focuses the direct ophthalmoscope on a retinal vessel, a useful trick to find the optic nerve is to follow a retinal vessel. The retinal blood vessels become larger near the optic nerve. Within the vascular branching pattern, the point of the "V" created by any bifurcation always "points" toward the optic nerve (Fig. 10–1). After visualizing the optic nerve, the clinician focuses the direct ophthalmoscope on the retinal vasculature. The optic nerve is approximately 1.5 to 1.9 mm in diameter, and a retinal vein on the surface of the nerve is approximately 125 μm in

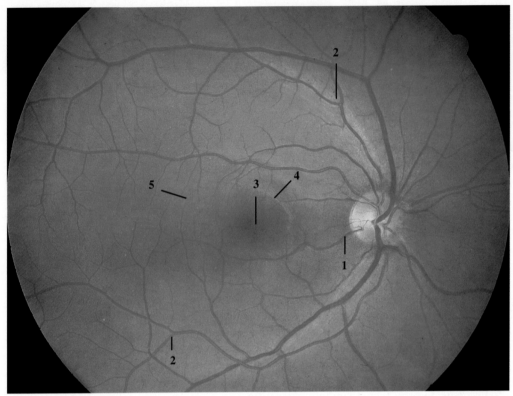

FIGURE 10–1 Normal fundus. A normal, pink optic nerve, cup-to-disc ratio of 0.1, normal arterial-to-venous diameter ratio of 7:10, and a cilioretinal artery (1) extending from the temporal border of the optic nerve and inferior to the fovea can be seen. Note that the branching points of the blood vessels "point" (2) toward the optic nerve. The foveolar reflex (3), fovea (4), and macula (an area approximately 5.5 mm in diameter, centered on the fovea) (5) also can be seen.

diameter. The arteries appear thinner and more orange-red, whereas the veins are larger and more crimson.

The normal ratio of arterial to venous diameter (A:V ratio) is approximately 7:10 or 8:10 (i.e., the retinal artery diameter is 70% to 80% of the apparent diameter of the adjacent vein). The A:V ratio is best judged by comparing vessel calibers *after* the initial branch point. As a rule, veins do not cross veins, and arteries do not cross arteries. Veins and arteries travel together in pairs and frequently cross over each other (arteriole-venule crossings).

Expertise with a direct ophthalmoscope is an important skill for a primary care physician to master. When the examining physician asks the patient to look directly into the light of the direct ophthalmoscope, the area with a slightly darker orange pigmentation and an absence of retinal vasculature is the fovea. Typically, this anatomic region is located mostly temporal and slightly inferior to the optic nerve. The small yellow reflex in the center of this area is the foveolar light reflex; it usually is present on examination in the normal eye. In children and young adults, a circular reflex of light identifies the foveal reflex, of about the same size as that of the optic nerve. The foveal reflex is formed by light reflecting from the internal limiting membrane of the retina at a circular area of peak thickness formed by the high density of ganglion cells that supply the fovea. The macula is a circular area 5.5 mm in diameter centered on the fovea (generally, the area within the temporal blood vessel arcades adjacent to the optic nerve) and is primarily responsible for central, critical visual function. Peripheral retinal structures and pathologic conditions located anterior to the equator of the globe require an indirect ophthalmoscope, a condensing lens (+20 diopter), and additional expertise.

The normal retina and blood vessel walls normally are transparent. The visible retinal vessel is actually an arterial or a venous "blood column." The normal orange-red color of the red reflex is produced by the vasculature of the choroid, retinal pigment epithelium, and choroidal melanocytes. The retina has two separate blood supplies. The central retinal artery supplies the *inner retina*, or the retinal layers toward the center of the eye. The *outer retina*, or the retinal layers toward the outer wall of the eye, is supplied by the highly vascular choroid. The high oxygen requirement of the photoreceptors, located in the outer retina, is provided by the choroid.

The fundus of lightly pigmented patients has a "blond" appearance, with readily visible choroidal vessels (Fig. 10–2). The fundus of darkly pigmented patients has a "brunette" appearance, with less apparent choroidal vasculature. Choroidal blood vessels are readily differentiated from retinal vessels. The retinal vasculature follows a typical branching pattern centered on the optic nerve; the choroidal vasculature demonstrates an *irregular* branching pattern of larger-caliber, poorly defined vessels. Retinal vessels pass anterior to choroidal vessels. A blood vessel that supplies the retinal circulation frequently arises from the choroidal circulation at the optic nerve; this is called a *cilioretinal vessel* (see Fig. 10–1). This vessel arises from the short posterior ciliary vasculature, rather than the central retinal artery, and offers an "accessory" supply to the distribution of the vessel.

A basic understanding of the cross-sectional anatomy of the retina helps in the identification of important pathologic states (Fig. 10–3). The inner retina contains the

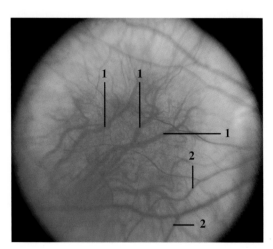

FIGURE 10–2 Fundus of eye in an albino with the absence of ocular pigmentation. The choroidal blood vessels (1) are readily visible. These are differentiated from the normal retinal vessels (2) by their size and branching pattern. Normal retinal vessels are seen emanating from the optic nerve and crossing over the choroidal vessels.

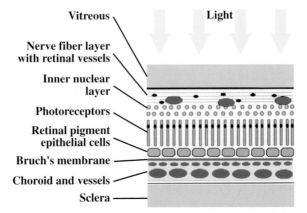

FIGURE 10–3 Cross-sectional schematic anatomy of the retina and choroid.

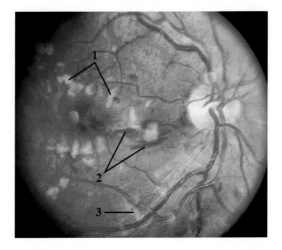

FIGURE 10–4 Multiple cotton-wool spots (1) in the perifoveal region in a young man with disseminated microemboli after bone marrow transplantation. Ischemia of the perifoveal capillaries is responsible for the cotton-wool spots. Multiple flame-shaped hemorrhages (2) in the nerve fiber layer also are present. The arcuate, whitish, radiating striae extending from the optic nerve next to the retinal vasculature (3) represent the light reflex from the normal nerve fiber layer.

nerve fiber layer and ganglion cell nuclei that extend their terminal axons through the optic nerve and chiasm to synapse primarily in the lateral geniculate nucleus of the brain, with some fibers extending to the midbrain to subserve the pupillary light reflex. The inner retinal layer also contains the retinal vasculature, originating from the central retinal vessels. Conditions that result in ischemia from the retinal vasculature manifest primarily in the nerve fiber layer and are seen clinically as opacification of the inner retina. Areas of axoplasmic stasis of the nerve fiber layer are seen clinically as fluffy white patches, also known as *cotton-wool spots* (Fig. 10–4). These whitish lesions follow the distribution of the nerve fiber layer. In the past, these lesions have been described as "soft exudates"—a misnomer, because a cotton-wool spot represents an infarction rather than an exudation.

Flame-shaped hemorrhages also occur in the nerve fiber layer. If a retinal vessel bleeds into the inner retinal layer, the blood intercalates with the nerve fibers in the manner of red paint spilled on the fibers of split wood, giving it a flame-shaped appearance. Pathologic conditions located in the deeper layers of the retina are more localized circular hemorrhages with fuzzy or blurry margins. These "dot and blot" hemorrhages commonly are seen in patients with diabetes mellitus or hypertensive retinopathy. Localized, yellow lipid exudates, or "hard exudates," form in the outer layers of the retina and remain more circular in contour and well localized.

Frequently, fluorescein angiography and, less commonly, indocyanine green angiography are used in the diagnosis and treatment of retinal disorders. Both dyes are extremely safe, water-soluble dyes that appear white or hyperfluorescent in photographs taken during dye circulation through the retinal and choroidal vasculature. Although fluorescein best images the retinal vasculature, indocyanine green is able to better image the choroidal vasculature. The differences between these dyes relate primarily to their light absorption and emission properties. A detailed examination at the capillary level is possible using these angiographic techniques. A disruption of the "blood-retina barrier" (analogous to the blood-brain barrier with intercellular tight junctions) results in leakage of the dye into the retina, which then appears irregular in the angiogram. In addition, areas of nonperfusion or ischemia appear dark or hypofluorescent on the angiogram.

Diabetic Retinopathy

Diabetic retinopathy is the leading cause of blindness in the Western world in people youger than 50 years of age. The current standard of care is for all patients with diabetes to be evaluated by an ophthalmologist annually. Patients with newly diagnosed type 2 diabetes mellitus should be scheduled for a baseline evaluation within weeks of diagnosis and should establish a long-term relationship with an ophthalmologist. The duration of type 2 diabetes mellitus is frequently indeterminate, and many patients will demonstrate some level of diabetic retinopathy at the time of diagnosis. Ophthalmologic referral is therefore more urgent.

Patients with type 1 diabetes mellitus are unlikely to have retinopathy at the time of diagnosis, and an ophthalmologic examination should be scheduled within 5 years of diagnosis and then annually. Although some studies have argued that cost effectiveness is optimized with screening every 2 years, *annual* examination is still recommended ("preferred practice patterns" of the American Academy of Ophthalmology).

Progression of diabetic retinopathy may accelerate during periods of strong hormonal influence such as pregnancy and puberty, so clinicians are advised to monitor patients closely during such periods. Most commonly, patients with diabetes have irreversible vision loss as a result of secondary complications that arise from injury to the retinal vasculature. Cataracts also may occur in the setting of diabetes and may be more challenging to manage than in eyes without diabetic retinopathy. The basic forms of diabetic retinopathy are proliferative diabetic retinopathy, diabetic macular edema, and macular ischemia.

Proliferative Diabetic Retinopathy

Proliferative diabetic retinopathy results from retinal ischemia. As perfusion to the retina is compromised, ischemic retinal tissue releases an angiogenic factor (vascular endothelial growth factor [VEGF]) that in turn stimulates abnormal new vessel growth,

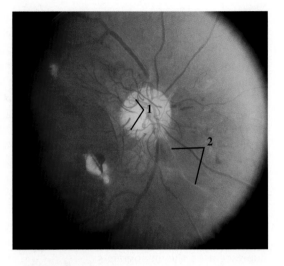

FIGURE 10–5 Fronds of neovascularization (1) on the disc are present in this right eye. Inferior and temporal, a cotton-wool spot has an adjacent hemorrhage. Native retinal arteries are narrowed and show evidence of sclerosis (2).

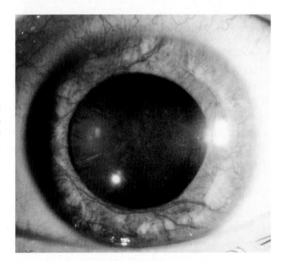

FIGURE 10–6 Dilated pupil of a patient with poorly controlled diabetes displaying advanced rubeosis with neovascularization of the iris. The vessels on the surface of the iris may occlude the normal drainage of aqueous fluid from the eye, leading to a severe form of neovascular glaucoma.

or *neovascularization*. VEGF also increases the permeability of retinal vessels and results in leakage and macular edema. Panretinal ischemia results in neovascularization emanating from the optic nerve or disc and is termed neovascularization of the disc (NVD), a high-risk condition (Fig. 10–5). Neovascularization may occur at any location elsewhere in the retina (NVE) but typically occurs along the vascular arcades. Neovascularization also may occur on the surface of the iris (NVI), imparting a red-brown color. The resultant condition is known as *rubeosis iridis*; these changes may lead to neovascular glaucoma, a severe form of glaucoma (Fig. 10–6). Almost any form of retinal neovascularization may be dangerous because the vessels grow into the vitreous gel, instead of providing needed vascularization of the retina. Movement or traction of the vitreous gel may cause shearing of these fragile vessels, leading to vitreous hemorrhage. Recurrent vitreous hemorrhage will lead to the formation of contractile,

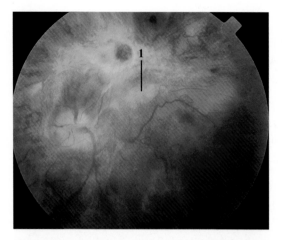

FIGURE 10–7 A large white sheet of fibrovascular tissue is present on the surface of the retina in this eye of a patient with diabetes. Contraction of the tissue distorts the retinal vessels and tractionally detaches the retina. The yellow substance deep to the fibrovascular tissue (1) is lipid, which results from chronic exudation of incompetent vessels. Surgical intervention (vitrectomy) is needed to remove the fibrovascular tissue and reattach the retina.

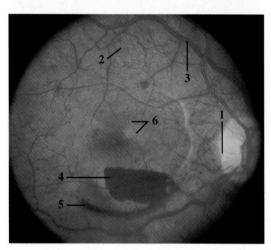

FIGURE 10–8 Proliferative diabetic retinopathy with high-risk characteristics. Neovascularization is present at the optic nerve (1) and along the vascular arcades (2). Retinal veins are engorged (3), and a preretinal hemorrhage (4) is present inferior to the fovea. This boat-shaped hemorrhage blocks the view of the retinal vessels. A more diffuse hemorrhage (5) is present in an arcuate pattern just inferior to the preretinal hemorrhage that represents a mild vitreous hemorrhage. A few small hard exudates are visible in the fovea (6).

fibrous scar tissue that may pull the retina toward the center of the eye, producing fractional retinal detachments (Fig. 10–7). Neovascularization can be differentiated from normal retinal vasculature by the characteristic growth pattern. New vessels typically are smaller and have more frequent branching points that grow in an irregular, haphazard manner (Fig. 10–8; see also Fig. 10–5).

Symptoms

- Some patients with severe proliferative retinopathy may have 20/20 visual acuity and be unaware of any visual symptoms.
- Vision may become blurry slowly or suddenly.
- Distortion of vision may occur (i.e., things may appear crooked or wavy).
- Floaters, possibly indicating vitreous hemorrhage, may be reported, usually in a pattern described as a "shower."
- Blind spots in the vision, or scotomata, may be noted by the patient.

Signs

- Neovascularization, or fine lacy blood vessels, are seen on the optic nerve, retina (see Figs. 10–5 and 10–8), or iris surface (see Fig. 10–6).
- Preretinal hemorrhages are boat-shaped hemorrhages that may be located anterior to the retinal vessels and block the view of these underlying vessels (see Fig. 10–8).
- Cotton-wool spots often are present (see Fig. 10–5).
- Venous beading, dilation, or engorgement is present.
- Dot and blot intraretinal hemorrhages are a common finding.
- Loss of the red reflex and resulting inability to view the fundus are possible with a vitreous hemorrhage.
- Areas of traction retinal detachment may be observed (see Fig. 10–7).
- Whitish fibrovascular tissue on the retinal surface may be seen in a distribution along the vascular arcades and above the optic nerve.

Differential Diagnosis

Considerations in the differential diagnosis include the following:
- Diabetes
- Vascular occlusions: central or branch retinal vein or artery occlusions
- Radiation retinopathy may appear identical to diabetic retinopathy
- Blood dyscrasias: sickle cell retinopathy (especially in patients with SC hemoglobin), anemias, leukemias, thalassemias, and hyperviscosity syndromes
- Retinal emboli
- Carotid disease, aortic arch syndrome, and carotid artery–cavernous sinus fistula
- Uveitis (e.g., sarcoidosis)

Workup

- To confirm the diagnosis of diabetes mellitus, fasting blood glucose level, oral glucose tolerance test, and hemoglobin A_{1C} are appropriate tests. If the diagnosis is confirmed, assessment of urine microalbumin by 24-hour urine protein assessment or random urine for albumin-to-creatinine ratio should be performed to evaluate for diabetic nephropathy.
- To address other possibilities in the differential diagnosis consider: complete blood count (CBC) with differential count, serum protein electrophoresis, angiotensin-converting enzyme level, chest x-ray, or vascular imaging studies (carotid ultrasound and echocardiography).

Treatment

- **Note:** The Diabetes Control and Complications Trial (DCCT) has shown that "tight" glycemic control decreases the progression of diabetic retinopathy, nephropathy, and neuropathy. The primary care physician's role is therefore critical in decreasing the incidence of vision loss from diabetic retinopathy in cases of both proliferative retinopathy and diabetic macular edema.
- Diabetic patients with neovascularization should be promptly referred to an ophthalmologist.

- Retinal laser photocoagulation destroys the peripheral retina and decreases the release of vasoproliferative growth factors from ischemic retinal tissue. Photocoagulation also creates multiple choroid-to-retina adhesions that limit the progression of a tractional retinal detachment.

Follow-up

- To minimize the risk of anticoagulation, the following considerations are important:
  - The guidelines for anticoagulation regimens in patients at risk for coronary artery disease, stroke, or other conditions are *not* altered by the presence of proliferative diabetic retinopathy. The risk of vitreous hemorrhage is no greater during anticoagulation therapy. However, a hemorrhage that occurs during anticoagulation may be more severe. Although many hemorrhages clear with time, others will require vitrectomy surgery. Anticoagulation recommendations generally should not change because of retinopathy, especially in life-threatening conditions requiring anticoagulation medication.
  - Ophthalmologic consultation is indicated to monitor the diabetic retinopathy when the patient is medically stable. For example, a diabetic patient taking anticoagulants for unstable angina is best seen by an ophthalmic consultant *after* appropriate cardiac care, rather than being seen first by the ophthalmologist to rule out proliferative diabetic retinopathy while anticoagulation therapy is delayed. Even if proliferative diabetic retinopathy is present, ophthalmologic treatment is deferred until the patient is medically stable.

Diabetic Macular Edema

The earliest detectable clinical alteration in the vasculature of a patient with diabetes is the formation of small 50-μm red dots on the retinal vasculature or microaneurysms (Fig. 10–9). Generally, the retinal vascular endothelium has "tight junctions" that form the inner blood-retina barrier, analogous to the blood-brain barrier. The microaneurysms represent proliferations of endothelial cells with increased permeability and an incompetent blood-retina barrier. Microaneurysms leak intravascular serum into the retinal tissue. The fluid may accumulate in the foveal area, leading to edema formation with decreased visual acuity. The proteinaceous and lipid portion of the serum may accumulate, leading to the formation of exudates (see Fig. 10–9). Alternatively, decreased visual acuity may result from ischemia or lack of perfusion to the fovea, usually due to loss of the capillaries in the foveal region.

Symptoms

- No symptoms may be noted. Diabetic patients may have normal vision and edema requiring laser treatment; therefore, all of these patients need ophthalmologic screening.
- Vision may be blurry unilaterally or bilaterally.
- Distorted or wavy vision may be described.

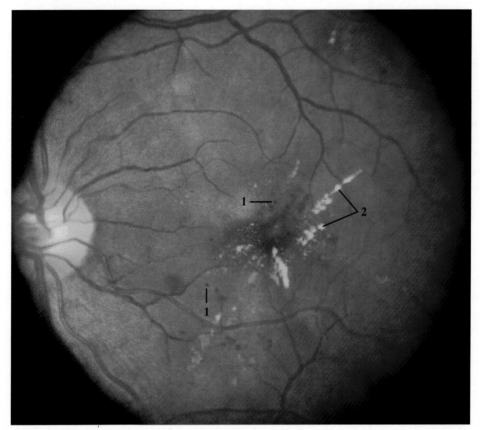

FIGURE 10–9 Clinically significant macular edema in this eye of an insulin-dependent diabetic patient. Multiple small red dots (microaneurysms) (1) are present throughout the macular area. Linear streaks of yellow deposits or hard exudates (2) are accumulations of lipid material from chronic leakage of the microaneurysms. Loss of the normal foveal light reflex with a more prominent yellow spot centrally suggests the presence of macular edema.

Signs

- Graying or a slight opacification of the retina results from edema in the macula.
- Microaneurysms usually are adjacent to retinal veins but may be found at any location in the retina.
- Dot and blot intraretinal hemorrhages occur.
- Cystoid changes or yellowing in the fovea may be observed.
- Hard exudates are dense yellowish lesions with discrete borders that may be isolated, linear, or stellate or form a "circinate ring" around leakage sites.

Differential Diagnosis

Considerations in the differential diagnosis include the following:
- Diabetes
- Vascular occlusions: central or branch retinal vein occlusions

- Hypertensive retinopathy
- Radiation retinopathy
- Choroidal neovascularization (subretinal neovascularization, usually associated with age-related macular degeneration [AMD])
- Macroaneurysms (larger retinal aneurysms associated with systemic hypertension)
- Epiretinal membrane

Treatment

- **Note:** As mentioned previously, the DCCT has shown that tight glycemic control decreases the progression of diabetic retinopathy. Therefore, the actions of the primary care physician are critical in decreasing the incidence of vision loss from diabetic macular edema.
- Patients should be referred to an ophthalmologist.
- Laser photocoagulation (based on Early Treatment of Diabetic Retinopathy Study [ETDRS] findings) is performed to decrease the further decline in visual acuity by reducing the amount of macular edema.

Hypertensive Retinopathy

Systemic arteriolar hypertension may affect the retinal vasculature in several ways. The traditional classification systems of hypertensive retinopathy were designed in the 1930s to 1950s and predate the current antihypertensive regimens now used to manage patients with hypertension. For this reason, the retinal vascular changes described in those classification systems are important to understand. Such classification systems rarely are used today, however, and the best measure of systemic arteriolar hypertension is the blood pressure cuff reading. Nevertheless, the appearance of hypertensive retinal vascular changes is a good indicator of "end-organ" damage and may give the clinician valuable information about long-term compliance with medication regimens or the effects of preexisting untreated damage from hypertension. Autoregulatory mechanisms are present in the retinal vasculature that limit the ability of a clinician to detect short-term or acute elevations in systemic arteriolar blood pressure.

The hallmark of hypertensive retinopathy is diffuse arteriolar narrowing. As stated earlier, the blood vessel walls are virtually transparent in the normal retina. The examiner sees the blood column, rather than the vessel wall. Chronic hypertension results in thickening of the vascular wall, with a concomitant narrowing of the vessel lumen and an apparent attenuation of the vessel. The normal A:V ratio of 0.8 (artery caliber 80% of the vein caliber) may change to 0.6 or less in patients with chronic hypertension. "Copper-wire vessel" is a dated term used to describe the yellowing of the linear light reflex seen on the surface of a narrowed arteriolar vessel using the illumination source of the older-style ophthalmoscopes. With the halogen light sources in current use, apparent color changes are minimized. "Silver-wire vessel" is a term used to describe a white retinal vessel with a minimal blood column or without a visible blood column. This term reflects the chronic changes that occur in the vessel wall that makes them less transparent. The ophthalmoscopic entities are more appropriately referred to as *arteriolar narrowing* (copper wire) and *sclerosis of the vessels* (silver wire).

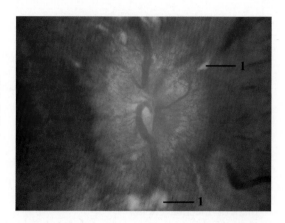

FIGURE 10–10 Swollen optic nerve caused by acute renal failure and accelerated systemic hypertension (blood pressure of 220/140 mm Hg). The condition was bilateral. The optic disc margins are blurry or fuzzy, with a loss of detail of the vessels as they pass over the disc. Multiple small cotton-wool spots (1) are present. The retinal veins are dilated.

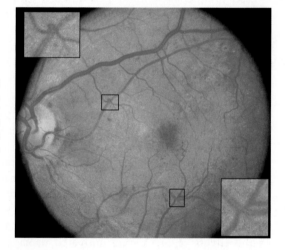

FIGURE 10–11 In this eye of a patient with diabetes and chronic hypertension, the A:V ratio is approximately 0.5, with significant arteriolar narrowing. Note the deviation or "humping" of the venules *(top inset)* as they cross over the arterioles. The artery crosses over the vein and causes "nicking" or attenuation of the venule *(bottom inset)* immediately under the crossing point.

Recently, an association of retinal vascular changes and an increased risk of congestive heart failure was discovered. Patients with acute or accelerated hypertension may exhibit a swollen optic nerve (Fig 10–10) with or without a stellate macular exudation that may be referred to as a *macular star* or associated cotton-wool spots.

Symptoms

- Vision may be normal, slightly blurred, or suddenly decreased.
- A blind spot in the vision (scotoma) may be reported.
- Double vision may occur.

Signs

- Arteriolar narrowing is diffuse in cases of chronic hypertension (Fig. 10–11) or a focal spasm in patients with acute hypertension.

- A:V crossing changes (where an arteriole crosses a venule) result from constriction of the common adventitial sheath at the crossing of an arteriole and a venule.
- Sclerotic vessels may be observed.
- Cotton-wool spots may be evident.
- Microaneurysms may be noted.
- Lipid exudation may occur and have a macular star configuration.
- Retinal edema may be present.
- Branch retinal vein or artery occlusion may occur.
- Macroaneurysm may cause exudation or rupture, producing acute vision loss from hemorrhage (subretinal, intraretinal, preretinal, or vitreous).
- Bilateral disc edema and swelling indicate accelerated hypertension or renal failure.
- Exudative retinal detachments indicate preeclampsia in pregnant patients.

Differential Diagnosis

Considerations in the differential diagnosis include the following:
- Diabetic retinopathy
- Atherosclerosis (e.g., carotid disease)
- Arteriosclerosis
- Accelerated hypertension ("malignant hypertension")
- Renal failure
- Radiation retinopathy
- Papilledema from increased intracranial pressure
- Pseudotumor cerebri
- Preeclampsia/eclampsia
- Systemic lupus erythematosus and other collagen-vascular diseases
- Pheochromocytoma
- Adrenal disease
- Anemia
- Coarctation of the aorta
- Other causes of systemic hypertension

Treatment

- Treatment is directed toward management of the underlying hypertension and systemic vascular or renal disorders. Chronic hypertensive retinopathy does not require specific ophthalmologic treatment. Acute hypertensive retinopathy with papilledema also is treated by prompt control of the systemic blood pressure and usually requires aggressive management, with imaging studies to rule out a central nervous system tumor.
- Patients with decreased vision, retinal macroaneurysm, branch retinal artery or vein occlusion, and an exudative maculopathy should be referred to an ophthalmologist for possible laser evaluation.
- For preeclampsia or eclampsia, the infant is delivered, and exudative detachments usually resolve post partum. Permanent visual loss from pregnancy-associated complications is uncommon and may result from retinal or occipital lobe ischemia.

Retinal Artery Occlusion

Retinal artery occlusion may involve the central retinal artery (CRAO) or a branch of the central retinal artery (BRAO). With unilateral involvement, vision changes may be obvious or noticeable only after the patient closes the uninvolved eye. Cilioretinal arteries supply a portion of the macula in up to 20% of eyes (see Fig. 10–1). Perfusion of the macula by a cilioretinal artery that arises from the choroidal blood supply may result in macular sparing despite an occluded retinal artery (Fig. 10–12). Retinal whitening will become less apparent with time. More commonly, CRAO will cause ischemia to the macula and sudden vision loss (Fig. 10–13). In an example of a BRAO, a soft, glistening, yellow embolus conforming to the blood vessel lumen, forming a Y-shaped obstruction (Fig. 10–14), probably is cholesterol (Hollenhorst plaque) from the carotid artery (Fig. 10–15). A hard, whitish plaque (Fig. 10–16) may represent a calcific embolus from an abnormal heart valve (Fig. 10–17).

Symptoms

- A sudden, painless, unilateral, near-complete loss of vision occurs in CRAO.
- A sudden, painless visual field loss that corresponds to the horizontal hemifield is found in cases of BRAO. For example, a superior BRAO causes an inferior visual field defect.
- In cases of amaurosis fugax, a transient loss of vision implies an impending CRAO or BRAO. Classically, patients describe a "curtain" descending over their vision that clears over several minutes.

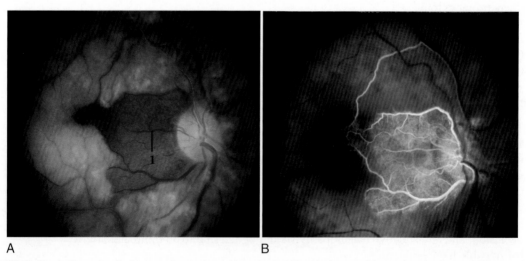

A B

FIGURE 10–12 **A,** Central retinal artery obstruction with a patent cilioretinal artery (1), sparing the fovea. Diffuse retinal whitening from the retinal ischemia occurs many hours after the arterial occlusion and may not be readily apparent at the onset of symptoms. The normal-appearing retina between the optic nerve and fovea is perfused by the centrally located cilioretinal arteriole. **B,** Fluorescein angiogram of the same eye. Note the dark appearance of the fundus resulting from lack of retinal artery perfusion. The cilioretinal arteriole is present in the center of the hyperfluorescent area.

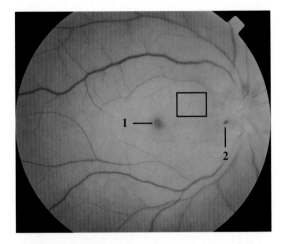

FIGURE 10–13 Right eye of a 75-year-old white man who experienced the sudden onset of decreased vision in that eye 1 day before this photograph was taken. Note the prominent "cherry-red spot" at the center of the fovea (1). No visible emboli are present, but the patient had a history of vascular disease. A small, flame-shaped hemorrhage is evident at the border of the optic nerve (2). Note the attenuation and "boxcarring" within the arterioles *(box)*.

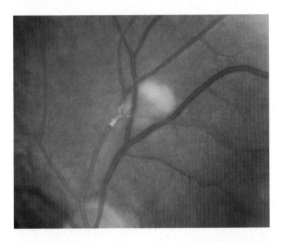

FIGURE 10–14 A Y-shaped embolus probably representing a cholesterol embolus from carotid disease. Note the cotton-wool spot peripheral to the arteriolar occlusion.

Signs

- A relative afferent pupillary defect is present.
- If a patient with retinal artery occlusion is seen within the first few hours of the onset of the disorder, retinal edema may not yet be present.
- An embolus may or may not be seen at the level of the optic nerve in cases of CRAO.
- An embolus may be seen at a branch point of an arteriole in cases of BRAO.
- A cherry-red spot represents ischemia and edema of the entire posterior retina; this spot develops within hours of occlusion and usually is prominent the next day. The red color at the center fovea results from perfusion of the choroid through the thinner retinal tissue and contrasts with the surrounding, ischemic retina.
- Arcuate retinal whitening corresponds to the retinal distribution of the occluded vessel.
- Segmentation, or "boxcarring," of the retinal vessels may be present.

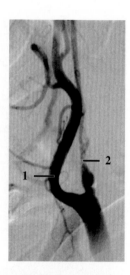

FIGURE 10–15 Carotid angiography of the carotid bifurcation. The external carotid artery is patent (1), whereas the internal carotid is severely obstructed (2).

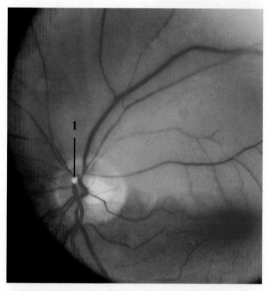

FIGURE 10–16 A highly refractile calcific embolus (1) is present on the optic nerve. A wedge-shaped area of retinal whitening corresponds to the distribution of the branch retinal artery occluded by the embolus.

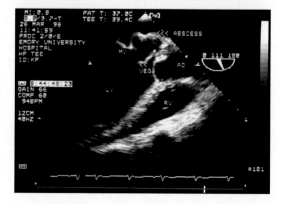

FIGURE 10–17 Transesophageal echography of the aortic valve reveals a dense vegetation (Veg) and an abscess.

- Cilioretinal sparing, or a pattern of normal retina surrounding a cilioretinal artery, may be observed.

Etiology

Possible causative disorders include the following:
- Carotid disease (atherosclerosis)
- Cardiac valvular disease
- Giant cell arteritis: jaw claudication, scalp tenderness, tongue pain, or polymyalgia rheumatica and its associated symptoms possibly present in older patients
- Thrombosis from hypercoagulable states, including pregnancy, oral contraceptive use, and various malignancies. Specific biochemical clotting abnormalities include antiphospholipid antibody syndromes including lupus anticoagulant, elevated plasma homocysteine (which can be hereditary or due to deficiencies of folic acid and/or vitamin B12), resistance to activated protein C (factor V Leiden mutation), prothrombin (factor II) gene mutation, and deficiencies of protein C, protein S, or antithrombin III.
- Cardiac myxoma
- Intravenous drug abuse and talc retinopathy (Fig. 10–18)
- Lipid emboli resulting from trauma
- Causes of disseminated intravascular coagulopathy (DIC) such as pancreatitis, amniotic fluid emboli, trauma, and sepsis
- Sickle cell anemia
- Polyarteritis nodosa
- Corticosteroid injections around the head and neck
- Retinal migraine
- Syphilis
- Cat-scratch disease (*Bartonella henselae* infection)
- Trauma
- Ophthalmic artery occlusion (involving the retinal and choroidal circulation)—a similar disorder in which vision usually is worse (typically with absence of any light perception) and total whitening of the retina occurs

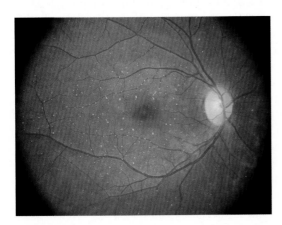

FIGURE 10–18 Multiple talc emboli from intravenous drug use.

Workup

- Evaluation is directed by the clinical examination, the age of the patient, and any known systemic medical associations.
- The examiner auscultates the carotid arteries and heart, listening for the carotid bruits or murmurs (e.g., aortic stenosis).
- If the patient is older than 55 years of age, the clinician should inquire about giant cell arteritis symptoms (see subsequent entry on laboratory evaluation; urgent erythrocyte sedimentation rate [ESR] and C-reactive protein determinations are indicated).
- A neurologic history and examination is performed.
- Carotid ultrasonography or angiography is performed.
- Cardiac echography is performed.
- Laboratory evaluation is modified for each patient and may include the following tests: a Westergren erythrocyte sedimentation rate (ESR), C-reactive protein assay, CBC with differential count, prothrombin time and partial thromboplastin time (PT/PTT) determinations, and hypercoagulation workup if indicated (antithrombin III, protein S, and protein C assays; evaluation for resistance to activated protein C [factor V Leiden mutation]; lupus anticoagulant panel; plasma homocysteine levels; serum protein electrophoresis; hemoglobin electrophoresis).

Treatment

- **Note:** Emergency ophthalmologic consultation is indicated to confirm or rule out a retinal artery obstruction.
- Despite the poor visual prognosis associated with this disorder, efforts are directed toward dislodging an embolus and moving it "downstream" to minimize the amount of retinal involvement. Several immediate maneuvers to dilate the retinal vascular system or decrease the intraocular pressure to dislodge the embolus are within the scope of the primary care provider. The following apply to the acute management of retinal artery occlusion:
  - An immediate ophthalmologic consultation is necessary.
  - For ocular massage, the clinician applies gentle but firm digital pressure on the globe, with the patient's eyelids closed, for 10 to 15 seconds. A rapid release of the pressure creates a transient, sudden decrease in intraocular pressure that may lead to dislodgement of the embolus. The clinician can repeat this procedure several times. If the patient has undergone recent ophthalmic surgery (within 1 month) or trauma with a hyphema or an open globe, massage is contraindicated.
  - In carbogen treatment, the patient rebreathes a mixture of 95% oxygen and 5% carbon dioxide, which may dilate the retinal vasculature. The patient rebreathes the mixture for 10 minutes every 2 hours in most cases. If no improvement occurs after two or three treatments, the treatment is discontinued.
  - Intravenous or oral acetazolamide (Diamox) in a dose of 500 mg is administered. In patients with a sulfa allergy, alternative drugs are used.
  - A topical beta blocker (e.g., timolol 0.5%) is administered.
  - Sublingual administration of nitroglycerin also may cause some vascular dilation.

○ Anterior chamber paracentesis is performed at the slit lamp. The ophthalmologist passes a 30-gauge needle on a tuberculin syringe through the cornea near the limbus into the anterior chamber. Removal of aqueous fluid immediately lowers the intraocular pressure. This may be the most effective method to dislodge an embolus. Potential complications include cataract formation from inadvertent lens touch, hyphema, and endophthalmitis.

○ For patients in whom an anticoagulation regimen is indicated, medical consultation is recommended. Treatment of embolic arterial occlusions should be similar to the protocol used for patients with stroke.

Follow-up

• All patients with artery occlusions require monthly ophthalmologic examinations for approximately 6 months after the initial event. The ophthalmologist determines the need for subsequent follow-up evaluation.

• Neovascularization of the retina or iris may occur and should be promptly treated with retinal laser photocoagulation by an ophthalmologist.

Retinal Vein Occlusion

As with retinal artery occlusion, retinal vein occlusion may involve either the central retinal vein (CRVO) or a branch of the central retinal vein (BRVO). The clinical findings include dilated venules and flame-shaped intraretinal hemorrhages in the involved distribution of the vein. CRVOs involve all four quadrants of the retina (Fig. 10–19), whereas BRVOs involve one quadrant, typically in an arcuate pattern corresponding to the occluded vein's distribution of drainage (Fig. 10–20). Venous occlusive events are relatively common in patients older than 60 years of age. As with artery occlusions, some patients may notice vision changes due to vein occlusions only when the uninvolved eye is covered. Unlike with artery occlusions, the onset of symptoms

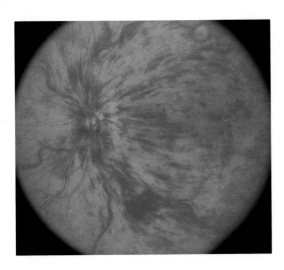

FIGURE 10–19 Central retinal vein occlusion in a patient with 20/400 visual acuity. Note the dramatic retinal hemorrhages in all four quadrants. The veins are dilated and tortuous. Diffuse cotton-wool spots suggest retinal ischemia. The optic disc is blurred with blood from peripapillary hemorrhage.

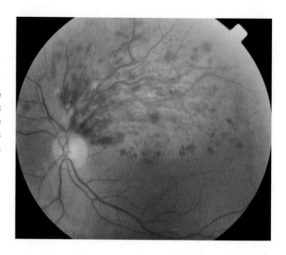

FIGURE 10–20 Branch retinal vein obstruction involving the superotemporal venule that drains in an arcuate, quadrantic distribution in the area of retinal hemorrhage. Note that the hemorrhages follow the nerve fiber layers and do not cross the horizontal raphe (midline). The vein in this quadrant is dilated and tortuous compared with the other veins.

usually is slower; however, symptoms may be noticed suddenly when the patient covers the unaffected eye. The mechanism of a CRVO is a vascular occlusion or thrombus that occurs in the venule at the exit site of retinal blood flow from the eye, within the optic nerve. BRVOs usually occur near the site of an arteriole-venule crossing. Chronic hypertensive changes of the vessel wall and constriction of the common adventitial sheath around both vessels at the crossing point lead to turbulent flow, thrombus formation, and venous occlusion. BRVOs commonly are associated with systemic arteriolar hypertension. The venous occlusion impedes the flow of blood from the retinal circulation. A severe obstruction is termed *ischemic*, whereas a partial obstruction is *nonischemic*. Vision loss from CRVO or BRVO may be from macular edema or macular ischemia.

Symptoms

- Sudden or gradual, unilateral, painless blurry vision or loss of vision is characteristic.
- Severe unilateral pain, redness, and loss of vision are reported. These findings may represent the neovascular glaucoma associated with retinal vein occlusions (RVOs)—informally called "90-day glaucoma," because it usually occurs 3 months after occurrence of an RVO.
- Unilateral visual field loss corresponds to a horizontal hemifield in cases of BRVO.

Signs

- A relative afferent pupillary defect most commonly occurs in cases of ischemic CRVO.
- A "blood-and-thunder" fundus is seen.
- Dilated and tortuous veins are noted.
- A flame-shaped hemorrhage is evident.
- Vitreous hemorrhage may occur.
- Cotton-wool spots are present.

- Macular edema is noted.
- Exudates are common.
- Neovascularization of the retina or iris can occur and usually is associated with glaucoma.

Workup

- The examiner evaluates the patient for systemic hypertension.
- Especially for patients younger than 50 years of age, systemic evaluation may be needed.
- A pregnancy test is performed.
- Information about oral contraceptive use is elicited.
- The possibility of other thrombotic events, including deep vein thrombosis, pulmonary emboli, and frequent miscarriages, and of a family history of thrombosis, is addressed.
- Laboratory evaluation is modified for each patient and may include beta-human chorionic gonadotropin (β-HCG) titer, Westergren erythrocyte sedimentation rate (ESR), CBC with differential count, PT/PTT determination, and hypercoagulation workup if indicated (antithrombin III, protein S, and protein C assays; evaluation for resistance to activated protein C [factor V Leiden mutation]; lupus anticoagulant panel; homocysteinuria testing; serum protein electrophoresis; hemoglobin electrophoresis).
- Testing is performed for thyroid eye disease and tumors, which may cause compression of the central retinal vein as it exits the eye.

Treatment

- Ophthalmologic evaluation is mandatory. The ophthalmologist should examine affected patients within 48 to 72 hours of diagnosis.
- A BRVO with macular edema may result in decreased vision. Laser photocoagulation helps treat macular edema and the neovascular complications. Use of intravitreal injections of triamcinolone (corticosteroid) is under investigation as a therapy to treat vision loss with both CRVO and BRVO.

Follow-up

- Patients with severe CRVO should be assessed every month for the first 6 months by the ophthalmologist to lower the risk of neovascular complications.
- Visual prognosis depends on the severity of the venous occlusion, level of retinal ischemia, and rate at which collateralization occurs. Neovascularization implies a worse prognosis, especially with the development of neovascular glaucoma. Some patients experience resolution of the venous occlusion with good visual acuity, whereas others suffer a significant loss of vision.

Sickle Cell Retinopathy

Paradoxically, the patients with the most severe retinal involvement are those with milder systemic disease—namely, those with hemoglobin SC (sickle cell and hemoglobin C) or S-Thal (sickle cell and thalassemia). These patients generally appear otherwise healthy, may have a negative sickle-prep test result, and are less likely to experience "sickle crisis." Approximate percentages of sickle patterns among African Americans are as follows: AS (sickle trait), 8.5%; SS (sickle cell anemia), 0.4%; SC (SC disease), 0.2%; and S-Thal, 0.03%.

Symptoms

- Vision may be normal or slightly blurred.
- A sudden or progressive, painless loss of vision may occur.
- Floaters are reported with vitreous hemorrhage.
- Flashes occur.
- A blind spot in vision (scotoma) may be present.

Signs

- Intraretinal and subretinal hemorrhage—producing the so-called salmon patch—occurs at the sites of vessel-wall blowout from a sickle obstruction of the arteriole (Fig. 10–21).
- A healed hemorrhage displays spiculated pigment migration, or a "black sunburst."
- Iridescent spots are retractile deposits of hemosiderin from a previous intraretinal hemorrhage.
- Vitreous hemorrhage may be seen.
- Retinal detachment occurs in rare cases.
- "Sea fans," or areas of peripheral neovascularization, are extremely difficult to see with direct ophthalmoscopy.
- Dilated vessels result from peripheral arteriovenous shunts.
- Peripheral neovascularization, gliosis, tractional retinal detachments, and ridges of proliferative tissue are possible findings. Using a direct ophthalmoscope, the examiner looks at the peripheral red reflex of both eyes (dilated) while standing several feet away from the patient. An asymmetrical red reflex is abnormal, and a white

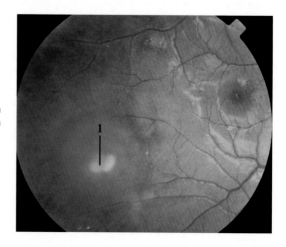

FIGURE 10–21   The right eye of an African American man with sickle cell disease. Note the normal fovea to the right, with a salmon-patch hemorrhage (1) inferotemporal to the fovea.

reflex in one eye strongly suggests a pathologic condition involving the peripheral retina.
- Comma-shaped capillaries of the conjunctiva may be observed.
- CRAOs or BRAOs can occur.

Etiology

- Lower oxygen tension in the peripheral retina causes sickling, with resultant vascular occlusion and peripheral retinal ischemia. Vasoproliferative factors are released from the ischemic retina and may induce peripheral retinal neovascularization with subsequent vitreous hemorrhages.

Differential Diagnosis

Considerations in the differential diagnosis are the same as those for proliferative diabetic retinopathy (see page 156).

Associated Factors and Diseases

- Patients of African or Mediterranean heritage have a higher incidence of sickle cell retinopathy.
- Patients with sickling disorders may have painful sickle crises.

Treatment

- Referral to an ophthalmologist is needed for a baseline peripheral retinal examination and annual examination. Patients with visual symptoms, vitreous hemorrhage, or retinal detachment require more urgent ophthalmologic evaluation, with frequent follow-up.
- Use of laser photocoagulation is controversial but may be beneficial in some circumstances.
- Retinal detachment requires prompt ophthalmologic evaluation for possible surgical repair.

Retinitis Pigmentosa*

Retinitis pigmentosa is a nonspecific term used to describe a large group of retinal degenerations, most of which are inherited. Some cases are sporadic, without any obvious inheritance pattern. Genetic defects affect genes that code for the photoreceptor proteins rhodopsin and peripherin and other retina-specific genes. Advances in molecular biology hold promise for future treatments of these conditions.

Symptoms

- Vision is normal or decreased.
- Night blindness (nyctalopia) may be a symptom. Patients may report difficulty adapting to the dark (e.g., when finding a seat in a darkened movie theater).

---

*Patient information on this subject may be obtained through Research to Prevent Blindness at www.rpbusa.org.

- Photophobia is common, especially with cone dystrophy.
- Shimmering or tiny blinking lights (photopsias) are noted.
- Blind spots in vision (scotomata) may be described.
- A peripheral visual field loss may be mild or severe.
- Color vision commonly is abnormal.
- Affected relatives may have similar symptoms.
- Progression may be slow or rapid, and age at onset of degeneration is highly variable.

Signs

- The fundus may appear normal.
- "Bone spicule" pigmentary retinopathy is observed (Fig. 10–22).
- Optic nerve pallor is common.
- Retinal vascular narrowing or attenuation is common.
- Cataracts may be present.
- Visual fields are constricted.
- The "golden ring" sign is presence of a yellowish-white halo surrounding the optic disc that is eventually replaced with pigmentation or atrophy.

Workup

- The retinal electric responses to various light stimuli in light-adapted and dark-adapted states are measured with studies such as an electroretinogram (ERG) or electro-oculogram (EOG).
- Formal visual field testing is performed.
- A family history is obtained. The severity of disease and prognosis may be similar to those in affected family members. In general, autosomal recessive cases are more severe, whereas autosomal dominant cases are less severe.
- Genetic studies and examination of family members are performed. Genetic consultation is encouraged.

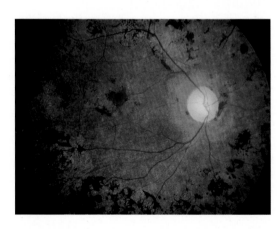

FIGURE 10–22   Eye of a 50-year-old African American woman with Usher syndrome (type II). She was deaf and had severe loss of vision (20/400). The peripheral retina displays the typical "bone spicule" pattern seen with retinitis pigmentosa. A central "bull's-eye" maculopathy also is present.

Differential Diagnosis

Considerations in the differential diagnosis include the following:
- Drug use (especially chloroquine, thioridazine [Mellaril], and chlorpromazine)
- Maternal infections such as syphilis, rubella, and toxoplasmosis, which may cause pigmentary retinal changes similar to those of retinitis pigmentosa
- Vitamin A deficiency (identical signs and symptoms)

Associated Factors and Diseases

- Patients with Usher syndrome (retinitis pigmentosa and deafness) may account for up to 50% of those who are both deaf and blind (see Fig. 10–22).
- Most patients (90% to 100%) with Bardet-Biedl syndrome have retinitis pigmentosa in addition to polydactyly, obesity, hypogonadism, and mental retardation.
- Kearns-Sayre syndrome involves retinitis pigmentosa, ptosis, chronic progressive external ophthalmoplegia, cardiac arrhythmia, heart block, defective mitochondria, and "ragged-red" fibers on muscle biopsy.
- Patients with Alström syndrome have retinitis pigmentosa, diabetes mellitus, obesity, deafness, renal failure, acanthosis nigricans, baldness, hypogenitalism, and hypertriglyceridemia.
- Many other genetic diseases are associated with retinitis pigmentosa.

Treatment

- The following considerations apply in cases of treatable or "pseudo–retinitis pigmentosa":
  - Patients with vitamin A deficiency initially may be seen for "pseudo–retinitis pigmentosa"; the deficiency is due to malabsorption conditions or malnutrition. Treatment consists of vitamin A supplementation. These patients usually are aware of the progressive loss of night vision.
  - Patients with Bassen-Kornzweig syndrome have abetalipoproteinemia, acanthocytosis, ataxia, and neuropathy. Treatment consists of vitamin A and vitamin E supplementation.
  - Refsum syndrome is a phytanic acid storage disease (elevated levels of serum phytanic acid). Treatment involves phytanic acid restriction (decreased ingestion of dairy products, meat, and fish oil).
  - Gyrate atrophy results from ornithine transferase deficiency. Treatment includes supplementation of pyridoxine with an arginine-restricted diet.
- For other common forms of retinitis pigmentosa, use of supplemental vitamin A palmitate (15,000 IU daily) is controversial. This treatment should be avoided in sexually active young women not using contraception because of the teratogenic effects of vitamin A treatment. For patients taking vitamin A supplements, monitoring of liver function with liver enzyme studies is indicated.

Age-Related Macular Degeneration

Age-related macular degeneration (AMD) is the leading cause of legal blindness in persons older than 55 years of age in the Western world. The cause of AMD is

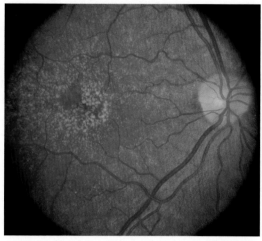

FIGURE 10–23 Extensive small or cuticular drusen in a 56-year-old African American man.

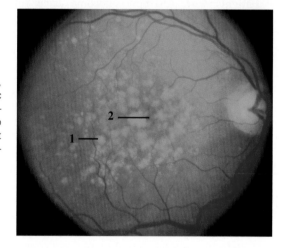

FIGURE 10–24 Multiple soft drusen (1), with numerous large, soft drusen (i.e., larger than the venule as it crosses the optic nerve), in a 72-year-old white woman with atrophic age-related macular degeneration. Pigment irregularities (2) also are evident in the foveal region. This patient would benefit from antioxidant vitamin therapy, as directed by the Age-Related Eye Disease Study (AREDS).

unknown; however, risk factors include older age, history of smoking, female gender, lighter pigmentation, high-fat diet, and, in some families, possibly a genetic component.

The most common abnormality seen in AMD is the presence of drusen, or yellowish deposits found between the neurosensory retina and the underlying retinal pigment epithelium (RPE). Drusen may occur in the earliest stages of AMD, even long before any noticeable vision loss has occurred. In fact, drusen commonly are seen at ophthalmoscopy in persons older than 50 years of age. Drusen may be small yellow bumps (Fig. 10–23) or larger soft-yellow deposits (Fig. 10–24). Drusen also may be localized to the foveal area or more peripherally located along the arcades. Deposits usually are multicentric and may be few in number or extensive.

The two common types of AMD are exudative (eAMD) and atrophic (aAMD), commonly referred to as "wet" and "dry" AMD, respectively. Vision loss occurs most commonly with aAMD, whereas more severe, sudden vision loss is more common with eAMD. In aAMD, geographic atrophy or loss of the retinal pigment epithelium leads to a depigmented appearance of the macula and loss of overlying photoreceptors. In eAMD, neovascularization originating from the choroidal vasculature extends between the RPE and neurosensory retina. The new vessels may leak or bleed, leading to fibrosis and scar tissue under the retina. The end stage of this process is formation of a large, fibrotic, circular or disciform scar that destroys the overlying retina.

Symptoms

- The onset of blurry vision may be gradual or acute.
- Wavy or distorted vision (metamorphopsia) may be noted.
- Intermittent shimmering lights (photopsias) may be described.
- A central blind spot (scotoma) may be a feature of AMD.

Signs

- Vision may be decreased.
- Amsler grid distortion may be found on testing. (An Amsler grid is a chart with horizontal and vertical lines that is used to detect distortion or blind spots within the central 10 degrees of the visual field [see Fig. 1–12].)
- Presence of multiple large, soft drusen with pigment mottling indicates a worse prognosis.
- A loss of normal pigmentation, with a yellow-white geographic area of atrophy, may occur.
- Subretinal (Fig. 10–25) or intraretinal blood or serous fluid may be present.
- Subretinal blood may appear greenish or gray.
- Serous (clear fluid) or hemorrhagic (dark red, black, or yellow) retinal detachment may occur.

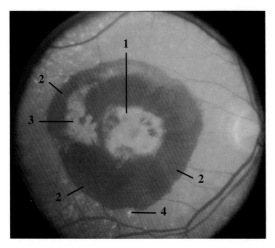

FIGURE 10–25 Eye of a patient with the exudative form of age-related macular degeneration (AMD). A circular, central, disciform fibrotic scar (1) and new-onset subretinal fluid (2) surrounding the subretinal hemorrhage can be seen. More yellow fibrosis is evident within the hemorrhage, temporal to the fovea (3). Note the surrounding yellow drusen (4), indicating AMD.

Workup

- Amsler grid testing is performed.
- Fluorescein or indocyanine green angiography may be helpful.
- Family members are evaluated if an inherited pattern is suspected.

Treatment

- High-dose antioxidant supplements (vitamins C and E, zinc with copper, and beta-carotene) are recommended for nonsmokers with defined levels (see Fig. 10–24) of AMD (smokers are advised to avoid the use of beta-carotene).
- For acute vision changes, the patient should be referred to an ophthalmologist within 24 to 48 hours.
- Laser photocoagulation may be performed.
- Ocular photodynamic therapy is recommended for certain forms of eAMD.
- Macular translocation and subretinal surgery are alternative treatments in selective cases.
- Antiangiogenic agents are currently in investigational stages, but use of these agents for eAMD probably will require either direct intraocular injection or periocular injection.
- Low vision aids—specifically, various forms of image magnification—often are used.

Prognosis

Photodynamic therapy is the primary treatment option for eyes with selective forms of eAMD as determined by angiographic categories, especially those including choroidal neovascularization with active growth in the subfoveal space. The process involves infusing a photoactivatable dye, followed by a long-wavelength laser that activates the dye, resulting in thrombosis of the neovascularization. Treatment rarely results in improvement of visual acuity but slows the deterioration and must be repeated multiple times. Current studies are examining the use of photodynamic therapy along with angiostatic agents and corticosteroids. Recently, new anti-angiogenic agents have been approved for eAMD.

Previous studies have shown the benefit of laser photocoagulation in selected cases of eAMD with neovascularization outside of the foveal region. The complications include a high rate of recurrence and development of a scotoma. Bilateral involvement is common, and surgical treatment is limited.

The Age-Related Eye Disease Study (AREDS) has shown that use of high-dose antioxidant vitamins for moderate stages of AMD decreases the risk of severe vision loss by approximately 20%. The use of these antioxidant vitamins in the very early stages of AMD has not been shown to decrease the progression to later forms, but current studies should help resolve this issue.

Roth Spots

Roth spots are retinal hemorrhages with a white center and may be caused by various systemic and ocular conditions (Fig. 10–26). The most likely source of the white center

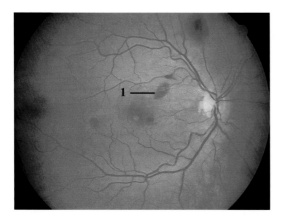

FIGURE 10–26   Eye of a patient with subacute bacterial endocarditis. A classic Roth spot, or white-centered hemorrhage, is present within the superotemporal arcade (1).

is a fibrin plug. Other possible causes include infective emboli and leukemic infiltrates. Treatment is directed at the underlying etiologic process. Vision often is normal.

Differential Diagnosis

Considerations in the differential diagnosis include the following:
- Septic emboli, possibly secondary to subacute bacterial endocarditis
- Diabetes with a resolving intraretinal hemorrhage
- Leukemic retinopathy
- Purtscher's retinopathy, which is associated with trauma, pancreatitis, and other causes of DIC
- CRVO or BRVO
- Pernicious anemia
- Sickle cell disease
- Systemic lupus erythematosus
- Collagen-vascular disease
- Anoxia (due to altitude sickness)
- Carbon monoxide poisoning
- Hypertensive retinopathy
- Birth trauma, with similar changes possibly occurring in the mother after delivery
- Physical abuse
- Intracranial hemorrhage

Cytomegalovirus Retinitis

Before availability of current pharmacologic treatment for human immunodeficiency virus (HIV) infection, cytomegalovirus (CMV) retinitis developed in approximately 30% to 40% of affected patients, usually after the T lymphocyte count dropped below 50 cells per mm^3. These patients require periodic dilated ophthalmoscopic examination. Retinal detachment affects approximately 25% to 40% of those with CMV retinitis. Therefore, CMV infection represents a source of morbidity in patients infected by

HIV. CMV retinitis also may occur in immunosuppressed persons, such as transplant recipients and patients with lymphoma or leukemia.

Symptoms

- Many patients have no symptoms.
- Floaters may be seen.
- Vision may be blurred or decreased.
- Blind spots in vision (scotomata) may be described.
- Flashes (photopsias) may indicate retinal detachment.
- **Note:** The appearance of any new visual symptoms in an HIV-seropositive patient requires a dilated ophthalmologic examination, especially when the CD4$^+$ counts are less than 50 cells per mm^3.

Signs

- Keratic precipitates that are stellate in shape are found on the corneal endothelium.
- Vitreous cells are present.
- Patchy areas of retinal whitening with areas of flame-shaped retinal hemorrhage that may occur posteriorly or peripherally (Fig. 10–27).
- The leading edge of retinal whitening often has satellite areas of punctate retinal whitening distal to the zone of white necrosis.
- The disorder progresses slowly but is considered "vision-threatening" when the affected area is near the optic nerve or macula.

Differential Diagnosis

Considerations in the differential diagnosis include the following:
- Acute retinal necrosis, or progressive outer retinal necrosis, a rapidly progressive retinitis with a poor prognosis that requires immediate treatment (varicella-zoster virus is the presumed etiologic agent)

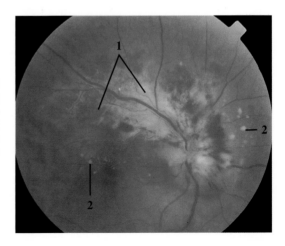

FIGURE 10–27 Sight-threatening cytomegalovirus-related retinitis involves the macula and optic nerve in this eye of a young man who was seropositive for human immunodeficiency virus (HIV). White, infected retina with intraretinal hemorrhage is present in the arcuate distribution of the nerve fiber layer (1). A small amount of lipid exudation near the fovea and nasal to the optic nerve also is seen (2).

- Toxoplasmosis, a more active vitritis, usually associated with an old chorioretinal scar
- HIV retinopathy, including cotton-wool spots and retinal hemorrhages
- Infectious causes such as tuberculosis, syphilis, *Pneumocystis jiroveci* infection, *Mycobacterium avium* complex infection, histoplasmosis, blastomycosis, coccidioidomycosis, and *Candida* and *Aspergillus* infections

Treatment

- For non–vision-threatening disease, ensuring compliance with anti-HIV medications is important.
- Initiation of oral valacyclovir at 1000 mg twice daily is indicated, with observation for signs of regression.
- Intravenous ganciclovir is used less often, owing to the availability of the oral prodrug (see preceding entry). The induction dosage is 5 mg/kg 2 times a day for 2 to 3 weeks, followed by intravenous maintenance therapy with 5 mg/kg daily. The primary side effect is neutropenia.
- With use of intravenous foscarnet, the induction dosage is 90 mg/kg 2 times a day for 2 to 3 weeks, followed by intravenous maintenance therapy with 90 to 120 mg/kg daily. Adequate hydration is essential to minimize the primary toxicity (nephrotoxicity). Nausea is common.
- With use of intravenous cidofovir, the dosage is 5 mg/kg weekly, in combination with oral probenecid (2 g given 3 hours before injection and 2 and 8 hours after injection). Dosages are modified if a change in renal functioning occurs.
- Reinduction may be required with progression of disease while the patient is receiving maintenance therapy.
- The combination of ganciclovir and foscarnet is used when CMV disease is unresponsive to monotherapy or if resistance is suspected.
- Intravitreal administration of ganciclovir, foscarnet, or cidofovir may be provided weekly by an ophthalmologist.
- An intravitreal ganciclovir implant necessitates surgery and does not provide a prophylactic effect against systemic or fellow eye CMV involvement. The implant must be replaced every 8 months. Intraocular drug levels obtained are five times higher than with intravenous treatment.
- The reader is advised to consult the Centers for Disease Control website, www.cdc.gov, for the most current treatment recommendations.

Follow-up

- Optimizing the immune status of the person at risk (whether immunosuppressed or HIV-infected) is the primary means of long-term control of CMV-related disease. Keeping the patient's $CD4^+$ count above 50 cells per mm^3 decreases the risk of CMV recurrence.
- If the retinitis can be controlled with medication, vision may remain normal. Sight-threatening disease occurs when the optic nerve or macula is involved.
- Retinal detachment also may cause sudden vision loss; surgical management is required in these cases.

- The risk of contralateral eye involvement with *active* CMV retinitis is approximately 20%.
- Primary care physicians should keep in mind that all antiviral therapies are virostatic. Should the patient discontinue systemic treatment, CMV retinitis probably will recur.

Toxoplasmosis

Toxoplasma gondii is an obligate intracellular parasite common among humans and animals (e.g., cats). Ocular toxoplasmosis is a potentially blinding, necrotizing retinitis that may recur.

Symptoms

- Vision is blurred or decreased.
- Wavy or distorted vision (metamorphopsia) may occur.
- Floaters may be seen.
- Pain is variable.

Signs

- Vitreous debris is seen.
- Iritis or cells are present in the anterior chamber.
- Yellow-white areas of retinitis are observed.
- The optic nerve is yellow-white and swollen (Fig.10–28).
- Retinal vascular infiltrates (due to periarteritis) may be observed.
- Old chorioretinal scars are found in the affected or fellow eye.
- Macular edema can occur.

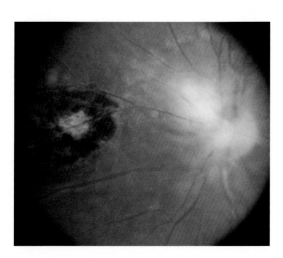

FIGURE 10–28 Left eye of a young man with elevated toxoplasmosis titers. Note the old, healed toxoplasmosis lesion *(black)* nasal to the optic nerve. The optic nerve has an area of active inflammation and reactivation of infection, with overlying vitreous involvement that obscures the disc margin.

Differential Diagnosis

Considerations in the differential diagnosis include the following:
- Uveitis
- Sarcoidosis
- Acute retinal necrosis, with herpes zoster infection the presumed etiologic process
- *Toxocara canis* infection, syphilis, and HIV infection

Treatment

Treatment of sight-threatening lesions—that is, those involving the macula and optic nerve or those with significant intraocular inflammation—is as follows:
- "Triple therapy" for 4 to 6 weeks:
  - Pyramethamine and folate
  - Sulfadiazine, sulfisoxazole, or Triple Sulfa
  - Clindamycin
- Alternatively, trimethoprim and sulfamethoxazole (Bactrim DS)
- Oral prednisone: 40 to 60 mg every day for 3 to 4 weeks, then tapering; used to limit the inflammation-mediated retinal destruction
- Oral atoquavone: 750 mg four times daily; has been suggested to kill the encysted form of toxoplasmosis

Postsurgical Endophthalmitis

Any invasive ophthalmologic procedure may result in endophthalmitis. This condition should be considered in the etiology of significant postoperative pain or inflammation.

Symptoms

- Pain is not always present.
- Reddening of the eye is apparent.
- Vision is decreased.
- Floaters are seen.

Signs

- Hypopyon, or layering cells in the anterior chamber, is observed (Fig. 10–29).
- Conjunctival injection is present.
- Hazy vitreous or obscuration of the posterior pole (vitritis) may be noted.

Treatment

- Either a vitreous culture with intraocular injection of antibiotics or, in more severe cases, vitrectomy surgery with intravitreal antibiotics is necessary.
- Immediate ophthalmologic referral is essential when endophthalmitis is suspected.

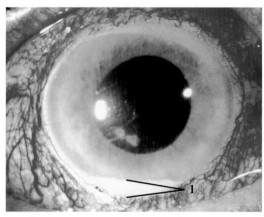

FIGURE 10–29 Endophthalmitis. Acute postoperative hypopyon in the inferior portion of the anterior chamber (1). Note the conjunctival injection in this painful, infected eye.

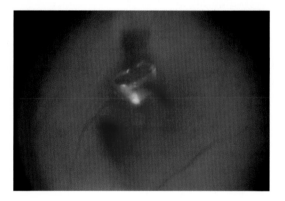

FIGURE 10–30 Intraocular metallic foreign body in a young man who was pounding a metal hammer on a metal post when he felt a sudden sharp pain in the eye. The small metal fragment may be difficult to see through an undilated pupil and is shown here surrounded with a small amount of vitreous hemorrhage. This fragment could be readily detected with a plain skull film or a computed tomography scan.

Trauma-Associated Endophthalmitis

 Failure of the emergency department physician or primary care provider to diagnosis or detect a retained intraocular foreign body may have significant medical-legal implications. Unfortunately, missed diagnosis in such cases can occur. These cases are considered ophthalmologic emergencies and should be referred immediately to an ophthalmologist. Similarly, any full-thickness, perforating, or penetrating wound to the eye (by definition, an open globe injury) necessitates urgent ophthalmologic referral.

Post-traumatic endophthalmitis should be suspected in all cases, particularly with trauma involving an intraocular foreign body, a dirty wound, or a history such as pounding metal on metal (Fig. 10–30). Any patient history suggestive of an intraocular foreign body necessitates radiologic imaging (usually with a skull film or computed tomography [CT] scan) to rule out the presence of foreign material in the eye. Many open globe injuries are treated with intravitreal and/or systemic intravenous antibiotics. Other accompanying injuries should be suspected in the setting of ocular trauma, such as neck, sinus, or central nervous system injuries.

Endogenous Endophthalmitis

Endogenous endophthalmitis results from septic emboli to the retinal or choroidal circulation. Patients usually are sick from the underlying sepsis and present with vitritis, focal areas of retinitis, and anterior chamber reaction. In the anterior chamber, a few cells to a layering of cells (hypopyon) may be present. Intravenous drug abusers, immunocompromised patients, and hospitalized patients with chronic indwelling catheters or central lines are at risk for endogenous endophthalmitis. Endophthalmitis due to *Candida* or other fungi usually appears as a small area of focal choroiditis or chorioretinitis that expands into fluffy white opacities that may extend into the vitreous. Infection may progress to complete opacification of the vitreous.

Intravitreal amphotericin and treatment of the systemic infection are indicated. Vitreous surgery may be required in severe cases. Vitreous cultures are helpful and may reveal the causative organism.

Posterior Vitreous Detachment

Posterior vitreous detachment occurs in most persons with time. The detachment usually occurs in the fifth to seventh decades of life. In highly myopic (very nearsighted) persons, development of a posterior vitreous detachment at an early age is likely because of the larger size of the eye. The vitreous is firmly adherent in the peripheral retina, less firmly adherent at the optic nerve and along the major retinal vessels, and weakly adherent along the surface of the retina. When the vitreous separates from the posterior retina, traction is transferred to the peripheral retina, where tears or breaks may occur.

Symptoms

- Patients report flashing lights.
- New floaters are commonly seen, sometimes stringy or circular.

Treatment

- Because the symptoms of a posterior vitreous detachment may herald a retinal detachment, indirect ophthalmoscopy by an ophthalmologist is required and should be performed within 24 hours of diagnosis.
- No treatment is indicated.
- Laser photocoagulation or cryotherapy may be used for any new retinal tears associated with symptoms.

Retinal Detachment

A retinal detachment occurs when fluid separates the neurosensory retina from the underlying RPE. A rhegmatogenous (from the Greek *rhegma*, meaning "breakage") retinal detachment typically occurs when the vitreous separates from the retina (posterior vitreous detachment), causing a tear or break (Fig. 10–31). Liquefied vitreous fluid then dissects the neurosensory retina from the underlying RPE, resulting in a

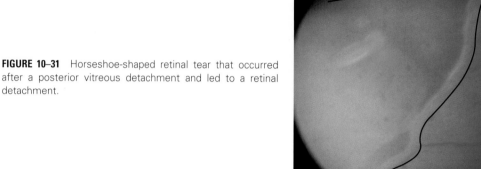

FIGURE 10–31 Horseshoe-shaped retinal tear that occurred after a posterior vitreous detachment and led to a retinal detachment.

detached retina. Serous or exudative retinal detachments occur following the leakage of fluid caused by a process occurring under the retina without a tear or break in the retina. The fluid leakage may be due to abnormal neovascularization, incompetence of the RPE barrier to fluid, tumors, or inflammation. A tractional retinal detachment results from scar tissue formation on the surface of the retina, leading to contraction with subsequent retinal distortion, elevation, and swelling. Tractional retinal detachments commonly occur with proliferative diabetic retinopathy as the result of repeated vitreous hemorrhage.

Symptoms

- Flashes are noted.
- Floaters are seen.
- A visual field loss occurs, which patients often describe as a curtain, shadow, or bubble of fluid.
- Vision is wavy or distorted (metamorphopsia).
- Vision is decreased.

Signs

- A relative afferent pupillary defect may be observed.
- The visual field loss is unilateral and may be sectoral, quadrantic, hemifield, or total.
- Retinal hydration lines, or rugae, have an appearance similar to that of ripples on a pond.

Workup

- Retinal detachments are difficult to diagnose with a direct ophthalmoscope. A simple technique using a direct ophthalmoscope allows the clinician to compare the red reflexes of the two eyes from a distance of several feet. Any differences in the quality of the reflex dictate further evaluation. An eye with a retinal detachment may have a lighter-colored reflex (yellow or orange) than in the fellow eye.

Treatment

- Patients should be referred for immediate ophthalmologic evaluation.
- Surgical intervention is necessary because untreated retinal detachments may lead to blindness in the affected eye.
- The cause of a serous retinal detachment should be determined, especially to rule out the presence of a tumor.

Epiretinal Membrane

A thin sheet of fibroglial tissue, or an epiretinal membrane, may form on the surface of the retina, often after a posterior vitreous retinal detachment. Contraction of the membrane wrinkles and distorts the retina (Fig. 10–32).

Symptoms

- Vision is decreased.
- Vision is wavy or distorted (metamorphopsia).
- Patients report difficulty reading with the affected eye.

Signs

- Amsler grid distortion is found on testing.
- A whitish, folded membrane is evident on the retinal surface (Fig. 10–32).
- The retinal vasculature is distorted.
- Macular edema may be present.

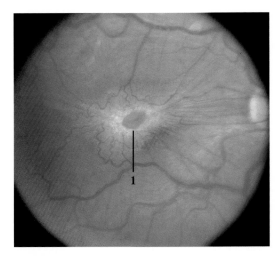

FIGURE 10–32 With contraction of the epiretinal membrane (1), the retinal elements are pulled centrally, with formation of accompanying wrinkles, folds, and vascular distortions.

Treatment

- Ophthalmologic referral is indicated.
- Occasionally an epiretinal membrane breaks free from the retina and vision spontaneously improves, but this is rare. If the patient's vision is minimally affected, no treatment is required.
- If vision is significantly affected, surgical removal of the membrane is necessary to improve the vision and distortion.

Follow-up

- The overall visual prognosis is good.

Vitreous Hemorrhage

Vitreous hemorrhage is the result of an underlying vascular process and occurs in many disorders. Because visualization of the retina may be impossible, ophthalmic ultrasonography may be necessary to determine the presence of an accompanying retinal detachment. Treatment is directed at management of the underlying etiologic process.

Differential Diagnosis

Considerations in the differential diagnosis include the following:
- Proliferative diabetic retinopathy
- Posterior vitreous detachment with an avulsed retinal vessel
- Retinal tear through a vessel (with or without a retinal detachment)
- Macroaneurysm
- Trauma
- Subarachnoid or subdural hematoma (Terson syndrome)
- Any retinal vascular lesion

Retinal Surgery

Advances in retinal surgery over the last 20 to 30 years have been dramatic because of the development of microsurgical techniques, wide-field viewing, and a better understanding of complex biologic processes. Many formerly blinding conditions, such as diabetic retinopathy, recurrent retinal detachments, and retinopathy of prematurity, are now managed more effectively. The two primary forms of retinal surgery are scleral buckling and vitrectomy surgery. The primary indication for surgery is a retinal detachment.

Standard scleral buckling surgery usually involves the placement of a solid silicone band around the equator of the eye to relieve the circumferential traction and support the retina in the region of the retinal tear (Fig. 10–33). The scleral buckle alters the internal fluid dynamics and decreases the rate of subretinal fluid accumulation. Either laser treatment or cryotherapy is used to form an adhesion (retinopexy) of the retina to the underlying choroid in the area of the tear. The combination of a buckle and

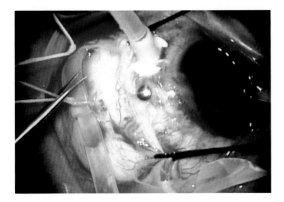

FIGURE 10–33 The external placement of a silicone scleral buckle. The element is sewn to the scleral surface. Note that black silk sutures are supporting the rectus muscles. The white infusion tubing and gold plug represent sclerotomy entry sites into the eye for vitreous dissection instrumentation.

the chorioretinal adhesion serves to repair most rhegmatogenous retinal detachments (80%). In certain situations, an intraocular gas bubble along with retinopexy may be used to reattach the retina. This technique is referred to as *pneumatic retinopexy*.

During vitrectomy surgery, the surgeon begins by making three small incisions in the sclera. One sclerotomy accommodates an infusion line; the other two are used to place instrumentation into the posterior segment of the eye. The surgeon views the inside of the eye through a surgical microscope that contains various lenses to help visualize the abnormal anatomy. Various instruments such as illuminated picks, scissors, endolaser probes, and forceps are used to perform delicate manipulation of the retina. Heavy liquids, air, gas, or silicone oil may be used to reattach the retina. Laser photocoagulation seals the retinal tear and may be used to treat ischemic retina (panretinal photocoagulation).

CHAPTER 11

Glaucoma

ALLEN D. BECK

Related Anatomy

Aqueous humor is produced by the epithelium of the ciliary body (Fig. 11–1). The aqueous flows past the lens, around the iris, into Schlemm's canal by way of the trabecular meshwork, and then into aqueous and episcleral veins. The trabecular meshwork is the site of the greatest resistance to aqueous outflow and is located at the junction between the cornea and the iris. This region of the eye is referred to as the *anterior chamber angle*.

Turnover of the entire volume of aqueous occurs approximately every 100 minutes. Intraocular pressure (IOP) is determined by the balance between production and outflow of aqueous humor. The range of normal IOP measurements is 10 to 21 mm Hg. An IOP measurement of 22 mm Hg or greater is considered abnormal. Diurnal variations in IOP are well documented for both normal and glaucomatous eyes. These pressure swings mean that the IOP may be in the normal range at certain times of the day in patients with glaucoma.

Damage from glaucoma is manifested by optic nerve cupping (Fig. 11–2). Loss of neurons and glial tissue causes glaucomatous cupping secondary to mechanical and ischemic mechanisms.

The damage to the optic nerve results in characteristic patterns of visual field loss (Fig. 11–3). Visual field loss in glaucoma classically respects the horizontal meridian. Visual acuity and the central visual field usually remain normal until late in the disease process.

Definitions and Epidemiology

The term *glaucoma* refers to a group of diseases with progressive optic nerve damage and visual field loss. In most cases of glaucoma the IOP is consistently above the normal range, although in some cases the IOP may always be within the normal range.

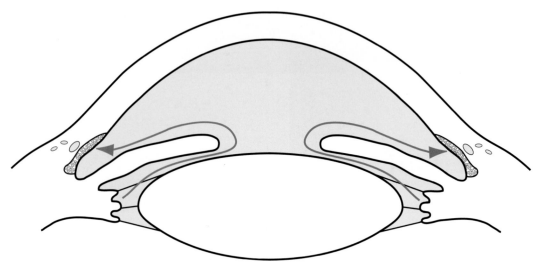

FIGURE 11–1 Anatomy of the anterior portion of the eye, demonstrating the flow of aqueous humor from the ciliary body to the trabecular meshwork.

The prevalence of glaucoma is approximately 0.5% of the total population. Elevated IOP without signs of optic nerve or visual field damage (ocular hypertension) occurs in approximately 1.5% of the total population. Glaucoma can be broadly categorized into open-angle glaucoma and angle-closure glaucoma. Most cases of glaucoma are of the open-angle type, in which the eye has a structurally normal outflow pathway (see Fig. 11–1). In angle-closure glaucoma, blockage of aqueous flow between the lens and iris causes a forward shifting of the iris and closure of the anterior chamber angle (Fig. 11–4). Patients with angle-closure glaucoma may experience acute symptoms of severe pain and blurred vision, whereas those with a chronic form of angle-closure glaucoma have slow elevation of IOP with no symptoms.

Open-Angle Glaucoma

Symptoms

- Patients usually have no symptoms, although decreased vision may be noted late in the disease course.

Signs

- IOP is elevated.
- Optic nerve cupping occurs (see Fig. 11–2).

Associated Factors and Diseases

- Increasing patient age is associated with a progressive increase in the prevalence of glaucoma.

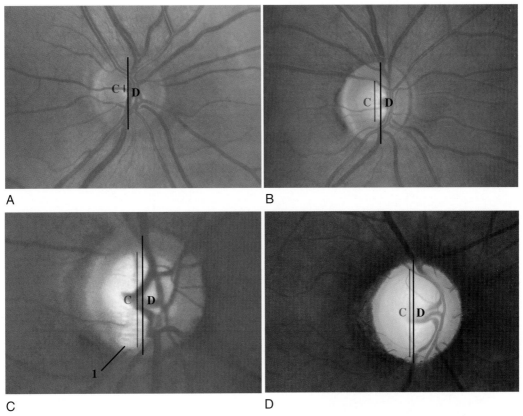

FIGURE 11–2 **A,** Normal cup-to-disc (C/D) ratio of 0.1. **B,** Likely normal C/D ratio of 0.5. **C,** C/D ratio of 0.8 vertically with inferior notching (1) of the nerve (glaucomatous change). **D,** C/D ratio of 0.90 vertically (glaucomatous change). C, cup; D, disc.

- Glaucoma is more prevalent, develops at an earlier age, and is more severe in African Americans than in white persons.
- A family history of open-angle glaucoma is associated with a fivefold to sixfold increase in the risk of glaucoma development.
- The prevalence of ocular hypertension in patients with diabetes mellitus is two to three times higher than in the general population. The possibility of an increased risk of ocular hypertension in patients with systemic hypertension has not been determined definitively.
- **Note:** Corneal thickness in patients with ocular hypertension plays an important role in the risk of developing glaucoma. Patients with thinner-than-average corneas are at higher risk, whereas those with thicker-than-average corneas are at lower risk.

Workup

- **Measurement of IOP** (see Chapter 1): The "gold standard" is Goldmann applanation tonometry. IOP is determined by measurement of the force required to flatten the central cornea. Fluorescein dye and a topical anesthetic are required, as is skill

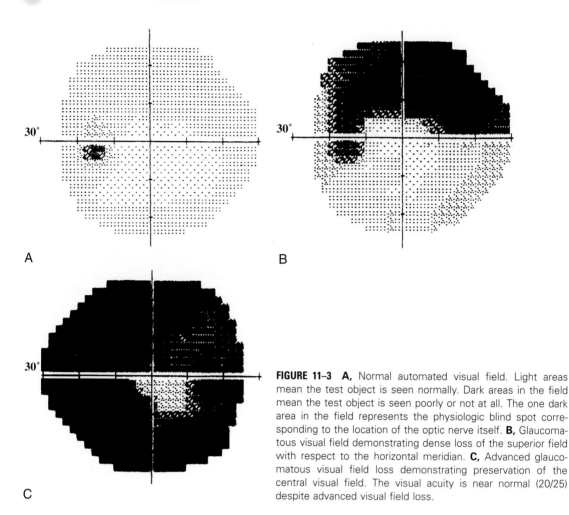

FIGURE 11–3 A, Normal automated visual field. Light areas mean the test object is seen normally. Dark areas in the field mean the test object is seen poorly or not at all. The one dark area in the field represents the physiologic blind spot corresponding to the location of the optic nerve itself. **B,** Glaucomatous visual field demonstrating dense loss of the superior field with respect to the horizontal meridian. **C,** Advanced glaucomatous visual field loss demonstrating preservation of the central visual field. The visual acuity is near normal (20/25) despite advanced visual field loss.

in interpretation of the fluorescent semicircles to determine the IOP directly, using a scale associated with this device.

- A relatively new device, the Tono-Pen, can be used more easily to measure IOP. Multiple applanation measurements are averaged by this instrument, which displays the IOP as a digital readout. Greater cost is one drawback to the Tono-Pen.
- **Pupillary examination**: A relative afferent pupillary defect may be present in asymmetrical cases of glaucoma.
- **Ophthalmoscopy**: Evaluation with a direct ophthalmoscope provides important diagnostic clues. Because the IOP may be in the normal range in a patient with glaucoma, the clinician who measures IOP and also examines the optic nerve is more likely to diagnose glaucoma correctly. A cup-to-disc ratio (see Fig. 11–2C and D) of 0.6 or greater is one sign of glaucoma. Asymmetry of 0.2 or greater in the cup-to-disc ratio and focal asymmetry in the neuroretinal rim also are highly suggestive.

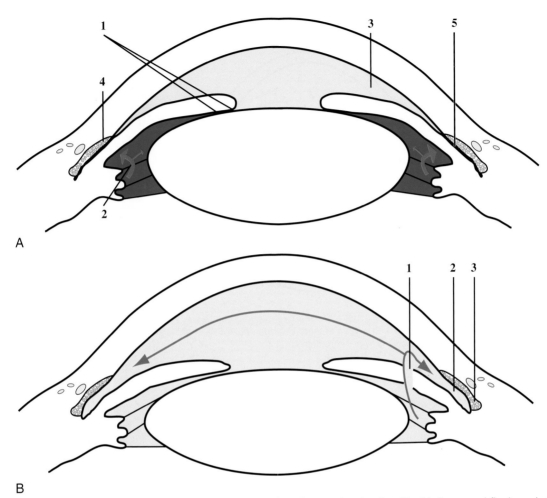

A

B

FIGURE 11–4 **A,** Pupillary block prevents flow of aqueous into the anterior chamber. The iris is pressed firmly against the lens (1), blocking aqueous flow (2) into the anterior chamber (3). The iris is pushed against the trabecular meshwork (4). The peripheral anterior chamber angle is thus closed (5), blocking aqueous outflow and raising the intraocular pressure. **B,** A small hole in the peripheral iris (1) is made with a laser (laser iridectomy), allowing aqueous to enter the anterior chamber of the eye. This opens the anterior chamber angle (2), so that aqueous can drain normally through the trabecular meshwork (3).

Dilation of the pupil with tropicamide 1% and phenylephrine 2.5% ophthalmic solutions greatly facilitates optic nerve evaluation.
- Eyes with a narrow chamber angle should not be dilated. (A simple penlight test for this condition is shown in Figure 11–5.)

Treatment

- Any patient with abnormal findings on optic nerve examination, an afferent pupillary deficit, or an elevated IOP measurement should be referred to an ophthalmologist for evaluation and possible treatment.

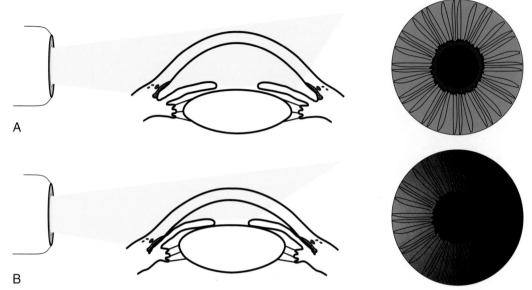

A

B

FIGURE 11–5 Use of the penlight to demonstrate a shallow anterior chamber. **A,** A penlight aimed obliquely to the eye will illuminate nearly the entire iris with a deep anterior chamber. **B,** With a shallow anterior chamber, only a portion of the iris is illuminated, with shadowing over the remainder.

- Treatment usually begins with medication:
  - ○ Medications work by one of two methods to lower IOP: decreasing the production of aqueous or increasing the outflow of aqueous. Medications that decrease aqueous production include topical beta blockers (levobunolol [Betagan], betaxolol [Betoptic], carteolol [Ocupress], metipranolol [OptiPranolol], and timolol [Betimol, Timoptic]), oral carbonic anhydrase inhibitors (acetazolamide [Diamox] and methazolamide [Neptazane]), topical carbonic anhydrase inhibitors (dorzolamide [Trusopt] and brinzolamide [Azopt]), and alpha-2 agonists (apraclonidine [Iopidine] and brimonidine tartrate [Alphagan P]). Medications that improve aqueous outflow include prostaglandin analogs (latanoprost [Xalatan], travoprost [Travatan], bimatoprost [Lumigan], and unoprostone isopropyl [Rescula]), topical miotic agents (pilocarpine [Pilocar] and echothiophate [Phospholine Iodide]), and epinephrine preparations (Epifrin and Propine).
  - ○ Eyedrops gain access to the systemic circulation by way of the nasal mucosa of the nasolacrimal system, and systemic side effects can be noted with these medications (see Chapter 17).
- Surgical options include the following:
  - ○ Open-angle glaucoma not responsive to medical therapy can be treated with laser and incisional surgery.
  - ○ Laser trabeculoplasty involves placement of multiple, low-energy burns to the trabecular meshwork, decreasing the IOP significantly in approximately 80% of cases.

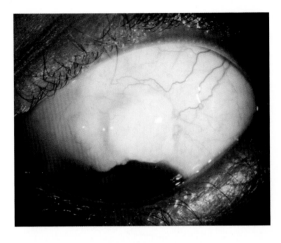

FIGURE 11–6 The whitish, elevated area on the superior portion of the eye is a filtering bleb in a patient with open-angle glaucoma.

- ○ Trabeculectomy bypasses the normal outflow pathway by the creation of a surgical fistula. An elevation of the conjunctiva known as a *filtering bleb* is a sign of a successful trabeculectomy (Fig. 11–6).
- ○ Conjunctivitis associated with a filtering bleb should prompt immediate referral to an ophthalmologist because of the risk of infection spreading inside the eye (endophthalmitis).

Acute Angle-Closure Glaucoma

Symptoms

- Vision is blurred, usually in one eye.
- Halos are seen around lighting fixtures (this symptom is almost always monocular).
- Intense ocular pain and photophobia are important symptoms.
- Vasovagal symptoms such as diaphoresis, nausea, and vomiting are possible.

Signs

- A *mid-dilated* pupil is seen (Fig. 11–7A).
- Conjunctival injection and lid edema are present.
- Corneal edema with blurring of the light reflex develops.
- IOP is markedly elevated, often to 60 to 80 mm Hg (normal range, 10 to 21 mm Hg).

Associated Factors and Diseases

- Women are affected three to four times more commonly than men.
- The peak age range for occurrence of angle-closure glaucoma is between the ages of 55 and 70 years.
- The disorder occurs in shorter, smaller, far-sighted eyes with narrow chamber angles (see Fig. 11–7B).

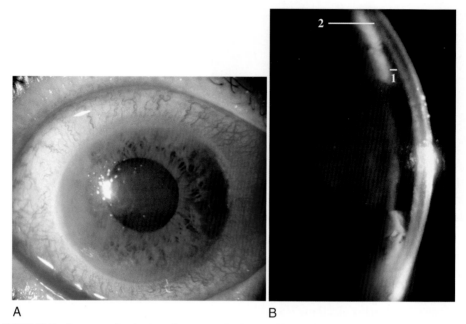

A   B

FIGURE 11–7 Acute angle-closure glaucoma. A, Acutely elevated pressure produces an inflamed eye with corneal edema (note fragmented light reflex) and a *mid-dilated* pupil. **B,** Slit lamp examination shows a very shallow central anterior chamber (space between cornea and iris) (1) and no peripheral chamber (2).

• Stress, a darkened room, and drugs that can dilate the pupil may precipitate an acute angle-closure attack. Many systemic medications with anticholinergic or sympatho-mimetic action carry a warning against use in persons with glaucoma. This caveat applies to patients with a narrow chamber angle only, not to patients with open-angle glaucoma. Because most glaucoma cases are of the open-angle type, these medications are rarely contraindicated in clinical practice. Consultation with the patient's ophthalmologist is recommended for the primary care physician if a question arises over a possible medication contraindication.

Treatment

• Acute angle-closure glaucoma represents an ophthalmic emergency and requires *immediate* referral to an ophthalmologist.
• Initial medical treatment to lower the IOP involves a topical beta blocker (e.g., Timoptic 0.5%, 1 drop), a topical alpha agonist (e.g., Alphagan P, 1 drop), a carbonic anhydrase inhibitor (e.g., Diamox 500 mg intravenously or two 250-mg tablets orally), and osmotic agents (e.g., oral 50% glycerin 2 to 3 mL/kg or intravenous mannitol, 1 to 2 g/kg given over 45 minutes; 500 mL of mannitol 20% contains 100 g of mannitol).
• In most cases, laser iridectomy (creating a full-thickness opening in the peripheral iris) reopens at least a portion of the angle, with subsequent marked lowering of the IOP (see Fig. 11–4A and B).

Follow-up

- After an acute angle-closure event, a portion of the angle may remain closed because of scarring of peripheral iris tissue to the cornea, causing chronic angle-closure glaucoma. Chronic angle-closure glaucoma also may occur without any symptoms, just like open-angle glaucoma. Treatment involves medications and incisional surgery such as trabeculectomy.
- Laser trabeculoplasty is not effective. Laser iridectomy may be recommended for persons with very narrow angles who are at significant risk for the development of either acute or chronic angle-closure glaucoma.

CHAPTER 12

Neuro-ophthalmology

TIMOTHY J. MARTIN

The subspecialty of neuro-ophthalmology encompasses disorders of the brain and cranial nerves that affect vision. Patients with neuro-ophthalmic disorders have presenting complaints of vision loss, diplopia (double vision), ptosis (eyelid droop), anisocoria (unequal pupils), or pain.

Disorders of the Afferent (Sensory) Visual System

The visual pathways extend from the front of the cranium (the eyes) to the most posterior aspect of the brain (the occipital cortex). As a result of this structural arrangement, patients with intracranial pathology often see the ophthalmologist first because of vision loss.

Measuring visual acuity is a key part of any eye examination, but other tests, such as plotting the visual field and examining for a relative afferent pupillary defect, may be just as vital in narrowing the differential diagnosis. In fact, the pattern of visual field loss often reveals the location of a lesion in the afferent visual system (Fig. 12–1).

Visual Field Loss Patterns in Optic Nerve Disorders

Over 120 million photoreceptors in the retina receive the image focused by the cornea and lens. Initial processing takes place in the retina, with approximately 1 million ganglion cells contributing axons to form the optic nerve. These axons traverse the innermost layer of the retina in a peculiar pattern; they arch above and below the sensitive fovea to form the optic nerve. The pattern of visual field loss in optic nerve disease reflects the course and organization of these nerve fibers, producing visual field defects that tend to be arcuate in shape and to respect the horizontal meridian (see examples in Figs. 12–2C, 12–5C, and 12–6B).

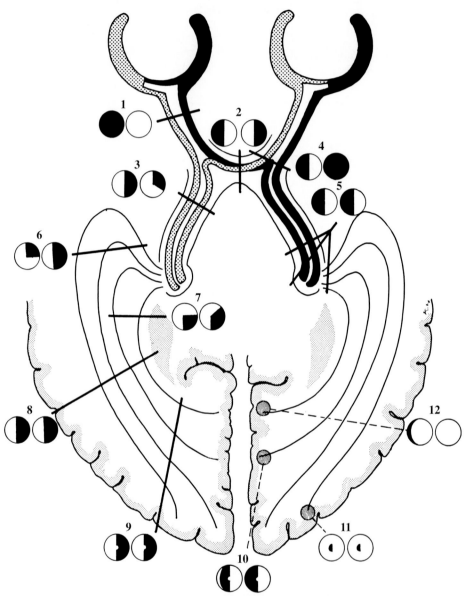

FIGURE 12–1   The visual system, with visual field defects resulting from lesions at various points in the visual pathway. Here, an optic nerve lesion affects the visual field of only one eye (1). Bilateral optic nerve lesions, however, are not uncommon. Lesions of the body of the chiasm tend to produce bilateral temporal visual field defects (2) (see also Fig. 12–9). Optic tract lesions (and all lesions posterior to the chiasm) produce defects that are homonymous (on the same side in both eyes) (3). Lesions at the junction of the optic nerve and the chiasm severely affect vision in the ipsilateral eye but produce an often asymptomatic temporal peripheral visual field defect in the contralateral eye (4). Complete homonymous hemianopic visual field defects are nonlocalizing; that is, they can occur anywhere from the optic tract to the occipital lobe (5 and 8). A unilateral homonymous hemianopia does not decrease visual acuity. Lesions in the temporal lobe produce superior homonymous defects (6). Parietal lesions cause inferior homonymous defects (7). Occipital lobe lesions are highly congruous (9 to 11). Be aware that bilateral occipital infarctions can profoundly affect visual acuity and visual fields bilaterally, with normal-appearing fundi and normal pupillary responses *(not shown)*. A lesion deep in the visual cortex can produce a visual field defect in the temporal visual field of one eye only (12).

Visual Field Loss Patterns in Lesions of the Chiasm and Posterior Visual Pathways

Axons from retinal ganglion cells that represent *right visual space* are routed through the chiasm to form the *left optic tract*, synapsing in the left lateral geniculate body (and vice versa for left visual space) (Fig. 12–1). Anatomically, this means that axons originating in the nasal half of the retina (which map the temporal visual field) cross in the chiasm to the opposite side. Therefore, mass lesions compressing the chiasm disrupt these crossing fibers, causing temporal visual field defects in both eyes. Lesions posterior to the chiasm (optic tract and posterior visual pathways) produce *homonymous* (on the same side in both eyes) visual field defects that respect the vertical meridian. From the chiasm posteriorly, corresponding axons from the right and left eyes that represent the same point in visual space move closer together as they converge on a common point in the occipital cortex. Thus, the more posterior a lesion is, the more *congruous* the resultant visual field defects become: the homonymous visual defects in each eye look more alike in shape and depth.

Optic Nerve Disorders

The optic disc is the proximal end of the optic nerve and can be observed with the ophthalmoscope. Optic nerve lesions may produce visible disc edema (swelling), infiltration, pallor, or pathologic cupping (from glaucoma). Lesions of the nerve more distant from the disc may not cause any observable optic disc abnormality acutely (such as with retrobulbar optic neuritis), but with time the normally pink neural rim turns pale.

Nonarteritic Anterior Ischemic Optic Neuropathy (NAION)

Symptoms

- A sudden, painless loss of vision occurs, frequently noted on arising in the morning.

Signs

- Patients usually are older than 40 years of age.
- The unilateral optic disc swelling often is segmental, and flame-shaped hemorrhages may be observed. Disc pallor is seen as the edema resolves over 4 to 6 weeks (Fig. 12–2A and B).
- An altitudinal (affecting upper or lower quadrants) visual field defect is common (Fig. 12–2C).
- A relative afferent pupillary defect is present if the fellow eye is unaffected.

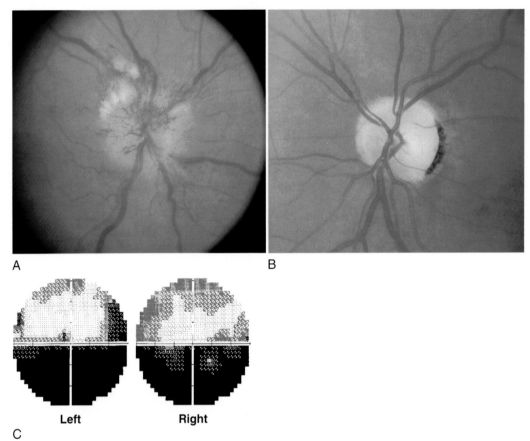

A   B

Left   **Right**

C

FIGURE 12–2 Nonarteritic anterior ischemic optic neuropathy in a 49-year-old man with diabetes. The patient initially presented with sudden, painless vision loss in his right eye. Approximately 2 years before, he had experienced a similar event in the left eye. **A,** Right eye shows optic disc edema, flame-shaped hemorrhage, and cotton-wool spot concentrated on upper half of the disc. **B,** Left, previously affected eye shows pallor of upper disc (sectoral pallor), with some pink still present inferiorly. **C,** Bilateral inferior altitudinal visual field defects were present (corresponding to superior optic disc events).

Etiology and Associated Factors and Diseases

- Vision loss results from hypoperfusion of the optic disc.
- Hypoperfusion may result from atherosclerotic or thrombotic processes affecting the arteries supplying the optic disc.
- Hemodynamic compromise is a potential cause, occurring in patients with hypotension or blood loss.
- The disorder is associated with hypertension, diabetes, coronary artery disease, and other vasculopathic conditions.
- Patients typically have a "crowded" optic disc configuration, with a small or absent physiologic cup.

Differential Diagnosis

Other optic neuropathies that need to be considered include the following:
* *Arteritic* anterior ischemic optic neuropathy (giant cell arteritis)
* Optic neuritis
* Infiltrative optic neuropathy
* Asymmetrical papilledema
* Compressive optic neuropathy

Workup

* Westergren erythrocyte sedimentation rate testing should be performed to look for evidence of giant cell arteritis.
* Medical evaluation for hypertension, diabetes, and anemia is indicated.
* Neuroimaging may be required in uncertain or progressive cases.

Treatment

* No treatment has been proved effective; intravenous and oral steroids are of uncertain help but are a consideration in patients with progressing vision loss or NAION in the better eye
* Daily aspirin may reduce the incidence of an episode in the fellow eye.

Follow-up

* Visual field testing should be performed at approximately 2 weeks and at 2 months to see if the clinical course is stable, as expected.
* Progression of visual deficits may require more extensive investigation such as neuroimaging.
* Mild improvement in the central vision may occur in about 50% of patients.
* Simultaneous or rapidly sequential anterior ischemic optic neuropathy (involvement of both eyes within a few months) suggests giant cell arteritis.

Giant Cell Arteritis: Arteritic Anterior Ischemic Optic Neuropathy (AAION)

Symptoms

* A sudden vision loss occurs in one or both eyes.
* Vision loss frequently is extreme.
* Systemic symptoms include headache, scalp and temple tenderness, myalgia, arthralgia, low-grade fever, anemia, malaise, weight loss, and anorexia. Jaw and tongue claudication are particularly suggestive of giant cell arteritis.
* Polymyalgia rheumatica may accompany or precede giant cell arteritis. Symptoms are morning stiffness and muscle aches, particularly in the neck and shoulders.

Signs

- The frequency of the disorder increases with each successive decade of life: Before the age of 50 years, it is very rare; at ages 50 to 59 years, it occurs occasionally. Most cases occur in patients 60 years of age or older.
- Optic disc pallor and swelling may be present on examination, or only minimal optic disc changes that do not reflect the profound vision loss may be noted (Fig. 12–3A).
- Temporal arteries often are firm, tender, or pulseless (Fig. 12–3B).
- The erythrocyte sedimentation rate is generally greater than 50 mm/hr but can occasionally be normal.
- Mild anemia commonly occurs.
- A third, fourth, or sixth cranial nerve palsy also may occur, as can vision loss from a central retinal artery occlusion.
- A relative afferent pupillary defect is present in unilateral cases.

Etiology

- Vision loss is caused by vasculitic occlusion of arteries to the optic disc.

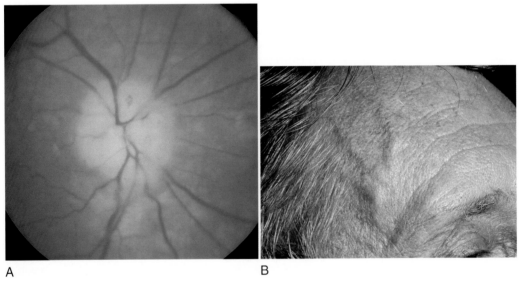

A   B

FIGURE 12–3 Arteritic anterior ischemic optic neuropathy (giant cell arteritis). The patient was a 73-year-old man who noted the progressive decline of vision in his right eye to no light perception over 2 days. He had experienced headaches and malaise for several weeks previously. Although his erythrocyte sedimentation rate was only 33 mm/hr, he was immediately hospitalized for high-dose intravenous corticosteroids for suspected giant cell arteritis. **A,** Pale swelling of the right optic disc, characteristic of arteritic anterior ischemic optic neuropathy. The left optic disc *(not shown)* is normal. **B,** The temporal artery was firm, pulseless, and tender. A temporal artery biopsy confirmed the diagnosis of giant cell arteritis.

Differential Diagnosis

Other diagnostic considerations in this setting include the following:
- NAION (when optic disc edema is present)
- Compressive optic neuropathy (especially with minimal optic disc signs)

Workup

- Measurement of the erythrocyte sedimentation rate should be performed immediately. Assay for C-reactive protein also is helpful.
- A temporal artery biopsy should be performed but is not required before institution of corticosteroid therapy (best if performed within 2 weeks of initiating corticosteroids).
- Neuroimaging may be needed if the diagnosis is uncertain.
- An ophthalmologic consultation should be obtained to aid in the diagnosis and management of vision loss.
- Chest x-ray imaging and determination of electrolyte and blood glucose levels are needed to evaluate existing medical problems that may be exacerbated by corticosteroid administration, such as tuberculosis, diabetes, and hypertension.

Treatment

- Corticosteroids are administered immediately: intravenous methylprednisolone 250 mg every 6 hours for 3 days with acute vision loss (followed by oral, daily prednisone) or prednisone 80 to 100 mg orally if giant cell arteritis is suspected but no vision loss has occurred.

Follow-up

- A second biopsy of the contralateral temporal artery or other tender scalp artery is recommended if the first biopsy results are negative but clinical suspicion remains strong.
- Long-term corticosteroid use (with slow taper, with periodic determinations of erythrocyte sedimentation rate) requires careful medical support to monitor the potentially serious side effects.

Optic Neuritis

Symptoms

- Vision loss in one eye occurs over several days.
- Pain with eye movement is common.
- Spontaneous recovery occurs over months.
- Patients may relate a history of transient neurologic disturbances.

Signs

- Patients usually are 15 to 45 years of age.
- Two thirds of patients initially have normal-appearing discs (with *retrobulbar* optic neuritis); one third have optic disc edema.

- Central visual field loss is common, but any disc-related visual field defect (such as altitudinal losses) may be present (Fig. 12–4).
- A relative afferent pupillary defect usually is present in the affected eye but may be absent if a previous event occurred in the fellow eye.
- Spontaneous, near-complete recovery from the visual deficit occurs within months in most cases.

Etiology

- Optic neuritis results from demyelination of the optic nerve, either with an idiopathic origin or occurring in association with multiple sclerosis.
- In some cases, the disorder is presumed to be of postviral origin.

Differential Diagnosis

With Normal Optic Discs
Other disorders that can cause poor vision, initially with relatively normal optic discs, include the following:
- Compressive optic neuropathy
- Vasculitis
- Carcinomatous meningitis
- Trauma
- Radiation-induced optic neuropathy
- Toxic or nutritional optic neuropathy (bilateral)

With Swollen Discs
In patients with swollen discs, the following possibilities should be considered:
- Anterior ischemic optic neuropathy
- Leber's optic neuropathy
- Hypertensive optic neuropathy
- Infiltrative or compressive optic neuropathy

Workup

- Ophthalmologic evaluation is required to rule out other ocular disease and to perform formal visual field testing.
- Magnetic resonance imaging (MRI) of the brain and orbits with contrast is needed to assist in determining treatment options (see Fig. 12–4B).
- Complete blood count (CBC), determination of electrolyte levels, and chest x-ray imaging should be performed if corticosteroid treatment is anticipated.

Treatment

- For patients with white matter plaques found on MRI, intravenous methylprednisolone (250 mg) every 6 hours for 3 days (with an optional 10-day oral corticosteroid taper) should be considered. This treatment has been shown to reduce future multiple sclerosis–related neurologic events, but only for the following 2 years. Intravenous methylprednisolone may hasten visual recovery but has not been shown to affect final visual outcome.

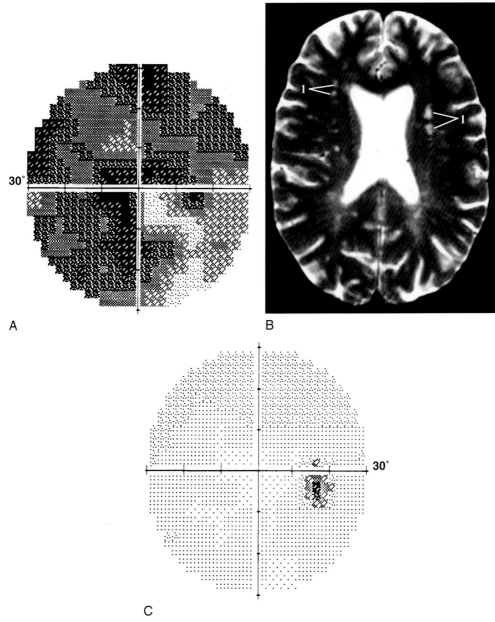

FIGURE 12–4 Optic neuritis. The patient was a 32-year-old woman who noted progressive decline in the vision of her right eye over 5 days, as well as pain with eye movement. The optic discs and fundus were normal, but a large relative afferent pupillary defect was present in the right eye. **A,** Initial visual field testing demonstrated significant visual field loss and a visual acuity of counting fingers only. **B,** MRI revealed periventricular white matter plaques (1) characteristic of multiple sclerosis. The patient was given high-dose intravenous corticosteroids. **C,** Results of visual field testing 3 months later were normal, and the visual acuity had improved to 20/20. Within 2 years, she experienced additional neurologic events consistent with multiple sclerosis.

- For patients without white matter changes found on MRI, intravenous corticosteroid treatment has no proven long-term advantage, but this treatment often is used to hasten recovery in "one-eyed" patients or those with severe vision loss.
- Oral corticosteroids must *not* be used alone, because they increase the incidence of recurrence of optic neuritis.

Follow-up

- Neurologic evaluation is needed to investigate the possibility of underlying multiple sclerosis and to assess subsequent treatment.
- Visual field testing is repeated at intervals to ensure that the course of the disease is consistent with optic neuritis. Failure of the patient to improve as expected necessitates additional workup.

Papilledema

The term *papilledema* refers to bilateral optic disc edema from elevated intracranial pressure but does not identify the underlying etiologic process. Both brain tumors and pseudotumor cerebri (idiopathic intracranial hypertension) produce papilledema in affected patients.

Symptoms

- Headache is common; nausea and vomiting also can occur.
- Brief, transient episodes of vision loss may occur with postural changes.
- Pulsatile tinnitus is common.
- Horizontal diplopia occasionally is present, resulting from paresis of one or both sixth cranial nerves.
- Other neurologic dysfunction may be present with an intracranial mass.

Signs

- Patients with pseudotumor cerebri are often obese females aged 12 to 40 years.
- Optic disc edema typically is present in both eyes (Fig. 12–5A and B).
- Patients initially may have relatively normal visual fields. Over time, chronic papilledema causes peripheral visual field loss (Fig. 12–5C).
- Visual acuity typically is not affected until very late in progressive cases.
- Unilateral or bilateral sixth cranial nerve paresis may occur.

Etiology

Elevated intracranial pressure is caused by the following:
- Intracranial mass
- Impediment to cerebrospinal fluid flow or absorption, as from dural sinus thrombosis, arteriovenous malformation, aqueductal stenosis, meningitis, and trauma (e.g., intracranial hematoma, subarachnoid hemorrhage)
- Idiopathic intracranial hypertension (pseudotumor cerebri) associated with obesity and some medications (vitamin A, some antibiotics such as tetracycline, and others)

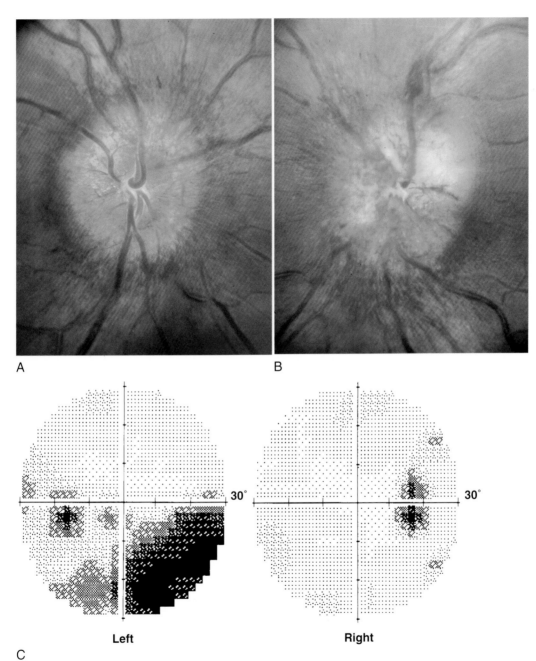

A

B

30°

30°

Left

Right

C

FIGURE 12–5   Idiopathic intracranial hypertension (pseudotumor cerebri). The patient was a 39-year-old woman who had experienced brief episodes of vision loss in both eyes, lasting seconds, and headache. MRI findings were normal, and lumbar puncture revealed an opening pressure of 400 mm of water. Right eye (**A**) and left eye (**B**) show papilledema (bilateral optic disc swelling from elevated intracranial pressure). **C,** Visual acuity was 20/20 in each eye, but visual field testing demonstrated enlargement of the blind spots bilaterally, and a visual field defect was evident in the left eye. This type of visual field defect ("nasal step") is characteristic of optic disc disease; it follows the nerve fiber layer pattern and respects the horizontal meridian.

Differential Diagnosis

Other disorders that can cause bilateral optic disc elevation include the following:
- Pseudopapilledema (anomalous optic discs)
- Bilateral optic neuritis
- Bilateral anterior ischemic optic neuropathy
- Amiodarone toxicity
- Bilateral infiltrative optic neuropathy (e.g., sarcoidosis, tuberculosis, metastatic cancer)
- Hypertensive retinopathy ("malignant" hypertension)

Workup

- Measuring the blood pressure is required, because severe hypertension can manifest with bilateral optic disc edema.
- Neuroimaging (MRI with contrast preferred) is performed immediately to look for a mass or dural sinus thrombosis.
- A lumbar puncture is needed to measure the opening pressure and to obtain cerebrospinal fluid for analysis if findings on neuroimaging are normal.
- Neurosurgery and neurology consultations are necessary for identified causes.
- Ophthalmology and neurology consultations are needed to confirm a diagnosis of pseudotumor cerebri, to monitor the clinical course, and for formal visual field testing.

Treatment

- Treatment of idiopathic intracranial hypertension (pseudotumor cerebri) includes the following:
  - Weight loss is very effective.
  - Acetazolamide (Diamox) is effective.
  - Topiramate (Topamax) is effective, especially in combination with acetazolamide.
  - Furosemide (Lasix) is less effective.
  - Neurosurgical shunting or optic nerve sheath fenestration may be needed in cases of visual field deterioration despite medical therapy.
- For other conditions such as a mass or dural sinus thrombosis, the etiologic process determines the treatment.

Follow-up

- Frequent, formal visual field testing is required in patients with chronic papilledema, because their visual acuity may remain 20/20 despite progressive peripheral visual field loss.

Other Optic Neuropathies

Infiltrative Disorders

- Lymphoproliferative cells (as in lymphoma and leukemia), infectious agents (as in tuberculosis), or inflammatory granulomas (as in sarcoidosis) may invade the optic nerve, resulting in an elevated, swollen appearance of the optic disc.

- Leukemic infiltration of the optic disc with visual loss constitutes a true oncologic emergency; prompt radiation treatment may preserve vision.

Toxic and Nutritional Disorders

- A slow, bilateral loss of central vision is characteristic, with mild pallor of the temporal aspect of the optic nerve.
- Alcohol abuse and a poor diet are common causes, suggesting nutritional and substance abuse consultation; folic acid and thiamine supplementation may improve vision.
- Other causes include pernicious anemia and heavy metal (lead) toxicity.
- Medications (e.g., ethambutol, isoniazid, streptomycin, digitalis) are sometimes implicated.

Leber's Optic Neuropathy

- A rapid, sequential bilateral loss of central vision occurs in young men and rarely in women.
- Mild disc swelling may occur acutely, with disc pallor developing over time.
- Mitochondrial DNA mutations in asymptomatic women are inherited by their children; however, usually the disorder manifests in males.

Optic Nerve Trauma

- Traumatic optic nerve injury may be caused by *direct trauma* from foreign bodies or bone fragments or *indirect trauma* from a blunt injury to the brow or cranium, even without fractures.
- The optic disc may appear normal at first, but pallor develops in 4 to 8 weeks.
- High-dose intravenous corticosteroids may be of benefit during the acute phase.
- Decompression of the bony optic canal has been advocated by some clinicians.
- In all cases the presence of associated ocular trauma (e.g., retinal detachment, penetrating injuries) must be determined.

Optic Disc Pallor

- Optic disc pallor is the final common pathway of almost all optic nerve insults.
- If the etiologic process is unknown, neuroimaging is required to look for compressive etiology (e.g., tumor).

Optic Nerve Head Drusen

- Hyaline material is present in the substance of the optic disc (in 1% of the general population).
- This rocklike yellow material forms irregularly shaped excrescences, which may be exposed on the disc surface in older patients (Fig. 12–6A).
- Peripheral visual field defects may occur; however, visual acuity is almost never affected (Fig. 12–6B).
- The occurrence is bilateral in 70% of patients.
- The drusen often are "buried" in young patients, making it difficult for clinicians to distinguish these elevated discs from discs with true edema (Fig. 12–7).

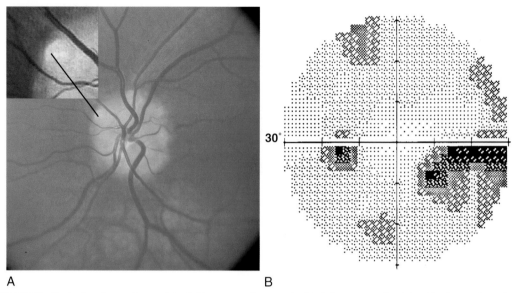

A   B

FIGURE 12–6   Optic disc drusen in an adult. **A,** Drusen can be seen in this left eye as yellowish-white lumps *(inset),* giving the disc margin a bumpy, scalloped appearance. **B,** Visual acuity is 20/20, but peripheral visual field loss (nasal step) is present.

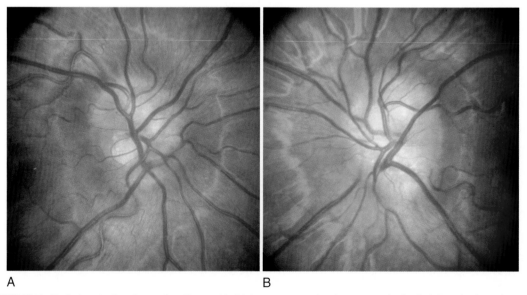

A   B

FIGURE 12–7   Buried optic disc drusen in a 7-year-old girl. In young people, drusen may be buried deep in the substance of the disc. The resulting disc elevation is difficult to distinguish from papilledema. **A,** Right eye. **B,** Left eye.

Optic Nerve Tumors

Symptoms

- Vision loss is slow and progressive.
- Proptosis (eye pushed forward) or double vision is possible.

Signs

- Gradual onset of optic disc pallor is typical, although the disc may appear normal early in the disease (Fig. 12–8C).
- Disc edema is possible in anterior lesions.
- Vascular shunt vessels may be noted on the optic disc.
- Optic nerve–related visual field defects demonstrate a slow, relentless progression (Fig. 12–8B).
- Nystagmus may be present in children.

Etiology

- In children, optic nerve glioma is most common; 90% of the tumors are diagnosed before the age of 20 years, and 25% are associated with neurofibromatosis. The clinical course with this tumor is slow in children. In adults, the tumor is very aggressive, resulting in blindness and death.
- Optic nerve meningiomas are more common in adults and originate from the optic nerve sheath or adjacent dural structures.
- Metastatic disease to the orbit may cause compression of the optic nerve.

Differential Diagnosis

Other disorders that may present in a similar fashion include the following:
- Optic neuritis (especially with vision loss and a normal fundus)
- Other optic neuropathies, including glaucoma
- Thyroid eye disease, which can cause optic nerve compression, proptosis, and diplopia

Workup

- Neuroimaging (computed tomography [CT] or MRI of both brain and orbits with contrast) is needed (see Fig. 12–8A).

Treatment

- Ophthalmology and neurosurgery consultations are required for definitive diagnosis and management.

Chiasmal Compression

As discussed at the beginning of this chapter, the visual field defect arising from a chiasmal lesion typically interrupts the crossing nasal retinal fibers to produce a

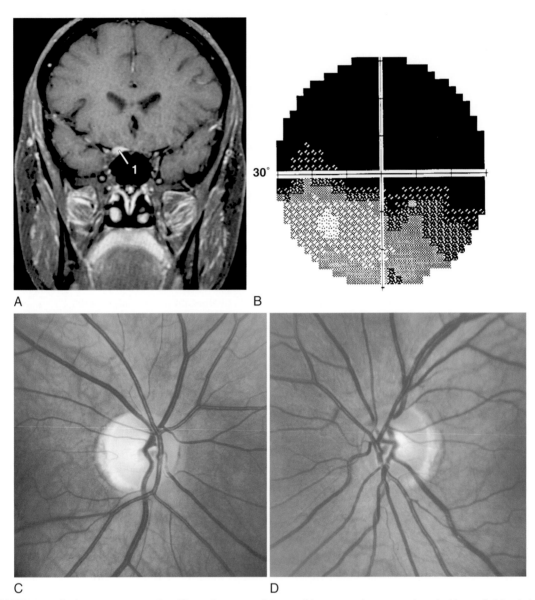

FIGURE 12–8 Optic nerve compression. The patient was a 32-year-old woman who reported gradual loss of vision in her right eye. **A,** MRI study shows an enhancing mass (1) abutting the right optic nerve, consistent with a meningioma. **B,** Resultant visual field loss in the right eye. **C,** Optic disc pallor in the right eye. **D,** Normal left optic disc.

bitemporal visual field defect (see Fig. 12–1). The most common cause is a mass lesion arising from the parasellar region.

Symptoms

- Slow, progressive vision loss may occur in one or both eyes.
- Headache sometimes occurs.
- Symptoms related to the pituitary dysfunction may be identified.

Signs

- Insidious optic disc pallor develops over time.
- Bilateral temporal visual field defects occur with chiasmal compression (Fig. 12–9B).
- The third through sixth cranial nerves may be affected by tumors that invade the cavernous sinus.

Etiology

- Chiasmal dysfunction usually is the result of compression by a mass lesion: pituitary macroadenoma (or apoplexy), meningioma, craniopharyngioma, or other suprasellar masses.

Differential Diagnosis

Other disorders that may produce bilateral temporal visual field defects include the following:
- Bilateral optic neuropathies, especially those affecting central vision and enlarging the (temporal) blind spot, such as Leber's and other hereditary optic neuropathies and toxic or nutritional optic neuropathies

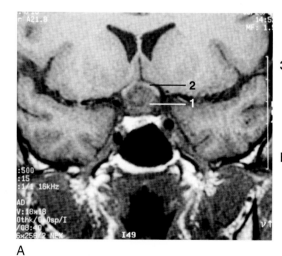

A

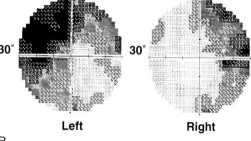

B

FIGURE 12–9 Craniopharyngioma with chiasmal compression. **A,** MRI study shows a mass (1) elevating and compressing the chiasm (2). **B,** Bilateral temporal visual field defects are present.

- Anomalous optic discs, in which abnormalities of the retina around the blind spot can produce temporal visual field defects
- Trauma to the chiasm

Workup

- Neuroimaging (MRI with contrast preferred) is performed, with attention to the sellar region (see Fig. 12–9A).

Treatment

- Neurosurgical consultation is necessary.
- Ophthalmic consultation is necessary for formal visual field testing to follow the progress of the disease, to monitor success of treatment, and to watch for recurrence.

Anisocoria

Anisocoria (unequal pupils) is caused by unequal pupillary motor inputs to the two eyes. Vision loss, even total blindness in one eye, does not cause anisocoria.

To evaluate anisocoria, the examiner first determines which pupil is abnormal by noting pupil size in darkness and in light. When the larger pupil is abnormal (does not constrict well), the degree of anisocoria is greatest in bright light (as the normal pupil becomes small). When the smaller pupil is abnormal (does not dilate well), the degree of anisocoria is greatest in darkness (as the normal pupil dilates). As a general rule, the pupil that reacts poorly to direct light is the abnormal pupil. Essential, or physiologic, anisocoria is common, with a small difference in pupillary size (generally less than 1 mm) remaining constant in light and dark. Previous trauma and eye surgery are common causes for different pupil sizes.

When the Larger Pupil Is the Abnormal One

Etiology, Associated Factors and Diseases, and Differential Diagnosis

- In third nerve palsy, a dilated pupil with ptosis and/or a motility abnormality suggests compression of the third cranial nerve (i.e., an aneurysm). Pupillary dilation in isolation, *without any other sign* of oculomotor nerve dysfunction, is unlikely to result from compression of the third cranial nerve.
- Adie's syndrome results from an often idiopathic insult to the ciliary ganglion in the orbit. The pupil responds to near focus (when the patient attempts to focus on a target inches from the nose), but the reaction to light is absent or very poor (Fig. 12–10).
- Pharmacologic causes of a dilated pupil include instillation of any anticholinergic or sympathomimetic compound into the eye (e.g., dilating drops, contamination from scopolamine patches, jimsonweed).

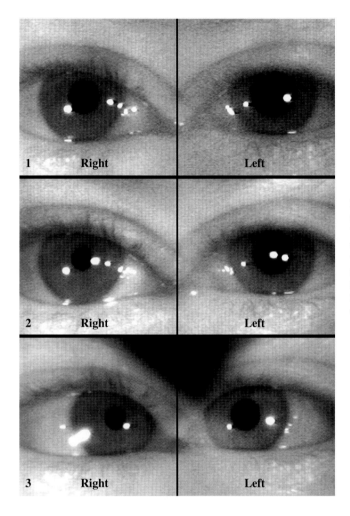

FIGURE 12–10 Adie's pupil. In room light, the anisocoria is evident (1). In bright light, the normal right pupil becomes small, but the affected left eye responds poorly (2). With a sustained near focus, however, the affected pupil does become smaller (3). This finding of a better response to a near stimulus than to a light stimulus is termed *light-near dissociation* and is characteristic of Adie's pupil.

- Because of possible non-neurologic causes such as eye trauma, iritis, angle-closure glaucoma, and eye surgery, patients with anisocoria should undergo an ophthalmologic evaluation.

Workup

- An ophthalmologist may use pharmacologic tests for cholinergic supersensitivity in Adie's pupil, with pilocarpine 0.125% producing marked constriction of the affected pupil and little effect on the normal eye. Pharmacologic dilation with anticholinergic agents can be identified with the use of pilocarpine 1%; this agent does not constrict the affected eye but produces marked constriction in the normal eye.

Treatment

- If a third nerve palsy is suspected as the cause of a dilated pupil, immediate referral to an ophthalmologist (a neuro-ophthalmologist if available), neurologist, and/or neurosurgeon is necessary to evaluate the possibility of an expanding aneurysm.

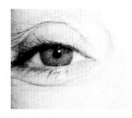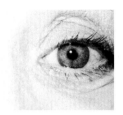

FIGURE 12–11   Horner syndrome. The mild ptosis (1 to 2 mm) and smaller pupil can be seen on the affected right side.

- If no sign of third nerve dysfunction is present, the patient should be seen again within a week; pharmacologic dilation should have resolved (unless repeated) and the examiner can recheck for any developing signs of third nerve dysfunction.

When the Smaller Pupil Is the Abnormal One

Etiology, Associated Factors and Diseases, and Differential Diagnosis

- In patients with Horner syndrome (oculosympathetic paresis), a 1- to 2-mm ptosis is virtually always present in addition to the miosis. Facial anhidrosis (unilateral lack of sweating) may be more difficult to identify (Fig. 12–11).
- Other causes of a small pupil such as eye trauma, iritis, angle-closure glaucoma, and eye surgery probably will be evident on ophthalmologic evaluation.

Workup

- An ophthalmologist may use pharmacologic tests to verify an oculosympathetic paresis in patients with suspected Horner syndrome. Cocaine 10% has a less potent mydriatic effect on the abnormal pupil than on the unaffected one. Hydroxyamphetamine does not dilate the affected pupil well in postganglionic lesions (from the superior cervical ganglion in the neck to the eye). Common etiologic processes for postganglionic lesions include cluster headache and carotid artery dissection, but postganglionic Horner syndrome often is idiopathic. Preganglionic lesions (affecting fibers from the hypothalamus, traveling through the brainstem, spinal cord, chest cavity, and neck to the superior cervical ganglion) frequently are serious (e.g., malignancy, stroke), requiring specialist evaluation and imaging of the brain, neck, and chest.

Treatment

- The underlying etiology determines treatment.

Disorders of the Visual Motor System

Third Nerve Palsy

The third cranial nerve (oculomotor nerve) is complex, innervating all of the extraocular muscles (including the levator palpebrae, which elevates the eyelids) except the lateral rectus and superior oblique muscles. It also innervates the pupillary sphincter.

Symptoms

- A ptosis typically is present and often is profound.
- Diplopia results if the drooping eyelid does not cover the pupil.
- Headache or periorbital pain often is present, depending on the etiology.

Signs

- The eye often is turned down and out.
- The ptosis may be mild or complete.
- Deficiencies in raising, lowering, or moving the eye toward the nose may be partial or complete (Fig. 12–12).
- A dilated pupil is an important sign, because it is more common with compression (aneurysm) than with ischemia.

Etiology

- An ischemic cranial mononeuropathy is a common cause in patients who are elderly or have conditions associated with increased risk for vascular problems, such as hypertension and diabetes.
- Vasculitis (giant cell arteritis) can cause ischemic cranial neuropathies.

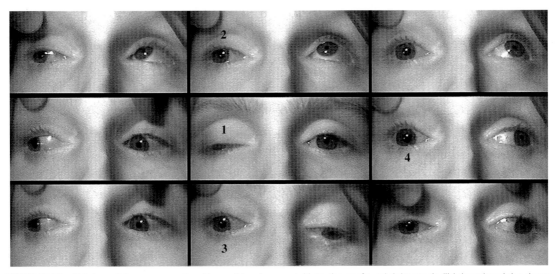

FIGURE 12–12   Third cranial nerve paresis with pupil involvement. Note the profound right ptosis (lid droop) and the down-and-out position of the right eye (1). Gaze positions demonstrate poor elevation (2), depression (3), and inability to turn the eye inward (adduction) (4). Note the dilated pupil in the affected right eye.

- Compression by aneurysm, tumor, or even uncal herniation can cause third nerve dysfunction.
- Head trauma is a common cause.

Differential Diagnosis

Other diagnostic considerations include the following:
- Ocular myasthenia gravis
- Thyroid eye disease
- Brainstem lesions

Workup

- MRI of the brain with contrast (and often MR angiography) is required in patients without obvious vascular risk factors.
- Cerebral angiography may be necessary in patients suspected to have an aneurysm, especially younger patients (younger than 45 years of age) and those with pupil involvement.
- An ophthalmologist who is confident in the diagnosis of a pupil-sparing third nerve paresis in a patient with vascular disease (with presumed ischemic mononeuropathy) may elect to simply observe if there is no evidence of giant cell arteritis.

Treatment

- The underlying etiology determines treatment.

Follow-up

- Patients with presumed ischemic mononeuropathy should return for follow-up evaluation within a week, to ensure that progression to pupil involvement has not occurred.
- Patients with ischemic mononeuropathy should recover in 6 to 12 weeks; further investigation is required for those who do not.

Fourth Nerve Palsy

The fourth cranial (trochlear) nerve innervates only the superior oblique muscle, but this muscle has a complex action. It can tilt, depress, and move the eye away from the nose.

Symptoms

- Vertical or oblique diplopia occurs.
- Objects may appear tilted.

Signs

- Patients may adopt a head tilt to minimize diplopia.
- The eye does not depress well when adducted (turned toward the nose) (Fig. 12–13).

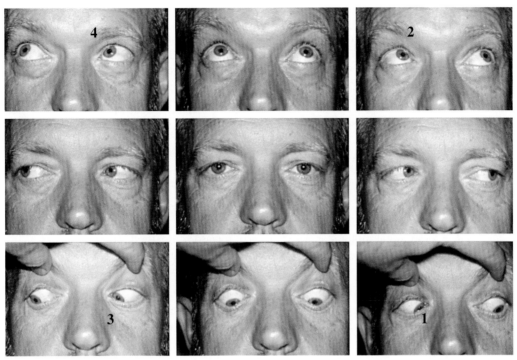

FIGURE 12–13 Traumatic right fourth cranial nerve paresis. Note that the right eye does not look as far down when the gaze is directed to the left and down (1). It also "overacts," or looks up too far, in upgaze (2). This often subtle finding is best appreciated on comparison with the normal responses of the opposite eye in adduction (3 and 4).

Etiology

- A fourth nerve palsy is common after head trauma.
- Congenital fourth nerve palsies are very common and may be discovered incidentally.
- Other than trauma, the most common acquired cause is an ischemic cranial mononeuropathy in patients with vascular disease.

Differential Diagnosis

Other diagnostic considerations include the following:
- Ocular myasthenia gravis
- Skew deviation (vertical misalignment after brainstem stroke)
- Thyroid eye disease

Workup

- Fourth nerve palsies are difficult to diagnose and monitor without careful measurement of the ocular alignment by an ophthalmologist.
- In patients at risk for ischemic events, only minimal workup (i.e., determination of erythrocyte sedimentation rate to look for giant cell arteritis) may be needed.

Treatment

- Treatment is directed toward alleviating symptoms. Prisms (stick-on Fresnel prisms or built-in prisms) are only occasionally helpful because of the torsion and gaze dependence of symptoms. A clip-on occluder (that fits on the patient's eyeglasses) helps eliminate diplopia by blocking the image from one eye.

Sixth Nerve Palsy

The sixth cranial (abducens) nerve exits the brainstem at the pontomedullary junction, climbs up the clivus, and travels through the cavernous sinus into the orbit to innervate the lateral rectus muscle.

Symptoms

- Horizontal diplopia is worse in gaze toward the palsied muscle.
- Headache or periorbital pain often is present for a few days at onset.

Signs

- An esotropia (eyes turned in) is present in primary position (front gaze).
- Testing side gaze reveals an abduction deficit (one eye does not move out well) (Fig. 12–14).
- Patients may adopt a head-turn position to minimize the diplopia.

Etiology and Associated Factors and Diseases

- Brainstem lesions from infarct, demyelination, or tumor (progressive symptoms) may cause a facial paresis ipsilateral to the sixth nerve deficit.
- Most isolated sixth nerve palsies result from lesions affecting the nerve after it exits the brainstem, from any of the following causes:
  ○ Ischemic cranial mononeuropathy (very common) in older patients with vascular disease
  ○ Trauma (common)
  ○ Intracranial hypertension (with associated papilledema)
  ○ Tumors of the cerebellopontine angle (possibly associated with hearing loss and ataxia)

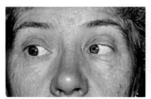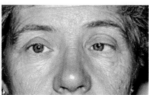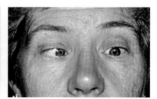

FIGURE 12–14 Left sixth cranial nerve paresis. Note the poor movement of the left eye in left gaze.

- ○ Cavernous sinus disease (e.g., tumor, carotid-cavernous fistula)
- ○ Postviral syndrome in children (tumor must be excluded)
- ○ Idiopathic (the cause is not identified in some cases)

Differential Diagnosis

Conditions that may mimic a sixth cranial nerve palsy include the following:
- Thyroid eye disease
- Congenital esotropia
- Ocular myasthenia gravis

Workup

- Ophthalmologic evaluation is necessary for measurement of the deficit and evaluation for associated signs such as papilledema.
- Determination of the erythrocyte sedimentation rate is performed to address the possibility of giant cell arteritis in elderly patients.
- Neuroimaging (MRI with contrast) is indicated in patients without obvious vascular risk factors, progression of symptoms, or other cranial nerve involvement.

Treatment

- The underlying cause determines treatment.
- For transient cases, use of an alternating clip-on occluder can prevent diplopia.
- For long-term cases, the ophthalmologist may consider prisms, botulinum injection (of antagonist medial rectus), and eye muscle surgery.

Carotid Artery–Cavernous Sinus Fistula

Symptoms

- Unexplained, persistent redness of the eye often is the first symptom.
- Double vision is common.
- Pulsating intracranial noises may be reported.

Signs

- Dilated, tortuous conjunctival vessels usually are found (Fig. 12–15).
- Dysfunction of the third, fourth, or sixth cranial nerve may be identified.
- Proptosis is common.
- A cranial bruit may be auscultated by the physician.
- A dilated superior ophthalmic vein often is seen on neuroimaging.
- Intraocular pressure may be elevated.

Etiology

- The disorder originates from an abnormal communication between the high-pressure arterial system and the low-pressure venous cavernous sinus.

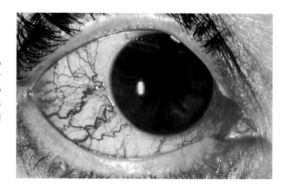

FIGURE 12–15 Right eye of a 64-year-old woman who presented with redness, proptosis, and elevated intraocular pressure in that eye. Diplopia and pulsatile tinnitus also were described. Her examination revealed dilated, tortuous ocular vessels, with subsequent angiography demonstrating a carotid artery–cavernous sinus fistula.

- The disorder can be *direct* (high flow), between the internal carotid artery and the cavernous sinus (e.g., with trauma or rupture of intercavernous aneurysm), or *indirect* (low flow), originating from the smaller vessels of the external or internal carotid arteries (e.g., congenital, spontaneous).

Differential Diagnosis

Disorders that can be confused with a carotid-cavernous fistula include the following:
- Thyroid eye disease
- Orbital or cavernous sinus tumor
- Orbital inflammatory pseudotumor
- Other causes of a red eye

Workup

- MRI or CT imaging of the brain and orbits with contrast is indicated to evaluate the orbital anatomy. These studies often will demonstrate enlargement of the superior ophthalmic vein and other venous structures connecting to the cavernous sinus.
- Bilateral internal and external carotid angiography will display the source of the fistula, which often is multiple and/or bilateral and can be contralateral to signs, and will delineate involvement of other vessels in the brain (which can cause intracerebral hemorrhage).

Treatment

- Indirect fistulas may spontaneously remit, frequently after diagnostic angiography.
- Therapeutic interventional radiographic procedures (e.g., placement of intravascular coils) may be required.

Follow-up

- Ophthalmologic consultation is needed to follow potential ocular complications of glaucoma or central retinal vein occlusion.

Ocular Myasthenia Gravis

Symptoms

- Variable ptosis or diplopia may be the initial reported symptom.
- Symptoms worsen as the day progresses.
- Symptoms diminish after the patient sleeps or rests.
- Generalized myasthenia results in weak chewing, swallowing, or breathing; fatigue of extremities also may be noted.

Signs

- Ocular motility measurements vary.
- Ptosis is variable, often with fatigue evident on sustained upgaze (Fig. 12–16).

Etiology

- The disease results from an autoimmune disorder of the neuromuscular junction.

Differential Diagnosis

Other disorders that can cause diplopia and/or ptosis include the following:
- Paresis of cranial nerves III (except pupil), IV, VI, and VII or supranuclear palsy
- Thyroid eye disease

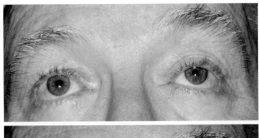

A

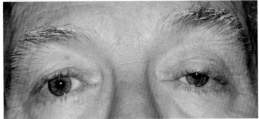

B

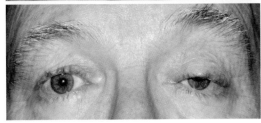

C

FIGURE 12–16 Ocular myasthenia gravis. The patient was a 69-year-old man with variable diplopia and a left ptosis. **A,** Eyelid position after resting (with eyes closed) for 5 minutes. **B,** Eyelid position immediately after 20 seconds of sustained upgaze. **C,** Further ptosis after continued fatigue.

- Ptosis from other causes (e.g., aging, trauma)
- Chronic progressive external ophthalmoplegia
- Paraneoplastic (Eaton-Lambert) syndrome

Workup

- An abnormal acetylcholine receptor antibody titer is specific for myasthenia.
- Edrophonium chloride (Tensilon) testing is only helpful if an obvious objective end point (such as an extreme ptosis) exists. Results of this test may be normal in patients with myasthenia.
- Repetitive nerve stimulation electromyography may be abnormal with systemic involvement.
- Single-fiber electromyography (of frontalis or orbicularis muscle) is sensitive and specific but technically difficult.
- Trial of pyridostigmine (Mestinon) may be unremarkable or equivocal.
- Patients with confirmed ocular myasthenia require a neurologic evaluation for systemic disease and a chest CT study to rule out thymoma.

Treatment

- Alternate occlusion of one eye prevents diplopia.
- Neurology consultant may consider pyridostigmine or low-dose (or alternate-day) prednisone administration.
- Thymectomy, even if the gland is normal in size, may be helpful in controlling the disease in some patients, although the effect may not be seen for 1 to 2 years.

Follow-up

- Neurologic follow-up is indicated to monitor for the development of generalized disease.

Acquired Nystagmus

Symptoms

- Oscillopsia ("oscillating" or moving environment) typically is present in acquired cases.
- Some patients simply report that vision is blurred.
- Patients may experience vertigo.

Signs

- Nystagmus ("shakiness") of the eyes is evident and may change with the position of gaze.

Etiology

The disorder can result from the following:
- Multiple sclerosis
- Peripheral vestibular (inner ear) disease

- Cerebellar or brainstem disease
- Drugs and medications (e.g., alcohol, lithium, anticonvulsants)
- Blindness from any cause

Workup

- A careful drug history is needed.
- Evaluation by a neuro-ophthalmologist and/or an otolaryngologist is indicated.
- MRI of the brain with contrast frequently is helpful.

Treatment

- The underlying cause determines treatment.

CHAPTER 13

Pediatric Ophthalmology*

ARLENE V. DRACK

Development of the Visual System

At birth the macula (the very center of the retina and the only place in which 20/20, detailed vision is possible) is not fully formed. Although infants perceive shape, color, motion, and gross pattern, true central fixation and detailed visual acuity do not develop until 3 to 4 months of postconceptional age (that is, gestational age at birth, plus number of weeks of life since birth). This is the reason newborns do not follow objects consistently or keep their eyes aligned perfectly. For babies born prematurely, it is important to calculate their postconceptional age when visual responses are evaluated.

The best stimulus for vision during the first weeks of life is a human face; babies usually follow a face (but not a toy) at about 6 weeks old. During these first months of life, as the macula thins and develops the potential for better acuity, the brain is learning to see. These first 3 to 4 months of life are the critical period of vision development; severe disruption of normal vision not corrected before 3 to 4 months of age results in lifelong visual deficit despite later treatment. The visual learning curve of the brain is steep, with development continuing at a rapid pace until the age of approximately 2 years. This is the period during which stereopsis (three-dimensional binocular depth perception) develops.

Fusion and stereopsis keep the eyes aligned and working together. The brain's development of vision continues until approximately 9 years of age. After this age, serious vision problems that began early in life can rarely be completely corrected.

---

*This chapter is dedicated to Mary Drack and Anya Emerson.

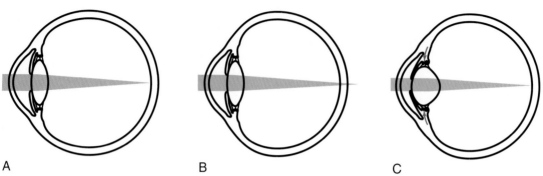

A   B   C

FIGURE 13–1 **A,** The normal eye, after developing full length, focuses on the retina without accommodation. **B,** An infant's eye focuses behind the retina without accommodation. **C,** An infant's eye focuses on the retina when the ciliary body contracts *(arrows)*, relaxing the zonules and thickening the lens (accommodation).

At birth a normal term infant is hyperopic, or farsighted, because the eye is relatively short. This means that when the ciliary muscle, which changes the lens shape to focus images, is completely at rest, images are focused behind rather than on the retina, and the image is blurred. To clear the image, the infant eye focuses (accommodates) to pull the image forward onto the retina (Fig. 13–1). Infants and young children have strong ciliary muscles and can accommodate to see well at distance and near. Near work takes more accommodative effort than far work. As the child grows, the eyes grow, and as the eyes elongate, the hyperopia decreases. Most normal eye growth occurs before the age of 2 years, with slow growth thereafter to approximately 13 years.

Infants who are more farsighted than normal may have difficulty as they grow older and their accommodative capacities decrease. Usually the difficulty manifests between 2 and 4 years of age as the acute onset of in-turning of the eyes (esotropia). Symptoms also may occur with reading in late adolescence or early adulthood.

Children who are less hyperopic than normal (i.e., those with eyes longer than the norm) may become myopic, or nearsighted, as they grow. A symptomatic decrease in distance vision usually becomes manifest at approximately 9 to 11 years of age in girls and slightly later in boys. Once myopia begins, it usually increases slowly throughout puberty and the early adulthood years.

Approach to the Pediatric Eye Examination

Vision represents a complex interplay between static anatomic structures and dynamic neurologic and physiologic processes. When an infant is born, the eyes are anatomically formed, but vision is truly a developmental sense. Events affecting the visual system during the first weeks, months, and years of life determine how fully vision potential will be realized, with earlier events playing the most important roles. Primary care providers, parents, and pediatric ophthalmologists are the guardians of this potential, and in many infants, without the intervention of all parties, the full potential for vision is lost.

Premature Infants

Babies born at approximately 24 weeks of gestation may have partially fused eyelids—a remnant of a normal developmental stage. The lids should open spontaneously over the ensuing weeks. Preterm infants born at less than 28 to 30 weeks of gestation have a membrane over the pupil, representing vestiges of the tunica vasculosa lentis, an embryonic vascular network that covers the lens and is continuous with the border of the iris. Presence of the membrane dulls the red reflex, but the condition resolves spontaneously by 36 to 40 weeks of gestational age. If the membrane does not regress normally, persistent pupillary membranes and anterior polar cataracts may result (Fig. 13–2).

The dilator muscle of the pupil is not well developed for several months after term; therefore, pupils may be small (miotic) and the anterior chamber shallow. The corneal diameter should be approximately 9 to 10 mm.

For premature infants before they reach term gestational age, the most important eye evaluation is an examination with the indirect ophthalmoscope by an ophthalmologist to detect retinopathy of prematurity (ROP). Primary care providers examining preterm infants can, however, look for reaction to light demonstrated by the infant's squeezing the eyes shut, a normal red reflex with direct ophthalmoscopy, and full spontaneous eye movements. An ophthalmologist should be involved in the care of all infants who weighed less than 1500 g at birth, were born at 32 weeks of gestational age or earlier, and selected infants with birthweights between 1500 and 2000 g with an unstable clinical course who may be at risk for ROP. The first ophthalmologic examination should be scheduled at 4 to 7 weeks after birth depending on gestational age at birth. The examination should take place at 31 weeks of postconceptional age or 4 weeks of post-natal age, whichever is later. Retinopathy of prematurity is the leading cause of pediatric blindness in the United States.

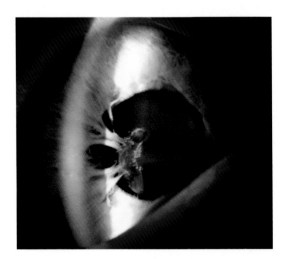

FIGURE 13–2 Failure of completion of any of the normal prenatal steps of ocular development results in congenital eye anomalies. Here, incomplete regression of tunica vasculosa lentis leaves a pupillary membrane and anterior lens plaque. Not all ocular anomalies are visually significant, but all children with such anomalies should be referred to an ophthalmologist for evaluation.

Term to 4-Month-Old Infants

A screening eye examination generally is part of all well-baby checkups, but because the eye and vision change so rapidly throughout infancy and childhood, the focus and assessment of each examination also must change.

Because the macula is not fully developed until 3 to 4 months of age, the eyes do not fixate well centrally and do not "lock onto" and follow objects before this age; variable crossing or drifting out of the eyes may be observed.

To test children in this age range, the examiner should have the parent hold the infant in a feeding position with the baby looking at the parent's face (Fig. 13–3). The parent then moves the head from side to side. The baby should grossly follow this movement with eyes or head and also should blink when a light is directed into the eyes.

Next, a gross inspection is made of the eyes and face. The lids, brows, and globes should look symmetrical. Any marked asymmetry is a warning signal, because the brain processes images from only one eye if the images from the two eyes are significantly different in any way.

Finally, the lights should be dimmed and the baby given a bottle, pacifier, or parent's finger to suck. Suckling usually elicits opening of the eyes. Normal infants may even have lid retraction and reveal visible sclera above and below the cornea. While the infant's eyes are open, the examiner uses a direct ophthalmoscope to look at the quality and symmetry of the red reflex. In blond or lightly pigmented infants, this reflex is truly orange-red. In more darkly pigmented infants, the reflex looks dull orange or whitish orange. This latter finding should not be confused with leukocoria, which is

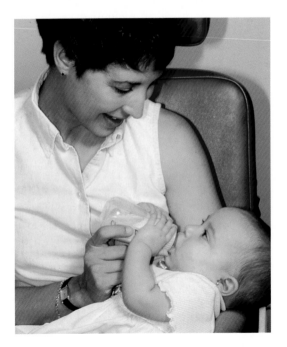

FIGURE 13–3 The best stimulus for infant vision is a parent's face. By 6 weeks of age the infant should look at the parent's face and move eyes and head to follow as the parent changes position.

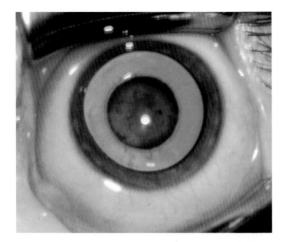

FIGURE 13–4 Blocking of the red reflex by a cataract as viewed with the direct ophthalmoscope. Note the uniform orange glow around the edges of the cataract. The opacity blocks the red reflex in the center of the pupil.

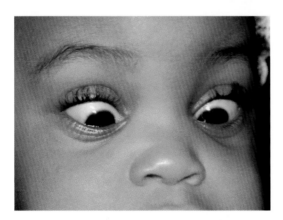

FIGURE 13–5 Sunsetting. Intermittent downward deviation of the eyes occurs when lights are dimmed.

a whitish appearance of the pupil on penlight or room light examination, usually differs between the two eyes, and generally is associated with the absence of any light reflex when the direct ophthalmoscope is used to check the red reflex. The key to judging responses as normal is symmetry and uniformity across the entire reflex (Fig. 13–4).

Sunsetting, a tonic or intermittent downward deviation of the eyes (Fig. 13–5), may be benign in babies, especially those born prematurely, if it is intermittent and persists for only a few weeks. If the sunsetting is constant or associated with poor feeding, nausea, vomiting, lethargy, bulging fontanelle, or abnormal head circumferences on a growth chart, or if it develops suddenly in an infant who never exhibited it before, it may be a sign of increased intracranial pressure and mandates immediate referral to an ophthalmologist and/or neurologist to prevent permanent brain and optic nerve damage or even death.

If the child is growing well and the fontanelle is flat, but the sunsetting is persistent, it often is a sign of periventricular leukomalacia or other pathologic brain conditions. The risk of cerebral palsy is high in such children, and referral to a pediatric ophthalmologist is indicated.

4-Month-Old Infants to Verbal Children

The initial examination is the same as outlined for younger infants; however, central, steady fixation and following of a toy should be elicited. Using one thumb to cover one eye while the hand steadies the head, the examiner should check for central fixation and following with each eye (Fig. 13–6). Each eye should independently lock onto the toy and follow it smoothly and fully. If the child will cooperate, an adhesive occlusive eye patch may be used. If attention is poor, the lights can be dimmed and a toy illuminated. Next, the lights are dimmed and a light source is held a few inches from the child's eyes in the midline. The examiner looks at the pupillary light reflex; it should be centered in each pupil (Fig. 13–7). If it is not, strabismus is present (Figs. 13–8 to 13–10). This method may miss an in-turning of the eyes (esotropia) if it is the result of accommodation, because a detailed target is needed to bring it out. If possible, the light is tapped on a toy to be sure the child is focusing and accommodating at near. This method also can miss intermittent exotropia, a drifting outward that occurs more with distance viewing. To diagnose intermittent exotropia, a toy or other object is presented at the end of the room and the location of the pupillary light reflex examined while the child's eyes are fixating at a distance. This abnormality can

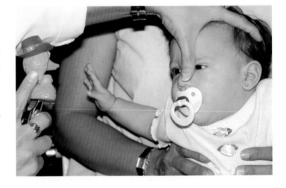

FIGURE 13–6 Checking fixation in infants aged 4 months to verbal development. Often, dimming the lights and making noises are necessary to get young children's attention on a toy. For young children, the thumb can be used to cover each eye in turn, for assessing fixation with the uncovered eye. Then the thumb is moved from one eye to the other (cover testing) to detect strabismus.

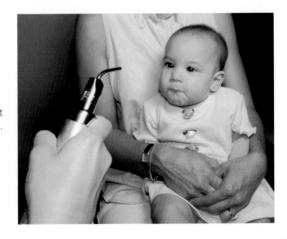

FIGURE 13–7 Checking for symmetrical pupillary light reflexes. Here a Fenhoff illuminator is used as a light source.

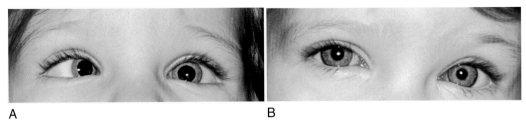

A   B

FIGURE 13–8   A, In this example of esotropia, the light reflex is off the center of the pupil in a temporal direction in the right eye. This child has congenital esotropia; both eyes are affected, but the fixating eye appears straight. **B,** Shortly after eye muscle surgery, the corneal light reflexes are centered on both pupils.

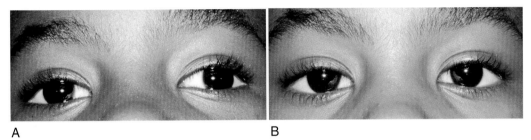

A   B

FIGURE 13–9   Intermittent exotropia. A, The light reflex is off the center of the pupil in a nasal direction in the left eye when this child fixates in the distance. **B,** At near distance, control is better in exotropia, eyes are straight, and corneal light reflexes are centered.

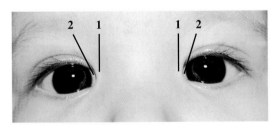

FIGURE 13–10   Pseudoesotropia. The eyes appear crossed because of large epicanthal skin folds (1) covering the sclera (2). This finding is normal before the nasal bridge develops fully. The corneal light reflexes are centered, proving the eyes are actually straight.

be difficult to elicit in the primary care office, so a suggestive history should prompt an ophthalmology referral.

The examination of the location of the pupillary light reflex to detect strabismus is the quickest and easiest method. Cover testing requires more practice and patience but is superior for detecting many types of strabismus (see Fig. 13–6). Fixation on a target is essential, and because children's attention spans are short, many toys for distance and near testing are needed. This is a standard setup in the pediatric ophthalmology office, but it may not be available for most primary care practitioners. Although children view these toys as simply being entertaining, accurate testing is impossible without them.

For cover testing, the child sits in the parent's lap. The clinician shows a toy at near distance and asks the child to touch or describe it to be sure fixation is occurring. One eye is rapidly covered; if the eyes are straight, no movement of the fellow eye should occur. The test is repeated for the other eye, thereby demonstrating constant deviations. If the child is older than 6 months of age, the test is repeated for distance. (Children younger than 6 months of age will not attend to distant targets.) Then the examiner again holds the target at near distance and slowly covers first one eye and then the other. If the eyes have no latent deviation, the uncovered eye should not move. If latent deviation (termed *phoria*) is present, the eyes shift back and forth as the cover is changed. The test is repeated for distance. Any child with a suspected deviation, latent or constant, should be referred to an ophthalmologist.

Verbal Children

Once children develop verbal abilities, the eye examination is much easier, but a few key points are worth noting. Corneal light reflex and cover testing should still be done as described. The major change is that objective measures of visual function, such as fixation and following, give way to subjective measures. As soon as children can speak well (usually by age 3 years), parents should be given a photocopy of the standard Allen or other calibrated pictures for practice at home with the child (Fig. 13–11). The first vision test in the office may not be accurate because of the child's unfamiliarity with the testing procedures.

The best way to test children before they know letters and numbers is to start with an Allen near card. An occlusive patch is then placed over one of the child's eyes. The examiner points to pictures on the card, starting at the largest and moving to the smallest, and has the child name them. The patch is changed to the other eye and the test repeated. Once the child is familiar with the symbols, keeping one eye patched, the examiner starts showing the cards in a flash card fashion while slowly walking backward to a distance of 20 feet. This pattern is repeated with the other eye. Children 3 to 5 years old may read the cards at only 15 feet instead of 20, but the distance should be the same for each eye and should improve on subsequent visits. The distance from the child and the figure size of the cards (20/30 for Allen cards) should be recorded. As an example, if the child sees the Allen distance (20/30) card at 20 feet, the vision is 20/30, which is normal for age. If the child sees it to only 10 feet, the vision is 10/30. This can be multiplied by 2 to obtain standard notation—in this case, 20/60. Vision should be at least 20/40 or 20/50 at a distance for children younger than 5

  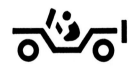

FIGURE 13–11   Allen figures. Several such standard figures are available. The 20/30 size is reproduced here; with this size, a normal child should be able to identify the figure at 20 feet. These figures are reproduced at actual size, so if a sharp photocopy that is well lit and placed at 20 feet is interpreted correctly, visual acuity is at least 20/30.

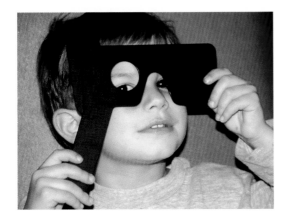

FIGURE 13–12   Vision testing. Children often peek around standard occluders, especially if their better eye is covered.

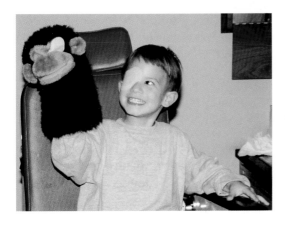

FIGURE 13–13 An adhesive patch prevents peeking during vision testing.

years, but 20/20 to 20/30 for all ages at near distance. A vision measurement less than this or any difference in values between the eyes suggests a need for referral. In children older than 5 years, distance vision should be 20/20. For Allen cards, cards should be identified all the way to 20 feet; most Allen cards test to only 20/30, because children young enough to be illiterate generally read at only 20/30, not 20/20 at distance.

Once children know numbers, a standard number chart can be used. Letters give the greatest accuracy, and once a child is old enough to read letters, attention usually is sufficient to cooperate with testing using a chart at the end of the room. Sometimes having a parent point to each letter helps with attention and accuracy.

The importance of using an adhesive occlusive patch rather than an occluder or covering eye with a hand or other device cannot be overemphasized. If one eye sees poorly, children will peek with the other eye in order to give the right answers (Figs. 13–12 and 13–13). Only an adhesive occlusive patch prevents this.

Photoscreening is a more recent technology available to primary care offices. Flash photographs of children's eyes are taken to detect opacities, refractive errors, and strabismus. Although extremely useful in many cases, especially refractive amblyopia, photoscreening should be used as a well-child screening test, not an examination technique for children in whom a problem is suspected, because certain disorders can be missed. All children with suspected ocular disorders should be referred to a pediatric ophthalmologist.

Red Reflex or Bruchner Test

Ideally, every child should have an examination of the red reflex at every well-child check-up. In the hands of an experienced examiner, this test can detect almost all major ocular problems of childhood. At a minimum it should be done at discharge from the hospital; once again before 3 months of age (to detect cataracts, which must be treated before 3 months to prevent blindness, and retinoblastoma, which if treated early need not result in loss of the eye or life); again at 6 months; and then again at all well-child visits.

The lights are dimmed, the infant is given something to suck on, and while standing at arm's length, the examiner uses the direct ophthalmoscope to look at both pupils at once and then one at a time. For most examiners, the ophthalmoscope should be set at 0, with the largest aperture open. If the pupils are small (miotic) or a good red reflex is not obtained, dilation of the pupils is recommended. For preterm infants up to 3 months of age, a weak concentration of cyclopentolate hydrochloride/phenylephrine hydrochloride (Cyclomydril) should be used, one drop in each eye, which is repeated in 5 minutes. Then the examiner waits 20 minutes for dilation. More darkly pigmented irides take longer to dilate, and in such eyes one additional drop in each eye may be required. The examiner must not exceed 4 drops in an hour. For term infants, cyclopentolate 0.5% and phenylephrine 2.5% eyedrops are used, one drop in each eye. After 6 months of age, cyclopentolate 1% and phenylephrine 2.5% are used, one drop in each eye. Again, light irides dilate in about 20 minutes; dilation of dark irides takes longer and may require another set of drops.

The risks with these doses of eye medications are few. Tachycardia and facial flushing may result, but these side effects usually are self-limited. These drops should be used with caution in children with cardiac disease or hypertension, and doses should be decreased for very lightly pigmented children. If all measures fail to get an infant to open the eyes, a lid speculum may be used (Fig. 13–14).

Ocular Disorders of Infancy

Conjunctivitis

Symptoms

• Usually no symptoms are noted, but in severe cases, irritability may be present.

Signs

• The disorder usually is bilateral but may be asymmetrical.
• Mild conjunctival injection is possible.
• A watery, mucoid, or mucopurulent discharge occurs.

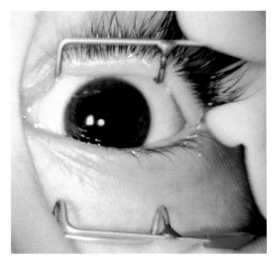

FIGURE 13–14 Use of a lid speculum. An assistant holds the child snugly, especially the child's arms. Keeping gentle pressure on both sides of the speculum with one hand to compress it, the clinician uses the other hand to elevate the upper lid and slide one lip under. Without allowing the speculum to spring open, the lower lid is pulled down and the other lip is slid under this lid. Next, pressure is removed from the speculum so that it will open the lids. A drop of proparacaine or tetracaine may be used in each eye before insertion. The procedure is not painful, but it is frightening to parents and child and reassurance is necessary.

- Eyelids may adhere when the child awakens.
- Eyelids may be erythematous or excoriated.
- Preauricular lymph node may be palpable.

Differential Diagnosis

Before 1 Week of Age
In infants younger than 1 week of age, diagnostic possibilities include the following:
- Toxic conjunctivitis from perinatal prophylaxis: The infant usually is initially seen with red lids and watery discharge.
- Infectious disorders (usually acquired in the birth canal): Most often staphylococci, *Chlamydia*, herpesviruses, and *Neisseria gonorrhoeae* are the infectious agents. The infant initially is seen with quiet lids and mucopurulent discharge, but symptoms can appear identical to those of toxic conjunctivitis. If discharge is purulent and excessive (so-called hyperacute), gonorrhea is possible. Emergency referral to an ophthalmologist is required, because blindness can result within 24 to 48 hours if the infection is not treated (Fig. 13–15). Systemic antibiotic treatment is also required.
- Children born at home may not receive appropriate prophylaxis and are at particular risk for infectious conjunctivitis.

After 1 Week of Age or with Community Exposure
In infants older than 1 week or those with community exposure, considerations in the differential diagnosis include the following:
- **Viral infections:** Especially with adenovirus or respiratory syncytial virus infections, massive lid swelling may be present in infants, simulating cellulitis. An enlarged preauricular node or upper respiratory infection often is present.
- **Nasolacrimal duct obstruction:** If the conjunctivitis is chronic and in particular unilateral, duct obstruction should be considered.

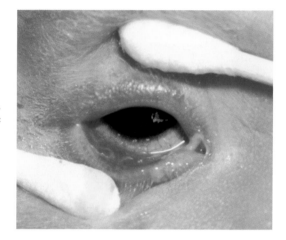

FIGURE 13–15 Hyperacute gonorrheal conjunctivitis. Immediate institution of topical and systemic antibiotic therapy is needed to prevent blindness.

- **Congenital glaucoma:** If manifestations include photophobia, an enlarged cornea, and, in particular, watery and chronic discharge, this disorder must be ruled out or confirmed. Congenital glaucoma necessitates immediate ophthalmologic referral and treatment.

Treatment

- In infants younger than 1 week of age with red lids and a watery discharge, toxic etiology is likely. All eye medications are ceased, conjunctival culture is obtained, and the infant is observed for 24 to 48 hours. If no improvement is seen after 48 hours or discharge is mucopurulent, antibiotic drops (e.g., polymyxin B/trimethoprim [Polytrim], 1 drop 3 to 4 times a day or erythromycin ointment 4 times a day) are administered. If one of these agents was used for prophylaxis, it should not be readministered, because it may have been a causative factor. If the infant's condition does not improve in 48 hours, routine bacterial cultures, as well as *Chlamydia* culture, should be performed. An ophthalmologist is consulted for these studies and further workup. Systemic antibiotics are required for *Chlamydia* infection due to the risk of pneumonia.
- If the discharge is hyperacute, Gram stain and culture (including chocolate agar) are indicated to look for gonorrhea; the infant receives presumptive treatment for gonorrhea with intravenous cefotaxime (Claforan) 50 mg/kg/dose every 12 hours for 7 days. The eyes should be irrigated with saline every 10 to 30 minutes, gradually decreasing to every 2 hours until the purulent discharge clears. Hospital admission and an ophthalmologic consultation should be done immediately. Gonorrhea can penetrate an intact cornea rapidly, causing blindness. The mother also is tested.
- If cultures, PCR assay, or stains reveal *Chlamydia* organisms, systemic as well as topical treatment is indicated because of the risk of pneumonia. The mother should also be tested.
- If *Haemophilus influenzae* is recovered, systemic treatment is given. Infection with this organism often proves refractory to topical treatment and is associated with a high risk for development of cellulitis and meningitis.

Nasolacrimal Duct Obstruction

Symptoms

- Usually no symptoms result from the obstruction, but patients may have irritation of the eyelids and conjunctiva if the condition is longstanding or bacterial super-infection is present (Fig. 13–16).
- Nasal stuffiness or respiratory distress if mucocele with nasal cyst is present.

Signs

- The obstruction usually is bilateral but asymmetrical.
- The tear lake usually is elevated, and the lashes look wet.
- With bacterial superinfection, a chronic mucopurulent discharge occurs, and the eyelids adhere in the morning. Later in the course, the periorbital skin becomes thickened and excoriated, and the conjunctiva becomes injected.
- A bluish mass beneath the medial canthal tendon on the side of the nose may be present with mucocele.

Etiology

- Most cases result from failure of the valve of Hasner to open; however, absence of the puncta or other anomalies of the system also may be factors preventing drainage (Fig. 13–17).
- The origin usually is idiopathic, and the disorder is very common.

Associated Factors and Diseases

- Infants with syndromes involving midface hypoplasia, clefting, craniosynostosis, trisomy 21, and mass lesions such as dermoids of the canthal area are at increased risk.

Workup

- To differentiate between conjunctivitis and nasolacrimal duct obstruction, the examiner presses a cotton-tipped swab firmly over the lacrimal sac while observing the puncta (Fig. 13–18). If a reflux of mucopurulent material is seen, the diagnosis is nasolacrimal duct obstruction, not solely conjunctivitis.

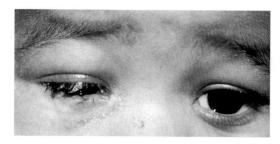

FIGURE 13–16 Chronic nasolacrimal duct obstruction with bacterial superinfection. This child has been treated with topical and systemic antibiotics without resolution. If nasolacrimal duct obstruction is present, infection will not clear without probing. Note skin changes. All signs resolved 24 hours after probing.

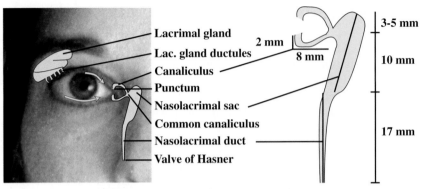

Lacrimal gland

Lac. gland ductules

Canaliculus

Punctum

Nasolacrimal sac

Common canaliculus

Nasolacrimal duct

Valve of Hasner

2 mm

8 mm

3-5 mm

10 mm

17 mm

FIGURE 13–17 Anatomy of the nasolacrimal system.

FIGURE 13–18 Differentiating nasolacrimal duct obstruction from conjunctivitis in the office. The examiner presses firmly on the nasolacrimal sac with a cotton-tipped applicator while the parent immobilizes the child; the presence of reflux of mucopurulent material from the puncta is determined. If reflux is present, the diagnosis is nasolacrimal duct obstruction.

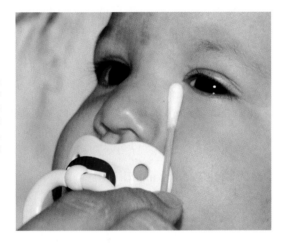

- To differentiate between nasolacrimal duct obstruction and congenital glaucoma, the clinician measures intraocular pressure and examines the corneas and optic nerves. If tearing does not respond to treatment within a few weeks and no reflux from the sac occurs with pressure, or if the patient keeps the eyes closed when exposed to light and/or has large hazy corneas, referral to a pediatric ophthalmologist is necessary.
- Examination of the nose is warranted in babies with mucocele, especially if there are any respiratory symptoms, to rule out associated intranasal cyst.

Treatment

- In approximately 75% of affected infants, the obstructed duct spontaneously opens within the first 6 months of life, so long as bacterial infection is not present. Thus, if the discharge is watery only, observation and daily massage over the lacrimal sac (rapid, downward pushing to pop open the valve of Hasner [Fig. 13–19]) are appropriate measures.

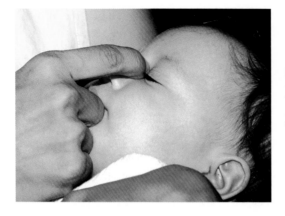

FIGURE 13-19 Home massage over the nasolacrimal sac to open obstruction. This maneuver should be done three to four times a day, followed by instillation of an antibiotic drop such as polymyxin B/trimethoprim (Polytrim). If the obstruction does not resolve after 2 to 3 weeks and discharge is still present, referral for probing is indicated.

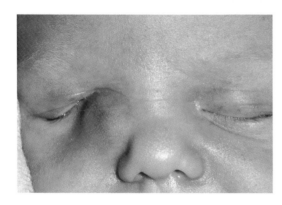

FIGURE 13-20 Dacryocele. These lesions usually are congenital and must be treated immediately by an ophthalmologist.

- After the age of 6 months, obstructions are far less likely to resolve, and the child should be referred to an ophthalmologist.
- With mucopurulent discharge, topical antibiotics (e.g., polymyxin B/trimethoprim [Polytrim] 1 drop 3 to 4 times a day) are administered for 1 to 3 weeks with massage and frequent cleansing of secretions. If the bacterial infection resolves, the system may open spontaneously.
- With a mass such as mucocele or dacryocele, rapid referral to an ophthalmologist is necessary (Fig. 13-20).
- If antibiotic drops do not clear the mucopurulent discharge in 1 to 2 weeks, the patient should be referred to an ophthalmologist, regardless of age. These children have severe obstructions with bacterial colonization, and the condition will rarely resolve unless probing is done. Constant bacterial infection in the lacrimal sac increases the risk of preseptal cellulitis.
- Nasolacrimal duct probing is 95% effective in opening obstructions if performed before 1 year of age. If performed before the child is 2 years old, probing is approximately 85% successful. Because spontaneous opening is unlikely after 6 months of age or in the presence of infection, and this procedure has a higher rate of success in some studies if done early, the treatment plan must be adjusted accordingly.

Probing can be performed in the ophthalmologist's office without anesthesia if the child is younger than 3 or 4 months of age. After this age, anesthesia is almost always necessary.

- Silastic tubing can be placed to keep the duct system open in older children and those in whom probing fails to open the duct.
- A balloon catheter procedure to widen the system may improve success in recurrent cases.
- Marsupialization of associated intranasal cysts may be necessary with mucoceles.
- Surgical creation of a passage between the tear lake, nasolacrimal sac, and nasal mucosa (dacryocystorhinostomy, or Jones tube placement) is reserved for older children or those in whom probing and Silastic tube placement do not resolve the problem. Such procedures are much more invasive and often can be avoided if early treatment is instituted.

Retinopathy of Prematurity

Symptoms

- No symptoms are present.

Signs

- The disorder is almost always bilateral but often asymmetrical.
- Pupils are small and immobile in the late stages, and iris blood vessels are enlarged.
- Most signs are seen only with the indirect ophthalmoscope. A ridge of abnormal vascular tissue grows from the retina into the vitreous. Blood vessels may become dilated and tortuous.
- If advanced stages are not treated, retinal detachment and blindness are likely. Leukocoria also may result if the detached retina comes to lie behind the lens.
- As children get older, strabismus (either esotropia or exotropia) can be seen as a late sequela.
- Microphthalmia (a small eye) and phthisis (a shrunken eye) can result after retinal detachment.

Associated Factors and Diseases

- Low birth weight, young gestational age, sepsis, and perinatal oxygen administration are risk factors for the disorder.
- All babies born at 32 weeks of gestation or before, weighing less than 1500 g, or with an unstable clinical course should be screened by an ophthalmologist familiar with retinopathy of prematurity at 31 weeks of postconceptional age or 4 weeks of postnatal age, whichever is later. If no retinopathy of prematurity is present, or the disorder resolves, these children still require follow-up with an ophthalmologist at approximately 3 months after discharge and throughout the first few years of life because of their increased risks of strabismus, high refractive error (i.e., need for glasses), amblyopia, optic atrophy, and retinal abnormalities.

Treatment

- Once the treatment threshold is reached, cryotherapy or laser therapy of the retina must be performed, usually within 72 hours. An ophthalmologist trained in management of retinopathy of prematurity makes the determination of threshold disease based on strict criteria. A 2003 study found benefit in treating earlier than the previous threshold designation from the original CRYO-ROP study. Another 2003 study found that strictly monitoring and limiting the oxygen babies receive in the neonatal care unit also may reduce the rate of severe retinopathy of prematurity. Future studies will better delineate the optimal amount of oxygen for premature babies. Up to 95% of infants with threshold disease who receive laser therapy retain vision, whereas before modern treatments were available, a majority developed blindness as a result of retinal detachment or scarring.
- Throughout life, glasses, patching, surgery, and other modalities may be needed to treat the sequelae of retinopathy of prematurity.

Congenital Anomalies

Intrauterine Infections

Infections that cross the placenta, such as toxoplasmosis, rubella, and infections due to cytomegalovirus, herpes virus, varicella virus, lymphocytic choriomeningitis virus (LCMV), and human immunodeficiency virus (HIV), often cause characteristic eye conditions. If an intrauterine infection is suspected, an ophthalmology consultation may help confirm the diagnosis. Vision often is affected, so early referral is essential.

Congenital Cataracts

Symptoms

- Vision is mildly to severely decreased.
- In severe cases in which essentially no vision is present, the infant may keep the eyes closed.
- When the condition results in a partial cataract, the infant may squint, especially in bright sunlight, to decrease the resultant glare.

Signs

- Leukocoria (white pupil) is present if the cataract is dense (Fig. 13–21).
- The red reflex is abnormal or absent.
- If the condition developed within the first 3 months of life, nystagmus may be present.

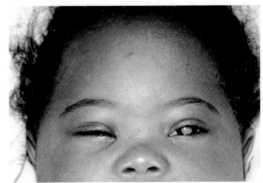

FIGURE 13–21 Leukocoria. This child has a unilateral cataract. Leukocoria is seen as a white pupil when viewed with a penlight or in room light.

Differential Diagnosis

Diagnostic possibilities include the following:
- Cataract
- Retinoblastoma
- Coats' disease (an exudative retinal detachment caused by vascular anomalies)
- Retinopathy of prematurity
- Chorioretinal coloboma (white sclera where retina should be)
- Corneal scar (Peters' anomaly)
- Retinal detachment

Associated Diseases

- Many genetic and metabolic disorders are associated with congenital cataracts. Some respond to dietary or other treatment. All infants with early-onset cataracts should have a genetic and/or metabolic evaluation.

Treatment

- Congenital cataract constitutes an emergency. The brain learns to see with the macula (the center of the retina where 20/20 vision is possible) most rapidly during the first 3 to 4 months of life. If vision is severely limited during this critical period of visual development, it cannot be restored completely. Thus, congenital cataracts must be surgically removed, and optical rehabilitation with contact lenses, intraocular lenses, or glasses must be in place *before* 3 to 4 months of age. Many patients can have near-normal vision if they receive prompt treatment. With treatment after this age, some vision may be restored, but the result often is in the 20/200 or legally blind range.
- An ophthalmologist determines the adequacy of the infant's visual stimulation in cases of partial cataract.
- *Persistent hyperplastic primary vitreous*, also called *persistent fetal vasculature*, is a type of congenital cataract that may result in a small eye and painful glaucoma.
- All infants should be screened for a red reflex before discharge from the nursery and at each well-baby checkup. If a cataract or other disruption of the red reflex is suspected, referral to an ophthalmologist is needed before the infant is 3 months old.

Congenital Ptosis

The lid is elevated primarily by the levator muscle, which inserts onto the tarsal plate of the eyelid, and by the orbicularis oculi muscle, which encircles the eye. The levator is innervated by the third cranial nerve. The lid also is partially elevated by Müller's muscle, which is innervated by sympathetic fibers. These fibers travel from the brain out through the spine, around the neck, over the lung, and then up around the carotid artery to innervate the pupil and muscle of the eyelid.

Symptoms

- If the ptosis is severe, vision is greatly decreased.
- If the condition is bilateral, the infant never opens the eyes or never focuses.

Signs, Etiology, and Differential Diagnosis

- A faintly defined or no lid crease may signal an abnormal insertion of the levator aponeurosis or absence of the entire muscle or insertion. Lack of a lid crease with normal function is common in Asian patients.
- One or both brows are often markedly elevated.
- The infant may keep a chin-up position (Fig. 13–22).
- Mild ptosis with a lid crease, a small pupil (miosis), a difference in iris color (heterochromia), and an inability to sweat (anhidrosis) on one side of the face are signs of Horner syndrome caused by sympathetic nerve interruption. In congenital cases, a history of brachial plexus injury or difficult delivery may help determine the etiology. If the history is not suggestive, workup for neuroblastoma and other anatomic abnormalities is indicated.
- If the lid is thickened or red, a hemangioma may be present.

Treatment

- Surgical correction often is necessary.
- If the ptosis is untreated, amblyopia and loss of vision often result. Ophthalmologic referral as soon after birth as possible is indicated.

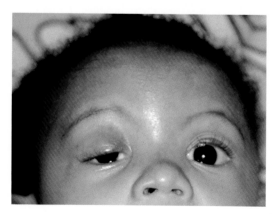

FIGURE 13–22   Congenital ptosis. Baby keeps the chin up to see. Note elevated brows and lack of right lid crease.

- If the condition is severe, surgical correction using a tarsal sling must be performed before the infant is 3 months of age.
- Often ptosis induces refractive error (e.g., myopia, astigmatism), which must be treated with glasses.
- Amblyopia may be severe and requires treatment with patching; if ptosis is asymmetrical, amblyopia is best treated before the infant is 3 months of age.

Congenital Glaucoma

Symptoms

- Vision is decreased.
- Photophobia is characteristic.

Signs

- Excess tearing occurs, especially during daylight or in bright light.
- The corneas are enlarged.
- Hazy or cloudy corneas cause a diminished corneal reflex.

Differential Diagnosis

- **Nasolacrimal duct obstruction:** Congenital glaucoma often is associated with blindness, whereas nasolacrimal obstruction generally is benign. Nasolacrimal duct obstruction often results in mucopurulent discharge and excess tearing over time. Even if no mucopurulent discharge is present on external examination, if gentle pressure is exerted on the nasolacrimal sac with a cotton-tipped swab, discharge often can be expressed. If this sign is not present and excess tearing continues for more than a few weeks, congenital glaucoma may be present. Simple nasolacrimal duct obstruction is not associated with photophobia; that is, in normal lighting, the infant should have the eyes open and be looking around the room. If the infant is reluctant to do this and keeps the eyes closed much of the time, either severe nasolacrimal duct obstruction with bacterial superinfection may be present or congenital glaucoma may be present. Simple nasolacrimal duct obstruction should not be associated with any cloudiness or abnormal appearance of the eyes. Congenital glaucoma may be associated with other congenital anomalies, especially Turner syndrome, Down syndrome, Rubinstein-Taybi syndrome, and Lowe syndrome.

Treatment

- Patients should be referred to an ophthalmologist.
- Medications, usually systemic or topical carbonic anhydrase inhibitors and topical beta blockers, may be used for short-term management to relieve pressure; however, they are rarely sufficient to preserve vision.
- Surgery is almost always needed. The approach to glaucoma, and the choice of procedures, are quite different in children than in adults, and consultation with a pediatric ophthalmologist or a glaucoma specialist familiar with glaucoma in children is

recommended. Despite better outcomes from new medications and surgical procedures, many children suffer lifelong vision impairment despite treatment.

Follow-up

- Most children need more than one operation, and concomitant problems such as amblyopia, high myopia, and strabismus almost always are present. Thus, families should be counseled that the condition is a lifelong ocular disorder requiring frequent follow-up evaluations.

Hemangioma

Symptoms

- Vision is decreased.
- In rare cases, respiratory or swallowing difficulties are noted if the hemangioma is extensive.

Signs

- Ptosis or an irregular lid with or without an elevated, reddish mass is observed (Fig. 13–23).
- Hemangiomas are most visually significant when they are located on the upper lid; however, they may occur on the upper and lower lids and below the eyes and can involve the scalp or, rarely, the airway.
- Capillary hemangiomas often are present at birth but may be very small. They generally begin to grow within the first months of life, continue to grow throughout the first 1 to 2 years, and then undergo slow regression.

Associated Diseases

- Multiple hemangiomas may be a sign of internal malignancy and systemic work-up may be indicated. Capillary hemangiomas are seen with greater frequency in premature infants than in full-term babies.

Treatment

- Referral to a pediatric ophthalmologist is necessary, even for small hemangiomas of the upper or lower eyelid or periorbital area, before the infant is 3 months of age

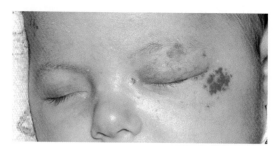

FIGURE 13–23 Capillary hemangioma of the eyelid.

because of the known association of this condition with severe amblyopia in the affected eye.

- Referral to an ophthalmologist is necessary at any age if the hemangioma enlarges, causes ptosis, or occludes the pupil.
- If vision is the same in both eyes and little or no induced astigmatism or myopia is present, observation usually is sufficient.
- In most cases, the induced refractive error differs between the eyes. Glasses are prescribed, and patching may be warranted to treat the amblyopia.
- If the hemangioma is on the upper lid or in another area in which it markedly interferes with vision and it is enlarging, it constitutes an ophthalmologic emergency. A course of systemic corticosteroids, usually prednisone at 2 mg/kg per day for up to 1 or 2 weeks, with a very slow taper thereafter, often achieves excellent results. Intralesional injection of corticosteroids also can be very effective, but severe complications such as central retinal artery occlusion have rarely been reported. Endocrinology referral may be advised to follow infants on steroids.

Follow-up

- Patients must be monitored by a pediatric ophthalmologist and a pediatrician.
- Long-term follow-up care is required until the capillary hemangioma regresses.

Port-Wine Stain

Symptoms

- No symptoms exist.

Signs

- A large, flat, purplish lesion is found on the skin of the face or scalp. Such lesions also may be present on other parts of the body.
- Glaucoma is likely to occur on the affected side, especially if the upper lid is involved.
- Seizures and developmental delay often are noted as well. When intracranial involvement of the hemangioma occurs with these signs, Sturge-Weber syndrome is diagnosed.

Treatment

- Because ipsilateral glaucoma occurs in approximately 50% of cases of port-wine stain (nevus flammeus) when it affects the upper eyelid, all children with the disorder should be referred for pediatric ophthalmologic consultation as soon as the lesion is detected. Magnetic resonance imaging (MRI) scan, computed tomography (CT) scan of the brain, and an electroencephalogram also may be indicated.
- Laser eradication of the lesion in some cases is now possible, but this treatment's effect on the incidence of glaucoma is not known. Generally, the laser treatment must be performed within the first 2 years of life to be successful; therefore, early referral is essential.

Congenital Esotropia and Exotropia

Variable, intermittent ocular misalignment is normal for the first 3 to 4 months of life; however, misalignment after 3 to 4 months of age is not normal. In addition, a constant misalignment of either or both eyes is always abnormal at any age. Children who have a constant deviation of one or both eyes should be referred to an ophthalmologist immediately. This finding may be a sign of a developmental anomaly or tumor in the eye. Congenital esotropia is a condition in which affected children have essentially normal eye movements for the first 3 to 4 months of life but exhibit crossing of the eyes before 6 months of age. Congenital exotropia is a condition in which one or both eyes deviate outward toward the ear.

Symptoms

- Early in the disease, double vision may occur.
- Decreased stereopsis (depth perception) is present throughout life.

Signs

- Strabismus, with one or both eyes turning in toward the nose (esotropia) or outward toward the ears (exotropia), is characteristic.
- Most patients with congenital esotropia are unable to abduct the eyes (look laterally) fully.
- Nystagmus occurs in a small subset of patients with congenital esotropia.
- A decreased ability to make eye contact and bond with parents is noted in some cases, which improves after treatment.

Differential Diagnosis

- Early-onset sixth nerve palsy or paresis may mimic congenital esotropia. This deficit often is caused by increased intracranial pressure and is associated with nausea, vomiting, lethargy, and increased head circumference.
- In premature infants, the development of esotropia may be related to neurologic causes: The disorder often is associated with periventricular leukomalacia and cerebral palsy. This type of esotropia may occur at the same age as for congenital esotropia, but the ocular misalignment varies throughout the examination.
- Congenital third nerve palsy is a possible cause of exotropia.
- If no other symptoms are present and the perinatal or birth history is normal, the condition can be an isolated finding in an otherwise healthy, normal infant.

Associated Factors and Diseases

- The risk of intracranial pathology is increased in congenital exotropia; therefore, neuroimaging often is indicated.
- Some children with severe esotropia have motor delays because they can never look straight ahead when they are holding the head straight. Their eyes are always pulled into the esotropic position. These children may turn the head to the side to attempt to crawl or walk and often gain developmental motor milestones rapidly after surgery.

Treatment

- Any patient with a constant deviation at any age, or any deviation constant or intermittent after 3 to 4 months of age should be referred for ophthalmologic evaluation.
- For patients with amblyopia, treatment immediately after diagnosis is most effective and usually involves patching and/or glasses.
- Stereopsis, the type of depth perception that results from the use of both eyes, can best be achieved in children with congenital esotropia or exotropia if surgery is performed before the age of 2 years. Approximately 65% of children need one surgical procedure to straighten their vision; 35% may require a second procedure. Ideally, the eyes should be straightened, regardless of the number of surgical interventions needed, before the patient is 2 years of age, to increase the chance of acquiring stereopsis. The value of stereopsis is twofold: (1) It allows the normal visual experience for the child, and (2) if stereopsis is achieved, the brain may work to keep the eyes straight throughout life. In children who do not have stereopsis, even if the eyes initially are straight, the risk for development of recurrent strabismus is greatly increased.
- Immediate referral of patients for ophthalmologic and neurologic evaluation is needed if acute crossing (esotropia) is associated with nausea, vomiting, lethargy, increased head circumference, and sunsetting of the eyes. These are signs of increased intracranial pressure.
- Parents need to be educated about the long-term nature of their child's treatment. Children with congenital strabismus often experience lifelong strabismus and stereopsis issues.

Nystagmus

Nystagmus may be a sign of a life-threatening neurologic disorder or blindness. Thus, any child who has nystagmus with the eyes in the primary position should be referred to a pediatric ophthalmologist.

Symptoms

- Vision is decreased.
- Vision in the dark may be decreased.

Signs

- A constant, jiggling movement of the eyes is evident. The eye movements may be horizontal, vertical, or rotary, or a combination of these.
- The disorder may be bilateral, unilateral, or asymmetrical.
- Compensatory head shaking or nodding is possible.
- Weight loss may occur.
- Failure to thrive may be associated with this disorder.
- Nystagmus may be present at birth but more commonly develops over the first few months of life.

Differential Diagnosis

Neurologic Abnormalities
Possible neurologic causes of nystagmus include the following:
- Hydrocephalus
- Diencephalic tumors
- Toxicity from a number of medications, including phenytoin (Dilantin)
- Arnold-Chiari malformation
- Other brain tumors and anomalies
- In rare cases, immaturity of the central nervous system (spasmus nutans), a benign condition possibly associated with head nodding and torticollis that is a diagnosis of exclusion, necessitating evaluation by an ophthalmologist or a neurologist
- Middle ear abnormalities (rare in infants)
- Any cause of severe visual deprivation in the first 3 to 4 months of life (which can lead to nystagmus)

Ocular Abnormalities
Potentially causative disorders involving ocular abnormalities include the following:
- Leber's congenital amaurosis (a congenital form of retinitis pigmentosa associated with blindness)
- Congenital stationary night blindness (a disorder in which glasses are needed and vision is extremely poor in dim illumination but that may be compatible with almost normal vision if glasses are worn and lighting is appropriate)
- Achromatopsia (a congenital abnormality of the retina associated with legal blindness and photophobia)
- Congenital motor nystagmus (a primary motor problem associated with decreased vision secondary to the nystagmus, potentially controllable with eye muscle surgery)
- Albinism (partial and complete)
- Optic nerve hypoplasia

Associated Factors and Diseases

- Sometimes the etiology of the nystagmus points to other associated congenital anomalies to investigate. For example, optic nerve hypoplasia may be associated with structural or functional pituitary abnormalities such as diabetes insipidus, deficiency of growth or thyroid hormone, or cortisol insufficiency. Albinism is associated with a high risk of skin cancer, and sunscreen must be worn at all times. In partial forms of albinism, children appear to have normal pigment, but they are lighter than family members.

Workup

- The focus of the complete eye examination is on possible refractive errors, retinal abnormalities, and other clues to an ocular diagnosis.
- An electroretinogram and visual evoked potential testing may be necessary.
- The head circumference is measured.

- If the findings on the electroretinogram are normal and no ocular clues exist, an MRI scan is obtained.

Treatment

Treatment depends on the underlying etiology.
- In patients with visual deprivation, treatment focuses on reversing the cause of the deprivation to lessen or eradicate the nystagmus. Ideally, treatment should be instituted within the first 3 months of life, but once nystagmus has begun, the condition probably has already persisted longer than 3 months. These conditions include very high refractive errors, untreated cataracts, vitreous hemorrhage, and congenital corneal anomalies. Nystagmus may lessen in severity if the condition is corrected.
- Inherited retinal conditions often have an associated refractive error. Glasses may optimize vision but will not completely correct it or eliminate the nystagmus. Affected children benefit from early intervention programs to help them meet their developmental milestones, so early diagnosis is critical.
- Although some neurologic conditions are obviously treatable (e.g., hydrocephalus, diencephalic tumors) and some are not, the underlying etiologic process must be known.
- In some cases of congenital motor nystagmus and, rarely, other types of nystagmus, specific positioning of the head may be associated with damping of the nystagmus. Children in whom such a "null point" has been identified should keep the head turned in the appropriate position to maintain optimal vision. If control of the nystagmus is achieved consistently at the null point, strabismus surgery can move the eye muscles into the most desirable position, to permit better vision with a normal head position.

Coloboma

Coloboma represents failure of closure of the fetal fissure during development of the eye in utero. Normally the optic cup collapses on itself, and the multilayered hemisphere grows closed around a central open space, with the inferonasal aspect being the last to close. Failure of complete closure results in only a partial circle of pigment for the iris and a defect in the optic nerve or inferonasal retina and choroid. White, bare sclera is visible inside the eye when a chorioretinal coloboma is present.

Symptoms

- No symptoms occur.
- Vision may be decreased.

Signs

- A keyhole or teardrop pupil is possible, with the open area located inferiorly or inferonasally.
- Leukocoria is possible if a large chorioretinal coloboma is present.

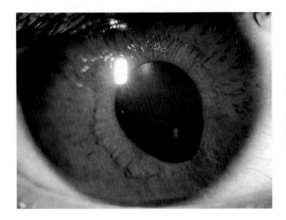

FIGURE 13–24 Very mild iris coloboma causing teardrop pupil. All affected children must have a complete eye examination to rule out associated chorioretinal coloboma, which may severely affect vision. This child also had a small retinal coloboma, but with glasses and amblyopia therapy, visual acuity improved from 20/200 to 20/30.

- In *forme fruste* presentations, the retinal coloboma looks like a small chorioretinal scar, and the pupil, instead of having a large keyhole or notch appearance, may simply be mildly larger or oval compared with the other pupil (Fig. 13–24).
- Nystagmus is possible if the defect is severe and bilateral.
- A small, malformed eye (microphthalmia) is possible.
- In some children, the CHARGE association—which consists of coloboma, *h*eart abnormalities, choanal *a*tresia, *r*etardation, *g*enitourinary anomalies, and *e*ar malformations—is evident.

Etiology

- Up to 22% of colobomas may be inherited in an autosomal dominant pattern, with extremely variable expressivity. Coloboma usually is an isolated anomaly in affected families.
- In some chromosomal disorders, coloboma may be part of a spectrum of malformations.

Treatment

- For patients with high refractive errors, glasses are needed. In these children, amblyopia often develops because of the asymmetry of the colobomas, and patching treatment is indicated. Immediate treatment is needed if cataract and glaucoma develop.
- Referral for pediatric ophthalmologic evaluation is indicated as soon as the coloboma is detected or suspected.
- Examination of the parents is necessary to identify any mild manifestations of autosomal dominant coloboma; the risk of recurrence is 50% for each subsequent child, and severity can range from a mild irregularity of the pupil to complete blindness.

Corneal Leukoma

Symptoms

- Vision is decreased.

Signs

- The cornea appears white or gray.
- The disorder is unilateral or bilateral.
- The opacity is central or peripheral.
- The disorder may be associated with a small, malformed globe (microphthalmia).
- The lesion may be elevated (corneal dermoid).

Differential Diagnosis

Considerations in the differential diagnosis include the following:
- A hazy cornea resulting from congenital glaucoma, with increased intraocular pressure causing cornea edema
- Peters' anomaly, a developmental abnormality of the cornea that results in corneal clouding
- Trachoma (more common in developing nations)
- Vitamin A deficiency (more common in developing nations but also can be seen in patients with pancreatic insufficiency or other malabsorption syndromes)
- Amniocentesis injuries
- Forceps injury, causing damage to the cornea and acute corneal edema with haziness
- Dermoid, a white elevated lesion on the cornea (Fig. 13–25) that also can occur under the skin in the brow area (Fig. 13–26), causing intense inflammation if traumatic rupture occurs
- Corneal ulcer in cases of congenital or neonatal herpes
- Sclerocornea, a rare developmental anomaly in which the cornea does not form and the entire front of the eye is white

Treatment

- Corneal leukomas always constitute an emergency, and immediate consultation with a pediatric ophthalmologist is essential.

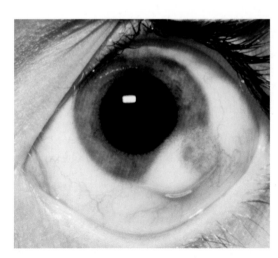

FIGURE 13–25 Corneal dermoid.

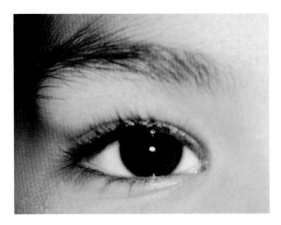

FIGURE 13–26   Temporal brow dermoid.

• Exact treatment depends on the type and cause but ranges from dilation of the eye with drops and patching of the fellow eye, to corticosteroid and antibiotic treatment, to corneal transplantation. Because corneal opacities produce dense, irreversible amblyopia if not treated within the first few months of the patient's life, referral is critical.

Retinoblastoma

Symptoms

• Usually, no symptoms occur; however, redness and irritation of the eye and eyelids may occur in advanced cases.
• Vision may be decreased.

Signs

• A white pupil (leukocoria) is present in patients with advanced retinoblastoma.
• Parents may notice an intermittent white reflex or "cat's eye" appearance early in the course, or a consistent difference between the eyes in the red reflex on flash photographs.
• Differing iris coloration (heterochromia) occurs in advanced retinoblastoma.
• Proptosis results if the tumor has spread into the orbit.
• The cornea is enlarged if glaucoma has developed.
• The patient is lethargic and experiences failure to thrive if a pineal tumor (trilateral retinoblastoma) or metastatic retinoblastoma is present.
• Multiple other abnormalities, including developmental delay, are associated findings if the retinoblastoma is precipitated by a large deletion of chromosome 13.
• Multiple other tumors occur in other family members or the affected child during life.

Differential Diagnosis

- The diagnostic possibilities are the same as those for leukocoria.
- Retinoblastoma needs to be confirmed or ruled out in any child who does not have a good red reflex or has any other signs of retinoblastoma. Referral for ophthalmologic consultation is essential. Because some tumors hug the wall of the eye and are not present in the visual axis, accurate diagnosis by a primary care physician using a direct ophthalmoscope, especially if dilating drops are not used, can be difficult or impossible. A parental history of seeing an intermittent white reflex, or "cat's eye," or of a consistent difference between the eyes on flash photographs, should be enough to prompt a referral.
  - **Note:** Photoscreening can miss retinoblastoma when the tumor is in certain locations.

Treatment

- If retinoblastoma is caught and treated early, the sight and life of the child may be saved.
  - For small tumors, laser treatment, cryotherapy, and radioactive plaque treatment, combined with chemotherapy in some cases, may restore vision or save the eye.
  - For orbital extension, radiation therapy and chemotherapy are often very successful.
  - For distant metastases, the prognosis is worse but chemotherapy and radiation therapy have a significant success rate.
  - For very advanced ocular tumors, removal of the eye (enucleation) is performed.
- In children who probably have the germline form of retinoblastoma (diagnosed or suspected because of a positive family history, bilateral tumors, positive result on DNA testing, or an early age at onset), close monitoring is essential throughout life to detect malignancies, especially sarcomas. The risk of all malignancies is increased.

Heterochromia

Symptoms

- No symptoms occur.

Signs

- Irides have different colors.
- Pupil on the side of the lighter iris is possibly smaller than normal, so pupillary size must be examined carefully.

Differential Diagnosis

- Heterochromia may represent a benign entity or be the harbinger of a life-threatening disorder.
- Nevus of the darker iris is possible if the pupils are of equal size.

- Waardenburg syndrome is a possible diagnosis if a white forelock of hair is present on the side of the lighter iris. Deafness often is an associated condition.
- Horner syndrome is possible if one pupil is miotic, especially if ptosis also is present on that side. (The two most common causes of Horner syndrome are birth trauma and neuroblastoma.)
- Heterochromia also can occur following inflammation or trauma, with retained intraocular foreign body, and with retinoblastoma.

Treatment

- Treatment depends on the etiologic process.
- All children with heterochromia should be referred for an ophthalmologic examination to determine whether the disorder is benign.

Ocular Disorders of Childhood

Conjunctivitis

Symptoms

- Itching is characteristic.
- Mild discomfort may be present.
- Rarely, vision is blurred.

Signs

- The disorder usually is bilateral but may be asymmetrical.
- Conjunctival injection is present.
- A watery mucoid or mucopurulent discharge is evident.
- Eyelids may adhere on the patient's awakening.
- A palpable preauricular lymph node may be present.
- Nodules or vesicles may be present on the conjunctiva.

Differential Diagnosis

- **Viral conjunctivitis:** In young children, a diffuse conjunctivitis often accompanies upper respiratory infections and many viral illnesses. Chickenpox and measles may have an associated conjunctivitis. Chickenpox lesions can occur on the conjunctiva and may be seen as small vesicles on the white part of the eye. These may become erythematous. A very red, painful eye in a patient with chickenpox may be a symptom of a more severe superinfection or intraocular inflammation and should be examined by an ophthalmologist immediately.

  The most common type of viral conjunctivitis is adenoviral conjunctivitis (see Figs. 5–3 to 5–6). The affected child generally presents with red, profusely watery eyes and a palpable preauricular lymph node. It often is contracted at day care facilities or from family members. Adenoviral conjunctivitis generally runs a 2-week course, with worsening symptoms during the first week and then slow improvement during the second week. It is contagious throughout the entire course. In some severe cases, a thick, white pseudomembrane forms on the inside of the lower and upper eyelids. Bleeding of the conjunctiva may occur. Some viral strains cause infiltrates of the cornea beginning 10 to 14 days after the acute infection; severely decreased vision may result, with some permanent scarring.

- **Herpes simplex conjunctivitis with corneal involvement:** All age groups can contract herpes simplex conjunctivitis. A dendrite (see Fig. 6–7) may be seen on the cornea. Vesicular lid lesions also are common.
- **Bacterial conjunctivitis:** In children, bacterial conjunctivitis is much less common than viral conjunctivitis (see Figs. 5–7 and 5–8). If it occurs on a chronic basis, nasolacrimal duct obstruction should be confirmed or ruled out.
- **Chronic conjunctivitis:** The chronic form of conjunctivitis should never occur in children. Persistence of symptoms for longer than a few weeks may signal toxic exposure, underlying iritis, nasolacrimal duct obstruction with dacryocystitis, or another disorder. Watery discharge and photophobia point to possible developmental glaucoma. Referral to an ophthalmologist is indicated in all cases.
- **Vernal conjunctivitis:** Found only in children and adolescents, vernal conjunctivitis is a type of allergic conjunctivitis and may be associated with other atopic disorders. The primary symptom is intense itching. The lids may be droopy and discolored from chronic eye rubbing. It generally is cyclic, occurring only at certain times of the year (e.g., spring). In children, the presenting manifestation usually is thickening of the conjunctiva around the limbus of the eyes, which can be excruciatingly uncomfortable. Prolonged treatment may be necessary. Children should be referred to an ophthalmologist at once if severe pain and discomfort are associated with conjunctivitis.

Associated Factors and Diseases

- After infancy, the chance that a red eye is caused by iritis rather than by simple conjunctivitis increases. Iritis can occur with viral illnesses such as coxsackievirus, chickenpox, and other acute viral conditions, and with juvenile rheumatoid arthritis and other inflammatory and infectious conditions. The conjunctiva appears diffusely pink, but usually no discharge is present. The pupil may be small (miotic), and photophobia is often present. Because untreated iritis can cause cataract, glaucoma, and permanent scarring in the eye, children with this constellation of signs should be referred to an ophthalmologist immediately.

Treatment

- No treatment modifies the course of viral conjunctivitis. Artificial tears, which may be obtained over the counter, generally are soothing to the eye in the early stages. Topical antibiotic drops are not administered unless signs of a bacterial superinfection (a thick, mucopurulent discharge and crusting and adherence of the eyelids) are noted. Use of antibiotics for viral ocular infections only increases resistant bacterial strains, causes increased irritation from the toxicity of the antibiotics to the cornea, and does not hasten the patient's recovery from the illness.

- For bacterial superinfection, antibiotic drops (e.g., polymyxin B/trimethoprim [Polytrim] ophthalmic drops 1 drop 4 times a day in each eye) are administered for 7 days. If the infection worsens on this regimen or recurs after the drops are stopped, the child should be referred to an ophthalmologist for appropriate culturing of the conjunctiva and workup.
- With no discharge, a small (miotic) pupil, and/or photophobia, iritis is a possible cause. Treatment involves the use of corticosteroids and cycloplegic dilating drops, so iritis should be diagnosed only with a slit lamp and treated by an ophthalmologist.
- Herpes conjunctivitis and keratoconjunctivitis can have the same symptoms and signs as for iritis, but if corticosteroids are given, loss of the eye can result. These diagnoses are more appropriately made by an ophthalmologist.

Ocular Trauma

Symptoms

- Symptoms vary and include pain, photophobia, decreased vision, and tearing.

Signs

- Lid swelling and ecchymosis are noted.
- Conjunctival injection is evident.
- Subconjunctival hemorrhage can occur.
- Blood in the anterior part of the eye (hyphema) may be observed.
- The pupil may be irregular in contour or peaked.
- A large or small, poorly reactive pupil may be present.
- A poor red reflex may be noted.

Differential Diagnosis

- On rare occasions, children try to conceal the actual events of an injury to avoid possible punishment. With unexplained pain, photophobia, or decreased vision, trauma should always be suspected.
- Children often have severe pain, nausea, vomiting, somnolence, and lethargy after intraocular bleeding. Layered red blood cells may be seen filling the anterior chamber (hyphema) just behind the cornea (see Fig. 16–16). Glaucoma may result and, if untreated, can cause permanent damage to the optic nerve. In children who have sickle cell disease or sickle trait, a hyphema is more likely to cause severe glaucoma.
- Any child who has suffered blunt trauma has an increased risk for development of glaucoma throughout life, even if glaucoma does not develop at the time of the initial trauma.
- Nonaccidental trauma, or the shaken baby syndrome, must be suspected in young children with trauma for which the history does not match clinical findings. Retinal hemorrhages may help confirm the diagnosis. The presence of typical retinal hemorrhages and/or perimacular retinal folds in an infant with lethargy, vomiting,

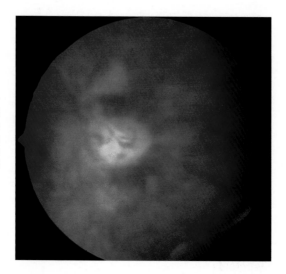

FIGURE 13–27 Retinal hemorrhage in the shaken baby syndrome. Visualization with the direct ophthalmoscope is not always possible. Extensive hemorrhage often breaks into the vitreous, requiring ocular surgery for removal and portending poor visual outcome. Vitreous hemorrhage correlates with poor neurologic outcome. Children with severe intracranial and intraocular damage may die of their injuries.

intracranial hemorrhage and a history that is not consistent with the severity of the clinical findings is suspicious and requires notification of authorities. Because retinal hemorrhages may not always be visible with the direct ophthalmoscope, consultation with an ophthalmologist is necessary for examination using indirect ophthalmoscopy (Fig. 13–27).

Treatment

- For severe blunt or penetrating trauma, the clinician places a protective shield over the eye, using a metal Fox shield or a paper or Styrofoam cup that has been cut so that the bottom can be taped over the eye. Excessive manipulation of lids by personnel unaccustomed to examining eyes can result in pressure on the eye and further damage. An immediate ophthalmologic evaluation is critical. Nonsteroidal anti-inflammatory agents decrease clotting and are contraindicated. The child is kept quiet until ophthalmologic evaluation is performed. Antiemetics are administered if the child experiences nausea, because vomiting worsens intraocular bleeding or may cause extrusion of ocular contents in the case of a penetrating injury.
- For penetrating trauma, a tetanus shot is administered if the child's tetanus vaccination schedule is not up to date. Treatment with a broad-spectrum intravenous antibiotic (ideally a fluoroquinolone, because these agents have the best vitreous penetration, although in very young children this class of drugs may be contraindicated) is initiated. Because of the possibility of surgical intervention, the child is allowed nothing by mouth that would delay an operation. If the trauma involves chemicals in the eye and no rupture, the clinician irrigates the eye with sterile saline solution, usually using 1 to 2 liters. This procedure is better tolerated if tetracaine or another topical ocular anesthetic is used initially. Determining the amount of the substance to which the eye was subjected is the first step; often only a small amount of toxic material entered the eye, and excessive irrigation may cause more abrasion

than the original injury. The pH may be tested with a standard pH strip on the conjunctiva to gauge the effectiveness of irrigation.

Follow-up

- Prevention is the best treatment, so children should be advised to wear polycarbonate safety goggles for sports and other high-risk activities. BB guns and paintball weapons are major causes of severe eye injuries in children. Bungee cords, golf clubs, and small sports balls such as racquet balls are other common causes of severe injuries.

Preseptal and Orbital Cellulitis

Symptoms

- **Preseptal cellulitis**: Erythema, warmth, and swelling of the eyelids are noted.
- **Orbital cellulitis**: Irritability, lethargy, decreased vision, high fever, and a more toxic appearance are present.

Signs

Preseptal Cellulitis

- The skin of the eyelids is red and swollen, with sharply circumscribed or diffuse areas of involvement.
- Conjunctival injection may be present.
- Mucopurulent discharge from the nasolacrimal system may occur if this is the source of infection.

Orbital Cellulitis

- All of the signs as described for preseptal cellulitis are present.
- Small or diffuse areas of infection may be associated with marked motility disturbance.
- Proptosis (a pushing of the eyeball forward because of a mass of infection behind the globe) may develop, depending on the location of the infection
- A large focus of pus accumulates near the optic nerve, causing the nerve to begin to lose function, a decrease in vision, a sluggishly reactive pupil, and a possible afferent pupillary defect.

Etiology

Cellulitis can result from the following:
- Ethmoid or maxillary sinus disease
- Lacerating trauma around the eye
- Bacterial infection with nasolacrimal duct obstruction
- Buccal mucosa infection
- Stye or chalazion
- **Note**: Because the orbital septum in children is extremely thin and does not provide a good barrier against infection from the anterior skin surface, preseptal cellulitis

may move rapidly posterior into the orbit, often into the subperiosteal space, causing an abscess. From this location, it may move back to the brain and cause a brain abscess and meningitis. The younger the child, the more rapidly this progression can take place.

Differential Diagnosis

Considerations in the differential diagnosis include the following:
- Retinoblastoma
- Ruptured dermoid tumor
- Orbital pseudotumor
- Leukemic infiltrate of the orbit

Treatment

- For children younger than 2 years of age, even if the cellulitis is preseptal, hospital admission for intravenous antibiotic administration and observation is recommended because of the rapidity with which the infection can move posteriorly. If the child is younger than 3 years of age, appears in a toxic state, or has an elevated white cell count and fever, a full septic workup, including lumbar puncture, is indicated. Broad-spectrum antibiotics are administered, particularly agents targeting gram-positive organisms.
- For children 2 years of age and older in whom the disease is clinically preseptal, oral antibiotics are administered; these patients are not hospitalized but are closely monitored with careful follow-up exams. If no response is observed within 48 hours or the clinical condition worsens at any point, the child is hospitalized and intravenous antibiotics are administered.
- In children with signs of orbital involvement, an immediate CT scan of the orbits is needed to detect an abscess or a nidus of infection. If a small subperiosteal abscess is noted, intravenous antibiotics initially are administered for up to 48 hours. In younger children, orbital cellulitis often resolves with intravenous antibiotic regimens, even when an abscess is present. If the patient's condition does not improve or worsens over the first 24 to 48 hours, surgical drainage of the abscess is needed.
- A lumbar puncture is indicated in septic patients before antibiotic administration begins.
- If a patient's mental status changes, a CT scan of the brain with contrast is indicated to confirm or rule out a brain abscess.
- Any immunosuppressed child with erythema around the eyelids should be immediately referred for ophthalmologic evaluation. Mucormycosis is a possible diagnosis, particularly in children with malignancies or diabetes mellitis. In general, mucormycosis is treated with surgical débridement; this disorder does not respond well to the administration of intravenous amphotericin alone.

Headache

Parents and physicians often assume that headaches are related to eye disease or eyestrain. This association is rare in children, but uncorrected refractive error should always be addressed.

Symptoms

- Headaches occur.
- Vision may be blurred or decreased.

Signs

- Usually, no signs are present.

Differential Diagnosis

- **Migraine:** Severe unilateral or bilateral headache, especially if associated with nausea or vomiting and relieved only by sleep, often is a migraine. The onset in most cases is in early childhood. The classic scintillating scotoma or wavy lines across the field of vision occur in only a minority of patients. A history of this phenomenon, however, is almost diagnostic for migraine. Often, a family history of migraine headaches is reported. Before the age of puberty, boys and girls experience migraines with equal frequency. After puberty, the incidence of migraines decreases in boys but increases in girls. Thus, a hormonal etiology is suspected.
- **Tension or stress headaches:** Often present in children, tension or stress headaches are generally not as prolonged as a migraine. They often occur toward the end of the day at school and are relieved by acetaminophen or aspirin. Children may associate them with reading, but questioning will often reveal that only one specific subject in school precipitates the headache.
- **Increased intracranial pressure:** If a headache is chronic and unremitting, does not subside with sleep or any medication, and is worse in the morning or associated with decreased vision, nausea or vomiting, double vision, or crossing of the eyes, increased intracranial pressure must be suspected. If the child is young enough, head circumference plots should be reviewed. In older children, a careful history is needed and physical examination performed for precocious puberty, ataxia, weight loss, and altered mental status and signs of craniopharyngioma and posterior fossa tumors. A funduscopic examination to detect papilledema (an elevation of the optic nerve, often with hemorrhage on the nerve [Fig. 13–28]) should be performed. If these signs or symptoms are present, the case should be referred to an ophthalmologist and/or neurologist or neurosurgeon as an emergency.

Treatment

- In cases of apparent migraine, triggers should be identified. These often include certain foods such as chocolate, uncorrected refractive error, skipping of meals, lack of sleep, and menstruation. If the headaches still persist once all triggers have been addressed, many appropriate medications are available. They must be used with care in children, and consultation with a pediatric neurologist may be indicated.
- In cases of milder, possibly tension-related headaches, stress-reducing activities are emphasized. Parents and children often perceive that the child's eyes are the source of the problem in tension headaches. The only ocular problems that cause headaches are uncorrected astigmatism of high degree, severe hyperopia in older children, iritis, and convergence insufficiency. If vision complaints accompany the headaches, examination by a pediatric ophthalmologist is warranted.

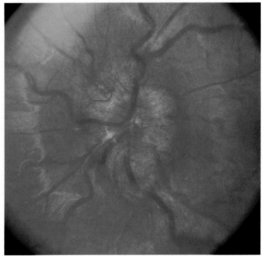

FIGURE 13–28 Elevated optic nerve head (papilledema) in a child who had a headache for 1 week, otitis media, and transverse sinus thrombosis from mastoiditis. Symptoms and signs resolved with serial lumbar puncture, antibiotic administration, and heparin therapy.

Styes and Chalazia

Symptoms

- Usually no symptoms are noted, but evidence of mild pain or discomfort may be present.
- In rare cases, vision is blurred as a result of induced astigmatism.

Signs

- An elevated, slightly tender, bright red nodule is present on the outer lid surface, or a very erythematous circumscribed area on the conjunctival lining of the inner eyelid is evident in the early stages (see Fig. 4–16).
- In later stages, the lesion becomes nontender but remains round and very firm, loses its reddish color, but does not disappear (see Fig. 4–17).

Differential Diagnosis

- In children, lesions of this type almost always are hordeola (styes), which is the acute phase, or chalazia, which is the chronic phase.
- In rare cases, basal cell or other types of cancer are present.
- In children with neurofibromatosis, a neuroma of the eyelid can develop.
- The lesions of molluscum contagiosum usually are much smaller than styes and have an umbilicated center.
- The lesions of tuberous sclerosis usually are not confined to the lids and can thus be differentiated.

Treatment

- For styes (hordeola), rapid institution of very warm compresses used for 15 to 20 minutes several times a day with or without topical erythromycin ointment in the eye often brings about resolution. Children who are predisposed to styes and chalazia get them repeatedly unless lid hygiene is practiced. This involves using commercially available eye scrub pads or baby shampoo on a warm, wet washcloth to scrub along the base of the eyelashes daily. The meibomian glands, which open near the base of the eyelashes, become plugged in persons who have thick secretions, causing the stye. In older children and adolescents in whom tetracycline may be used safely without damaging the teeth, a regimen of oral tetracycline or doxycycline usually is very effective when recurrent hordeola are resistant to daily lid scrubs.

- For chalazia, warm soaks, antibiotics, and scrubs usually are not effective. Chalazia must be removed by an ophthalmologist. In older, cooperative children, this procedure can be performed in the office setting with use of local anesthesia. For very young children, removal requires anesthesia in the operating room. Large chalazia can cause refractive errors, specifically astigmatism. Thus in young children, these lesions should be treated aggressively, and if vision is decreased, an ophthalmologic consultation is needed.

Strabismus

The peak occurrences of benign esotropia are before 6 months of age (congenital) and between 2 and 4 years (accommodative). Congenital exotropia is rare; intermittent exotropia is quite common. It often is seen fleetingly in the first year of life; in one third of affected children, the episodes of exotropia increase in frequency during early childhood and adolescence.

Symptoms

- Double vision and loss of depth perception are initial symptoms. Very young children usually are not aware of either symptom. Blindness (amblyopia) evolves slowly in many cases if strabismus is not treated.

Signs

- The pupils of the eye are misaligned.
- In esotropia, one or both eyes are deviated inward.
- In exotropia, one or both eyes are deviated outward.
- In hypertropia, one eye is deviated upward.
- In some types of strabismus, one or both eyes cannot move fully in one or more directions.

Differential Diagnosis

Considerations in the differential diagnosis depend on the form of strabismus.

With Acute Acquired Esotropia
- Increased intracranial pressure causing sixth nerve palsy or paresis
- Acute viral sixth nerve palsy
- Accommodative esotropia
- Undetected congenital esotropia

With Acute Acquired Exotropia
- Acute third nerve palsy
- Intermittent exotropia with a breakdown of fusion
- Undetected congenital exotropia

With Vertical Misalignment of Eyes
- Acute fourth nerve palsy
- Decompensated congenital fourth nerve palsy
- Partial third nerve palsy
- Dissociated vertical deviation in a child who had a congenital horizontal misalignment
- Other congenital eye muscle syndromes

Treatment

- All patients with strabismus should be immediately referred to an ophthalmologist.
- Treatment varies with the form of strabismus.

Esotropia
○ If the cause is sixth nerve paresis from increased intracranial pressure, normalization of intracranial pressure, either medically or accomplished with neurosurgery, generally results in resolution of the sixth nerve palsy within 6 months. Amblyopia therapy is needed during this time. Any sixth nerve palsy that does not resolve within 6 months after the insult requires eye muscle surgery.
○ Viral sixth nerve palsies usually disappear spontaneously once the underlying illness resolves; however, amblyopia therapy during and after the paresis often is necessary in young children.
○ Accommodative esotropia is the most common cause of eye crossing in children 2 to 4 years of age and usually is caused by uncorrected hyperopia (Fig. 13–29). These children require cycloplegic refraction by a pediatric ophthalmologist and must wear their spectacles all the time. As the eye grows, the hyperopia often decreases. In some children, the prescription strength can be decreased over time with monitoring by serial examinations, and glasses may not be required for straight eyes by approximately 9 years of age. If the glasses are not worn, permanent esotropia requiring surgical correction and amblyopia causing blindness of one eye usually result. Some children also require a bifocal to correct crossing at near distance. Contact lenses, rather than spectacles, may be used in some cases but are difficult to manage in young children. Refractive surgery in young children with this condition is controversial and is currently under study.

Exotropia
○ Intermittent exotropia may be treated with eye exercises, glasses, or surgical correction, depending on the patient's age, frequency of deviation, magnitude of deviation, refractive error, and other considerations.
○ Third nerve palsy exotropia is extremely difficult to treat. Surgery often can improve cosmetic alignment, and intensive patching therapy for amblyopia is required, but normal movement of the eyes and use of the eyes together usually cannot be achieved.

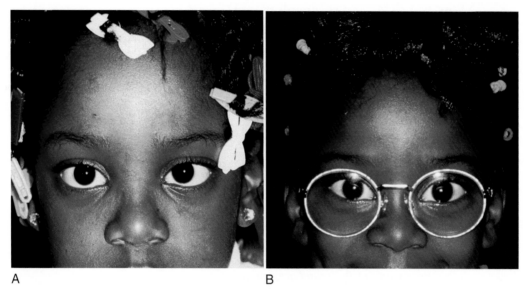

A   B

FIGURE 13–29   **A,** Accommodative esotropia. In this child, fixation with the right eye is preferred; the pupillary light reflex is temporal to the center of the pupil in the left eye because it is crossing in. Vision was not normal even in the right eye because of severe hyperopia. **B,** After the child started wearing spectacles with full hyperopic correction, the eyes are straight (i.e., pupillary light reflexes are centered), corrected vision is 20/20 in each eye, and stereopsis (depth perception) returned to normal. Such good outcome is possible only if glasses are quickly prescribed once crossing begins.

Hypertropia

○ Acute fourth nerve palsy may be a viral entity or a disorder secondary to an intracranial pathologic disease. Prompt referral to an ophthalmologist is recommended.

○ Decompensated congenital fourth nerve palsy should be treated if the child demonstrates a significant head tilt. The treatment of choice is surgery. Exercises do not help this condition, although concomitant exercises for the foreshortened neck muscles may be necessary. Rarely, surgical correction of the torticollis is necessary if the neck does not straighten after the eye muscle surgery has been performed. In other vertical muscle palsies and abnormalities, correction is more complex and beyond the scope of this chapter.

Amblyopia

Symptoms

- Vision is decreased in one eye, typically to the range of legal blindness (20/200).
- The amblyopia is bilateral in some cases.
- When the disorder is unilateral, children rarely complain or notice the visual deficit.

Signs

- In some cases, no signs occur. The eyes appear normal. Visual acuity is found to be decreased on standardized testing, provided that the fellow eye is completely occluded to prevent peeking.
- Strabismus is possible, with the poorly seeing eye turning inward in very young children and outward in older children. Decreased stereopsis can be detected on standard testing for the condition.
- In rare cases, an afferent pupillary defect is present in the affected eye.

Differential Diagnosis

The diagnostic possibilities depend on whether vision is decreased in one or both eyes.

With Severely Decreased Vision in One Eye
- Amblyopia
- Refractive error
- Abnormality of the retina or optic nerve
- Cataract
- Malingering

With Bilateral Decreased Vision
When the deficit is bilateral, the visual acuity often is reduced in both eyes to the 20/200 range; nystagmus is present if the deficit occurred within the first 3 months of life and absent if the deficit occurred later.
- Bilateral refractive errors
- Bilateral amblyopia
- Bilateral optic nerve or retinal dysfunction

Treatment

- The mainstay of treatment is early correction of the underlying cause, followed by patching of the better eye under a strictly prescribed regimen appropriate for the child's age.
- Deprivation amblyopia is seen in patients with congenital cataracts, hemangiomas of the eyelid, severe congenital ptosis, and corneal leukomas. If this condition is present at birth, it must be completely corrected, including optical correction, before 3 to 4 months of age for the child to have any potential for normal vision. This type of amblyogenic factor generally must be picked up by the pediatrician on the baby's nursery exit examination or at a well-baby checkup.
- Amblyopia resulting from uncorrected refractive error is a very common type of amblyopia that often is undiagnosed until the child is too old for the most effective treatment. This condition is missed because the refractive error occurs in only one eye or because the refractive error is much greater in one eye than in the other. The brain favors the better-seeing eye unless spectacles or contact lenses are prescribed. Usually the eyes stay straight and appear normal. Only careful testing for a difference in brightness on the red reflex test, with photoscreening, or reading of an eye chart in verbal children with complete occlusion of the better eye can detect

this type of amblyopia. Spectacle or contact lens correction is sufficient if the condition is detected early and the amblyopia is mild. If the amblyopia is detected later, patching of the fellow eye also must be instituted. If both eyes have equal, high refractive errors and glasses are not worn before the age of 8 or 9 years, vision will never be perfect because of bilateral refractive amblyopia.

- Strabismic amblyopia is caused by the underlying esotropia, exotropia, or vertical deviation. Because the brain cannot process two images at once, it ignores one image, and one eye loses the ability to see. Again, timing of diagnosis and treatment is critical. If strabismus is present from birth and amblyopia begins very early, complete correction is not possible unless treatment is started within the first months or years of life. If the strabismus begins between 2 and 4 years of age and is rapidly corrected, no amblyopia may result. The longer the amblyopia is untreated, the more severe and harder to reverse it becomes. Generally, refractive and strabismic amblyopia can be effectively treated up to the age of 9 years, whereas deprivation amblyopia does not have a good outcome after a child is 4 months to a year old in most cases. Strabismus must be treated before children reach 2 years of age for them to have the best chance of regaining stereopsis. Despite these guidelines, some children have better outcomes than expected, even at advanced ages. Therefore, if parents and child are interested in treatment, it may be attempted even after the age for optimal outcome.
- Organic amblyopia results from an anatomic abnormality of the eye, such as dragging of the retina in retinopathy of prematurity, coloboma, and optic nerve hypoplasia. The potential for vision in the eye is not 20/20; however, amblyopia therapy must be instituted shortly after birth for the patient to attain the best possible vision.

Refractive Errors

Symptoms

- Vision is decreased.
- Eye strain sometimes occurs.
- Diplopia may be present.

Signs

- Squinting is observed.
- Blinking of the eyes is excessive.
- The child rubs the eyes.
- The child performs poorly on tasks requiring good distance vision at school.
- The child has poor tolerance for extended periods of reading.

Differential Diagnosis

Although refractive errors are the cause of decreased vision in a majority of cases, other diagnostic possibilities include the following:
- Midline brain tumors that compress the optic chiasm
- Tumors of the optic nerves

- Optic neuritis
- Iritis
- Retinal degenerations
- Corneal dystrophies
- Developmental cataracts

Workup

- Any child who fails a vision screening test or whose parents have noted evidence of decreased vision should be referred for a complete ophthalmologic examination and cycloplegic refraction. This test objectively measures refractive errors and does not rely on a child's answers to a vision test. It also allows for close examination of the optic nerve and retina. Because many progressive disorders result in few signs initially, all children who have decreased vision that is not immediately improved to normal with spectacles should be monitored closely for the development of neurologic and other signs.
- An ophthalmologist should determine the need for glasses in infants using the retinoscope and dilation with cyloplegic drops.

Treatment

- Not all refractive errors in children need to be treated. Unless associated with esotropia, small amounts of hyperopia do not mandate treatment. Minimal myopic correction or correction for small amounts of astigmatism need not be instituted until children begin school.
- High refractive errors are associated with bilateral amblyopia and developmental delays, particularly delayed walking. In these children, spectacle correction should be immediate.
- Because the natural developmental desire is to see clearly, glasses are readily accepted and worn by infants if the refractive error significantly interferes with vision. Even small infants keep them on and search for them if the glasses markedly improve vision and fit comfortably. Often an infant who has been wearing glasses appropriately will become less tolerant of wear, which usually indicates that the prescription should be changed and mandates another referral to the pediatric ophthalmologist. The eye grows very rapidly during infancy, and lenses may need to be changed every 3 to 6 months for the first 2 years of life. Slightly less frequent changes in lenses are needed over the next couple of years. After a child is 4 years of age, yearly examinations are usually acceptable.
- Refractive errors have a genetic basis, although they usually do not follow simple mendelian inheritance patterns. Thus if parents have high refractive errors, children should be seen at an early age to rule out or confirm refractive errors. All children who wear glasses should be questioned about sports participation and should have a separate pair of prescription wrap-around safety goggles for sports.
- Topical medications that may slow the progression of myopia have shown efficacy in animal models and are in clinical trials, but such agents are not yet available commercially.

• Laser refractive surgery in children with a unilateral high degree of myopia has been performed and is under study but at present is not widely recommended for children younger than 18 years of age.

Inherited Retinal and Corneal Degenerations

Many retinal degenerations such as retinitis pigmentosa are hereditary. Decreased night vision often is an early symptom. Photophobia can occur during childhood in cases of inherited corneal dystrophies and some cone retinal dystrophies. Congenitally deaf children have an increased risk of retinitis pigmentosa (the combination of this disorder plus deafness constitutes Usher syndrome) and require close ophthalmologic follow-up. Any child with a family member who has significant early-onset vision problems requires a baseline examination early in life and again if symptoms occur. DNA blood tests are now available for some inherited eye disorders.

Syndromes Affecting Vision

Approximately 25% of the U.S. population is nearsighted (myopic), and although myopia begins in childhood, it usually is of low to moderate degree and increases slowly throughout adolescence. If high myopia or rapidly progressive myopia is present before 6 years of age, an underlying syndrome should be sought. Homocystinuria, Marfan syndrome, Weill-Marchesani syndrome, and sulfite oxidase deficiency are associated with lens subluxation, which causes high myopia. These disorders can be life-threatening. Stickler syndrome is a disorder of autosomal dominant inheritance that includes cleft palate, early arthritis, partial deafness, and high myopia. High hyperopia and astigmatism may be associated with albinism. Retinal dystrophies may be associated with many different metabolic and genetic syndromes with such associated findings as developmental delay, extra toes and fingers, and deafness, among others. Any child with a very high refractive error, especially myopia, or decreased vision not correctable by spectacles, should undergo a complete workup by a pediatric ophthalmologist and by a geneticist if indicated.

CHAPTER 14

Orbital Disease

TED H. WOJNO

Related Anatomy

The bony orbit is a four-sided pyramid with the apex pointed posteriorly (Fig. 14–1). The medial orbital wall is composed mainly of the ethmoid bone. The lateral wall is composed of the zygomatic bone anteriorly and the greater wing of the sphenoid bone posteriorly. The superior wall is composed of the frontal bone, whereas the inferior wall is formed by the maxillary and zygomatic bones. The optic foramen transmits the optic nerve and the ophthalmic artery. The superior orbital fissure transmits the third, the fourth, the ophthalmic division of the fifth, and the sixth cranial nerves.

The four rectus muscles are involved in horizontal and vertical movements of the globe (Fig. 14–2). The superior and inferior oblique muscles are involved in the globe's torsional movements, and the orbital fat cushions and supports the globe. The pink lacrimal gland is located just under the superolateral orbital rim. The clinician can easily visualize this structure, which is responsible for reflex tearing, by retracting the upper lid superolaterally and having the patient look inferonasally (Fig. 14–3). The lacrimal drainage system begins with the puncta and canaliculi, which join to enter the lacrimal sac (Fig. 14–4). The sac empties into the nasolacrimal duct, which passes through the medial wall of the maxillary sinus and empties into the nose under the inferior turbinate.

Preseptal Cellulitis

For preseptal cellulitis in children, see Chapter 13.

Symptoms

- Warm, erythematous, tender swelling of the lids may extend over the nasal bridge to the opposite side.

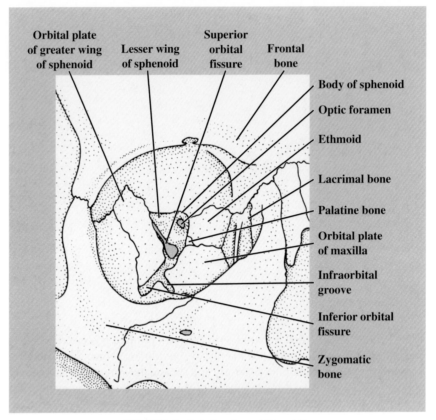

Orbital plate
of greater wing
of sphenoid

Lesser wing
of sphenoid

Superior
orbital
fissure

Frontal
bone

Body of sphenoid

Optic foramen

Ethmoid

Lacrimal bone

Palatine bone

Orbital plate
of maxilla

Infraorbital
groove

Inferior orbital
fissure

Zygomatic
bone

FIGURE 14–1 Anterior view of the orbit.

Signs

- A low-grade fever and elevated white blood cell count are usual findings.
- Vision, pupillary reflexes, and extraocular movements are normal.
- Blood culture results are negative unless the organism is *Haemophilus influenzae* or *Streptococcus pneumoniae*.

Etiology

- An upper respiratory tract infection or sinusitis can result in the disorder. The most common causative organisms in adults are *Streptococcus* species, *Staphylococcus aureus*, and mixed flora.
- Lid trauma (blunt or perforating) can lead to preseptal cellulitis. The most common causative organisms are *Streptococcus pyogenes*, *S. aureus*, and fungus (if organic material was involved).
- The disorder can result from superficial lid infections such as a stye (hordeolum) or impetigo.
- Conjunctivitis can cause the disorder.

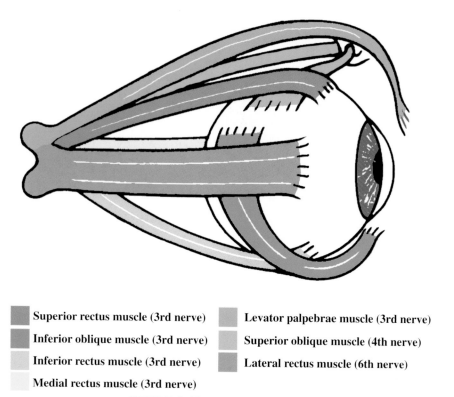

Superior rectus muscle (3rd nerve)

Inferior oblique muscle (3rd nerve)

Inferior rectus muscle (3rd nerve)

Medial rectus muscle (3rd nerve)

Levator palpebrae muscle (3rd nerve)

Superior oblique muscle (4th nerve)

Lateral rectus muscle (6th nerve)

FIGURE 14–2 The extraocular muscles.

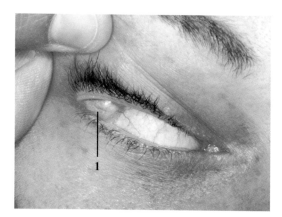

FIGURE 14–3 The normal lacrimal gland (1).

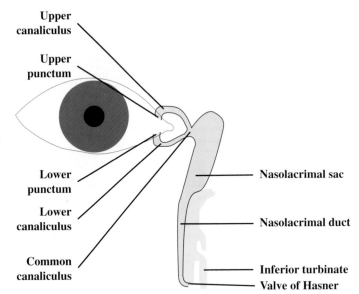

FIGURE 14–4 The nasolacrimal excretory system.

Upper canaliculus

Upper punctum

Lower punctum

Lower canaliculus

Common canaliculus

Nasolacrimal sac

Nasolacrimal duct

Inferior turbinate
Valve of Hasner

- Dacryocystitis can lead to the disorder.
- In rare cases, septicemia results in the disorder.

Differential Diagnosis

Considerations in the differential diagnosis include the following:
- Orbital cellulitis
- Orbital pseudotumor
- Carotid artery–cavernous sinus fistula

Workup

- A CBC is performed.
- Culture of material obtained from an open wound, purulent nasal drainage, conjunctival discharge, or any weeping vesicles is performed.
- Computed tomography (CT) scan of orbits and sinuses is performed if indicated.
- Blood cultures are performed if *H. influenzae* or *S. pneumoniae* infection is suspected.

Treatment

- In cases of mild to moderate preseptal cellulitis without localized abscess, an oral broad-spectrum antibiotic (e.g., amoxicillin/clavulanate [Augmentin] 500 to 875 mg two times a day) is administered. If the patient is allergic to penicillin, oral erythromycin (250 to 500 mg four times a day) is given.
- In cases of severe preseptal cellulitis, an intravenous broad-spectrum antibiotic (e.g., cefuroxime [Zinacef] 750 mg to 1.5 g three times a day) is administered. If the

patient is allergic to penicillin, intravenous clindamycin (300 mg four times a day) and intravenous gentamicin (1 mg/kg three times a day) are administered.

- **Note:** Antibiotic dosages should be adjusted in the presence of renal impairment. Peak and trough levels of gentamicin are used to adjust dosage. Blood urea nitrogen (BUN) and creatinine levels are followed closely.
- In cases of localized abscess formation, an oral or intravenous broad-spectrum antibiotic is administered, depending on the severity of the abscess. Incision and drainage with or without a placement of a drain may be performed, depending on the severity of the abscess.
- For lesions with extensive crusting, after incision and drainage, or in cases of penetrating injury, a topical broad-spectrum ophthalmic ointment such as polymyxin B/bacitracin (Polysporin) is used.

Follow-up

- The focus of follow-up is on preventing the development of orbital cellulitis.

Orbital Cellulitis and Abscess

For orbital cellulitis in children, see Chapter 13.

Symptoms

- The symptoms are the same as those for preseptal cellulitis. Orbital involvement can lead to vision loss and double vision.

Signs

- A low-grade fever and elevated white blood cell count are usual findings.
- Proptosis, restricted motility, sluggish pupillary reflex, and decreased vision are noted (Fig. 14–5).

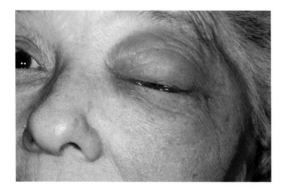

FIGURE 14–5 Orbital cellulitis resulting from ethmoid sinusitis.

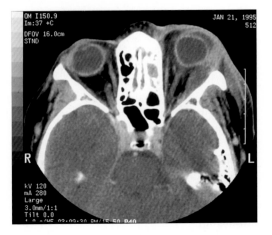

FIGURE 14–6 An axial computed tomography scan of the head obtained in the patient in Figure 14–5 shows diffuse infiltration of the left orbital structures.

Workup

- Workup is the same as that for cases of preseptal cellulitis.
- A funduscopic examination may reveal retinal hemorrhages, venous congestion, and disc edema.
- A CT scan displays diffuse infiltration of orbital fat that may progress to abscess formation (Fig. 14–6).
- Blood culture results usually are negative.

Etiology

- Underlying causes are the same as those for preseptal cellulitis.
- Surgical procedures that violate the orbital septum such as strabismus, retinal detachment repair, and orbital surgery can lead to the disorder.

Differential Diagnosis

- Considerations in the differential diagnosis are the same as those for preseptal cellulitis.

Treatment

- An intravenous broad-spectrum antibiotic (e.g., cefuroxime [Zinacef] 750 mg to 1.5 g three times a day) is used. If the patient is allergic to penicillin, intravenous clindamycin (300 mg four times a day) and intravenous gentamicin (1 mg/kg three times a day) are used.
- **Note:** Antibiotic dosages should be adjusted in the presence of renal impairment. Peak and trough levels of gentamicin are used to adjust dosage. Blood urea nitrogen (BUN) and creatinine levels are followed closely.
- Surgical drainage is needed for a large abscess or small abscess that does not resolve after 2 or 3 days of intravenous antibiotic therapy.
- Sinus drainage is performed if appropriate.

Follow-up

- The focus of follow-up is on preventing development of cavernous sinus thrombosis.

Nasolacrimal Duct Obstruction

Symptoms and Signs

- Tearing occurs.

Etiology and Associated Factors and Diseases

- Previous nasal or sinus disease, surgery, or trauma can lead to stenosis of the nasolacrimal duct.
- The disorder can have an idiopathic origin.
- In rare cases, a tumor also may be present.

Differential Diagnosis

- Tearing secondary to ocular irritation should be ruled out or confirmed.

Workup

- Probing and irrigation of the nasolacrimal system are performed to confirm the presence of an obstruction.

Treatment

- If the patient and the physician feel that the symptoms warrant intervention, a surgical fistula is created by connecting the lacrimal sac to the nasal mucosa, thus bypassing the obstructed nasolacrimal duct (dacryocystorhinostomy).

Dacryocystitis

Symptoms

- Tearing, pain, and mucopurulent drainage occur in dacryocystitis (infection of the lacrimal sac).

Signs

- Tearing, swollen lacrimal sac, and mucopurulent drainage are evident (Fig. 14–7).
- In rare cases, preseptal cellulitis occurs.

Etiology

- Nasolacrimal duct obstruction can lead to infection of the lacrimal sac.

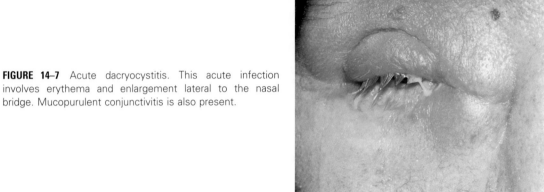

FIGURE 14–7 Acute dacryocystitis. This acute infection involves erythema and enlargement lateral to the nasal bridge. Mucopurulent conjunctivitis is also present.

Differential Diagnosis

- An ethmoid mucocele should be ruled out or confirmed.

Workup

- Digital pressure over the lacrimal sac may cause reflux of the mucopurulent material.

Treatment

- In cases of acute dacryocystitis, an oral, broad-spectrum antibiotic (e.g., amoxicillin/clavulanate [Augmentin] 500 to 875 mg two times a day) is administered. If the patient is allergic to penicillin, oral erythromycin (250 to 500 mg 4 times a day) is used.
- Incision and drainage are appropriate interventions if a large abscess has formed.
- Dacryocystorhinostomy or dacryocystectomy is performed when the infection is quiescent.
- In cases of chronic dacryocystitis, dacryocystorhinostomy or dacryocystectomy is performed.

Dacryoadenitis

Symptoms

- Lateral lid swelling, pain, and tearing are features of dacryoadenitis (inflammation of the lacrimal gland).

Signs

- The lacrimal gland is swollen, tender, and erythematous (Fig. 14–8).
- Inferonasal globe displacement occurs.

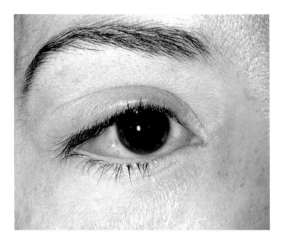

FIGURE 14–8 Acute viral dacryoadenitis. The superior temporal lid is erythematous, and the lid margin is S-shaped as a result of the underlying enlargement of the lacrimal gland.

Etiology

- Commonly, the inflammation is idiopathic.
- Less common inflammations include sarcoidosis, vasculitis, and Sjögren syndrome.
- Uncommonly, bacterial and viral infections (e.g., mononucleosis, mumps, herpes zoster) can lead to the disorder.

Differential Diagnosis

- Tumor of lacrimal gland should be ruled out or confirmed.

Workup

- Signs of bacterial or viral infection are sought.
- Signs of other inflammatory disorders are sought.
- A CT scan or an MRI study of the orbits is performed.
- A biopsy of the lacrimal gland is undertaken if indicated.

Treatment

- In cases of idiopathic inflammation, oral corticosteroids are administered.
- In cases of a specific inflammation the underlying disorder is treated.
- In cases of infectious agents the following apply:
  - Oral, broad-spectrum antibiotics (e.g., amoxicillin/clavulanate [Augmentin] 500 to 875 mg two times a day) is used for bacterial infection. If the patient is allergic to penicillin, oral erythromycin (250 to 500 mg 4 times a day) is administered.
  - In cases of viral infection, the underlying disorder is treated.

Follow-up

- A biopsy of the lacrimal gland is performed if the condition fails to resolve with appropriate therapy.

Canaliculitis

Symptoms

- Tearing, pain, and mucopurulent discharge are characteristic.

Signs

- Swelling and erythema are noted over the involved canaliculus (Fig. 14–9).
- Mucopurulent discharge results when digital pressure is applied over the involved canaliculus.

Etiology

- Infectious organisms that can lead to the disorder include *Actinomyces* species (most common) and *Streptomyces* species, which often are associated with stones in the canaliculus (dacryoliths).

Differential Diagnosis

Diagnostic possibilities include the following:
- Dacryocystitis
- Tumor

Treatment

- Curettage of the canaliculus is performed by an ophthalmologist to remove the stones.
- Surgical incision of the canaliculus (canaliculotomy) is performed to remove the stones.
- Nasolacrimal duct probing and irrigation confirm patency of the distal system.

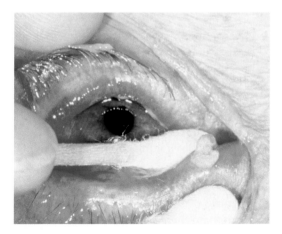

FIGURE 14–9 Canaliculitis manifests with conjunctivitis, inflamed and pouting punctum, and expressible discharge from the canaliculus.

Follow-up

* The focus of follow-up is on monitoring for recurrences, which are uncommon if the canaliculus was incised.

Thyroid Eye Disease

Symptoms

* In mild cases, irritation, burning, foreign body sensation, and tearing are characteristic.
* In moderate cases, double vision, aching discomfort, and blurred vision may be reported by the patient.
* In severe cases, symptoms progress to visual loss and pain from corneal ulceration.

Signs

* The onset is gradual.
* Lid retraction occurs, with superior or inferior scleral show (Fig. 14–10).
* The patient is unable to close the eyes (lagophthalmos).
* The disorder usually is bilateral, although often asymmetrical.
* Ocular motility is restricted (Fig. 14–11).
* Exophthalmos is evident (Figs. 14–10 and 14–12).
* Conjunctival blood vessels are dilated, especially over medial and lateral rectus muscles.

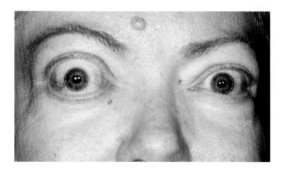

FIGURE 14–10 Exophthalmos and lid retraction are characteristic features of thyroid eye disease. Note the dilated conjunctival blood vessels over the medial and lateral rectus muscles.

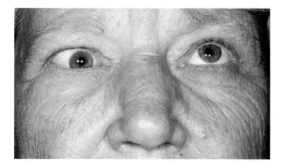

FIGURE 14–11 Severe ocular motility disturbance may result from thyroid eye disease. The patient is attempting to look up.

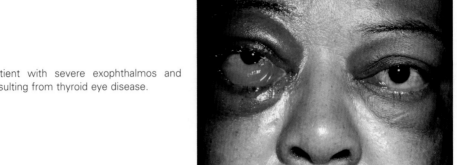

FIGURE 14–12 A patient with severe exophthalmos and orbital congestion resulting from thyroid eye disease.

- Swelling of the conjunctiva, lids, and brows is noted.
- A loss of visual acuity, visual field, and color vision occurs.

Etiology

- A thyroid abnormality can lead to ophthalmic disease.
  - Patient may be hyperthyroid, hypothyroid, or euthyroid when the orbital disease occurs.
  - Some patients have autoimmune thyroiditis (Hashimoto's disease).
  - Ophthalmic disease may precede or follow glandular disease by many years.
  - Most commonly, ophthalmic disease develops shortly after the patient undergoes treatment for hyperthyroidism.

Differential Diagnosis

Considerations in the differential diagnosis include the following:
- Conjunctivitis
- Orbital pseudotumor
- Myasthenia gravis
- Orbital tumor

Associated Factors and Diseases

- Ophthalmopathy remains active for an average of 2 years and much longer in some patients.

Workup

- A complete battery of thyroid tests is needed.
- Careful monitoring of the patient's thyroid status is performed if the findings on thyroid tests are normal.
- A CT scan or an MRI study is needed if the ophthalmic diagnosis is not completely confirmed (Fig. 14–13).

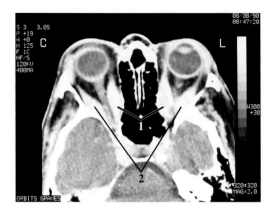

FIGURE 14–13 An axial CT scan of the head obtained in the patient in Figure 14–12 shows fusiform enlargement of the medial (1) and lateral (2) rectus muscles in both eyes, producing compressive optic neuropathy at the orbital apex.

- A thorough ophthalmologic examination and computerized visual field testing are performed to diagnose early visual loss and other sight-threatening conditions. Visual loss is caused by compression of the apical portion of the optic nerve (compressive optic neuropathy) by enlarged extraocular muscles.

Treatment

- In mild cases, artificial tears are used for lubrication.
- In moderate to severe cases, the following considerations apply:
  - The head of the bed is elevated to reduce congestion.
  - Oral prednisone (20 to 100 mg/day) is used to treat congestion, inflammation, and compressive optic neuropathy. Unfortunately, when the dosage is reduced, the ophthalmopathy flares again quickly. Oral prednisone usually is a temporizing therapy.
  - Orbital irradiation is performed for congestion, inflammation, and compressive optic neuropathy. This may shorten the overall course of the disease or decrease the severity. This therapy begins working in 1 month, and it may cause radiation retinopathy.
  - Orbital decompression is performed for congestion, compressive optic neuropathy, and exophthalmos. Beneficial effects may be noted within days. Ocular motility disturbances may worsen. Long-term side effects include sinusitis and facial paresthesias.
  - Eye muscle surgery (strabismus surgery) to correct double vision is performed after the disease is quiescent.
  - Repair of lid retraction is performed after the disease is quiescent or during the active phase if severe exposure is present.

Follow-up

- Ophthalmologic examination is needed every 3 to 6 months during the active phase and yearly thereafter to monitor for ophthalmopathy, which may recur.
- Visual field testing is performed as needed to exclude the possibility of compressive optic neuropathy.

Orbital Pseudotumor

Symptoms

- The acute variety, in which the onset occurs over hours to a few days, is the common form and involves severe pain, proptosis, visual loss, restricted ocular motility, malaise, and fatigue.
- The subacute to chronic variety, in which the onset occurs over weeks to months, is the uncommon form.
- Symptoms experienced depend on the location and rapidity of onset. In general, the more acute the onset, the more dramatic the symptoms.

Signs

- The disorder usually is unilateral.
- See Box 14–1 for classification.

BOX 14–1 Classification of Orbital Pseudotumor

Diffuse

- Generalized orbital involvement is characteristic (Figs. 14–14 and 14–15).

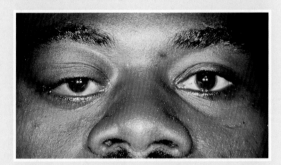

FIGURE 14–14 Diffuse orbital pseudo-tumor. The patient was a 30-year-old man who had a 2-day history of pain, proptosis, motility restriction, and visual loss involving the right eye.

BOX **14–1**   **Classification of Orbital Pseudotumor** (Continued)

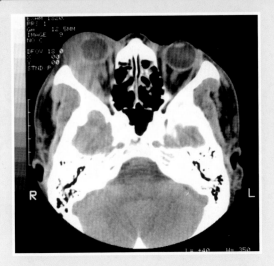

FIGURE 14–15   An axial CT scan of the head obtained in the patient in Figure 14–14 shows diffuse orbital inflammation on the right side.

Posterior Tenonitis

- The inflammation is restricted to the posterior half of the connective tissue surrounding the globe (Tenon's capsule) (Figs. 14–16 and 14–17).

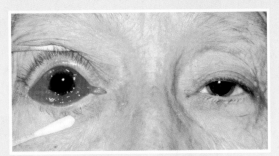

FIGURE 14–16   Orbital pseudotumor, posterior tenonitis. The patient was an 86-year-old woman who had a 3-day history of pain, lid and conjunctival swelling, and visual loss involving the right eye.

BOX **14–1** **Classification of Orbital Pseudotumor** (Continued)

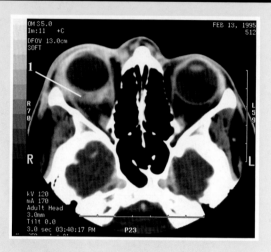

FIGURE 14–17 An axial CT scan of the head obtained in the patient in Figure 14–16 shows that the inflammation is restricted to the posterior Tenon's capsule (1) of the right eye.

Orbital Myositis

• The inflammation is restricted to one or a few extraocular muscles (Figs. 14–18 and 14–19).

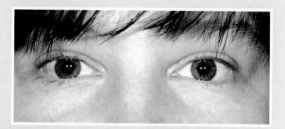

FIGURE 14–18 Orbital pseudotumor, myositis. The patient was a 30-year-old woman with a 1–week history of double vision and pain in the left eye.

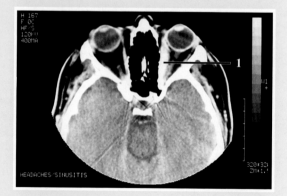

FIGURE 14–19 An axial CT scan of the head obtained in the patient in Figure 14–18 shows orbital myositis involving the left medial rectus muscle (1).

BOX 14–1 Classification of Orbital Pseudotumor (Continued)

Dacryoadenitis
• The inflammation is restricted to the lacrimal gland (Figs. 14–20 and 14–21).

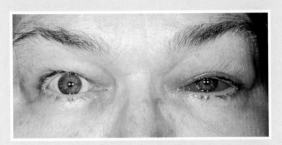

FIGURE 14–20 Orbital pseudotumor, dacryoadenitis. The patient was a 64-year-old woman with a 1–month history of pain, swelling, and erythema of the left eye unresponsive to oral antibiotics and topical corticosteroid drops.

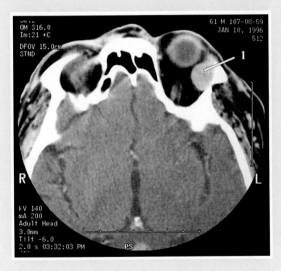

FIGURE 14–21 An axial CT scan of the head obtained in the patient in Figure 14–20 shows enlargement of the left lacrimal gland (1).

Etiology
• The origin of the disorder is idiopathic.

Differential Diagnosis
Diagnostic possibilities include the following:
• Thyroid eye disease
• Specific orbital inflammation (e.g., sarcoidosis, vasculitis)
• Orbital cellulitis
• Orbital tumor

Workup

- A biopsy often is necessary, because orbital pseudotumor is a diagnosis of exclusion. Polymorphous inflammatory cell infiltrate with a variable degree of fibrosis is a characteristic finding on examination of the biopsy specimen.
- A CT scan or an MRI is indicated.
- The diagnosis of orbital pseudotumor is made when other causes of these symptoms are highly unlikely.

Treatment

- Prednisone (80 to 120 mg/day) is administered and tapered over 4 to 8 weeks. This corticosteroid regimen usually gives rapid (1 to 3 days) and permanent resolution of symptoms.
- Low-dose orbital radiation (20 to 30 Gy) is an acceptable alternative if the patient relapses after corticosteroids are tapered (uncommonly) or if the patient cannot take corticosteroids.
- Immunosuppression may be needed with cyclophosphamide (Cytoxan), azathioprine (Imuran), or cyclosporine if the patient fails to respond to corticosteroids and radiation therapy, which is a rare occurrence.

Follow-up

- The disorder rarely recurs.

CHAPTER 15

Systemic Disease and Therapies

EMMETT F. CARPEL

Systemic Diseases

Certain systemic diseases are characteristically associated with ocular manifestations or carry an increased risk of ophthalmic complications.

Ankylosing Spondylitis

Ankylosing spondylitis is an immune-mediated disease with arthritis as its major manifestation. The rheumatic changes involve the sacroiliac and vertebral joints. The incidence of the disorder is higher in males than in females. The ocular manifestation is anterior uveitis.

Symptoms

- Vision is decreased.
- Pain is characteristic.
- A burning sensation is reported.
- Brow ache also occurs.
- Light sensitivity is noted.

Signs

- Perilimbal injection is evident.
- Cells and flare usually are seen on slit lamp examination.
- Pupils may be small.

Treatment

- Patients should be referred to an ophthalmologist.
- Cycloplegia and topical corticosteroids are used for anterior uveitis.
- The ocular prognosis generally is very good.

Behçet's Disease

Behçet's disease is a systemic vasculitis of small blood vessels with major mucocutaneous and ophthalmic manifestations. The diagnosis is based on presence of oral ulcers, which are the most consistent clinical sign, genital ulcers, uveitis or retinitis, and characteristic skin lesions (erythema nodosum). Arthritis and neurologic involvement also are features of this disease.

Symptoms

- Pain, redness, and light sensitivity accompany anterior uveitis if present.
- Vision is decreased if the retina or optic nerve is involved.

Signs

- In cases of anterior uveitis, conjunctival injection, anterior chamber cells and flare, corneal cellular precipitate, and an accumulation of white cells in the anterior chamber (hypopyon) are seen on examination.
- Retinal vasculitis occurs.
- Optic nerve atrophy can occur (Fig. 15–1).

Treatment

- Patients should be referred to an ophthalmologist.
- Cycloplegia and topical corticosteroids are administered.
- Systemic immunosuppression may be necessary for retinal or systemic vasculitis.

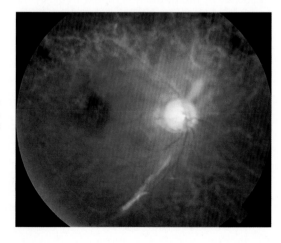

FIGURE 15–1 End-stage retinal disease in Behçet's disease, resulting from recurrent retinal vascular occlusive episodes. Note markedly attenuated retinal vessels, fibrosis, and optic atrophy.

- Systemic corticosteroids, cyclosporine, azathioprine, and a combination of azathioprine and cyclophosphamide have been used for treatment.
- The prognosis is poor even with aggressive treatment. Severe vasculitis may lead to a loss of vision.

Dermatomyositis

Dermatomyositis is a collagen-vascular disease that primarily involves the skin and muscle. It is an immune complex–mediated vasculopathic disorder and may occur with other collagen diseases such as rheumatoid arthritis, systemic lupus erythematosus, scleroderma, and polyarteritis nodosa. Muscle weakness, especially of the proximal limb muscles, may develop over weeks or may be of acute onset. Muscle pain may be present.

Symptoms

- Usually no ocular symptoms are noted.
- Pain, redness, and light sensitivity accompany anterior uveitis if present.

Signs

- A heliotrope discoloration of upper eyelids often is present in patients with telangiectasia (Fig. 15–2).
- Periorbital and conjunctival edema are reported.
- Anterior uveitis is rarely found.
- Retinopathy may manifest as cotton-wool spots.
- Hemorrhages, variable pigmentation of the fundus, and optic atrophy caused by occlusive vasculitis are rare findings.

Treatment

- No specific ocular therapy is necessary unless anterior uveitis is present.
- The ocular prognosis generally is good.

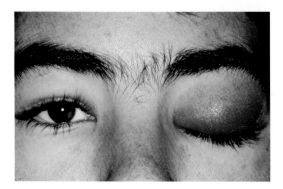

FIGURE 15–2   The violaceous discoloration on the upper lid is a heliotrope rash, a manifestation of telangiectasia, in this case associated with dermatomyositis.

Diabetes

Diabetes is a metabolic vasculopathy in which permanent visual loss is possible and typically results from retinal vascular disease. (For a more detailed description of diabetic retinopathy, see Chapter 10.)

Symptoms

- Patients have no symptoms until retinopathy is advanced.
- A sudden change in visual acuity occurs; most often, the patient becomes nearsighted.
- A sudden, painless visual loss is associated with vitreous hemorrhage from retinal neovascularization.
- A gradual visual loss often is due to cataracts or macular edema.
- A sudden, painful visual loss is associated with neovascular glaucoma.

Signs

- A change in the refractive error occurs (i.e., glasses need to be stronger or weaker).
- Small, poorly reactive pupils (pseudo–Argyll Robertson pupils) are observed.
- Cortical spokes (Fig. 15–3) or snowflake-type cataracts are evident.
- Retinal hemorrhages, exudates, microaneurysms, neovascularization, and vitreous hemorrhage may be other findings (see Chapter 10).

Ehlers-Danlos Syndrome

Symptoms

- No ocular symptoms are present.
- Vision loss may result as a complication of angioid streaks.

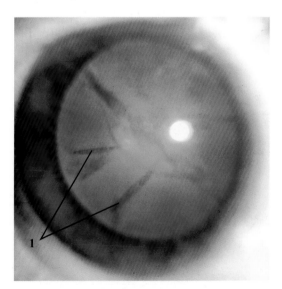

FIGURE 15–3 Spokelike clefts in the lens cortex (1). Cataracts may occur at an earlier age in patients with diabetes than in the general population.

Signs

- Angioid streaks are found in the retina adjacent to the optic disc (Fig. 15–4). Retinal bleeding may occur as a result of these streaks. Other causes of angioid streaks include sickle cell disease, Paget's disease of the bone, lead poisoning, and other collagen or connective tissue disorders such as Weill-Marchesani syndrome and pseudoxanthoma elasticum.

- Extreme thinning of the cornea (keratoglobus) can occur with Ehlers-Danlos syndrome type VI (Fig. 15–5).

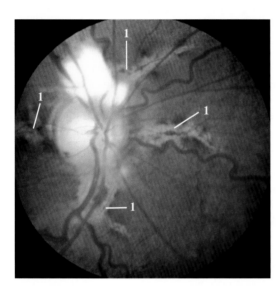

FIGURE 15–4 Ehlers-Danlos syndrome: Angioid streaks (1). These irregular, hypopigmented lines are a result of degeneration and breaks in Bruch's membrane. Angioid streaks also are seen in pseudoxanthoma elasticum, sickle cell disease, and Paget's disease (osteitis deformans).

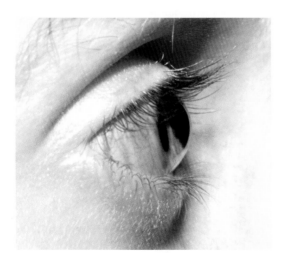

FIGURE 15–5 Ehlers-Danlos syndrome: Blue sclera. This syndrome is characterized by poor cross-linking of collagen, resulting in joint hypermobility, skin hyperextensibility, easy bruising, and a propensity toward tissue rupture. The apparent blue coloration of the sclera results from thinning of the sclera.

Treatment

- No specific ocular treatment exists. With sudden visual loss resulting from subretinal neovascular membrane associated with angioid streaks, laser photocoagulation may be indicated.
- Patients with extremely thin corneas (keratoglobus) must wear safety glasses at all times, because minor trauma can result in globe rupture and blindness.

Human Immunodeficiency Virus Infection

The human immunodeficiency virus (HIV) is a retrovirus that destroys the cells of the body's immune system, resulting in a host of systemic and ophthalmic problems.

Molluscum Contagiosum

Molluscum contagiosum is characterized by the presence of nodular, umbilicated lesions often up to 2 to 3 mm in diameter (see Fig. 4–18). This condition occurs more often in HIV-infected patients, and lesions are seen on the eyelids in many cases. They can cause a chronic conjunctivitis. Treatment usually focuses on evacuating the contents of the crater, but simple excision probably is a more definitive treatment.

Herpes Zoster Ophthalmicus

Herpes zoster ophthalmicus is seen with increased frequency in young adults with HIV infection, and it may be the initial sign of HIV infection. It typically begins with a rash or vesicles in the distribution of the fifth cranial nerve (see Fig. 6–9). Signs of ocular involvement include corneal inflammation, glaucoma, and uveitis. The eye abnormalities may progress as the skin lesions resolve. (For treatment, see Chapter 6.)

Kaposi's Sarcoma

Kaposi's sarcoma is a bluish-purple vascular tumor frequently seen on the eyelid or conjunctiva in HIV-infected patients. These lesions usually are painless and discrete and may appear as flat patches, elevated papules, or raised nodules. When the lesions occur on the conjunctiva, the disorder initially may manifest as a hemorrhagic conjunctivitis, most commonly occurring inferiorly (Fig. 15–6). Treatment options include surgical excision, cryotherapy, radiotherapy, and chemotherapy, or no treatment may be implemented.

Cotton-Wool Spots

Cotton-wool spots are the most common ocular finding in early HIV-related retinopathy. The lesion is a nerve fiber layer infarct caused by a microvasculopathy. HIV-related cotton-wool spots appear identical to such spots seen in patients with diabetes or hypertension (see Fig. 10–10). Distinguishing between cotton-wool spots and very early cytomegalovirus retinitis may be difficult; observation leads to the correct diagnosis. No specific treatment of cotton-wool spots is indicated.

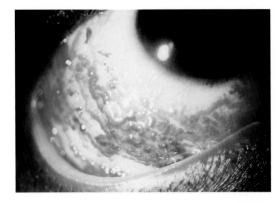

FIGURE 15–6 Kaposi's sarcoma mimics subconjunctival hemorrhage or hemangioma, but the nodularity and thickness of the vessels are distinctive.

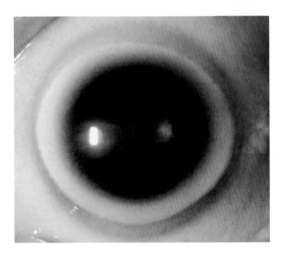

FIGURE 15–7 Arcus senilis. A heavy deposition of lipid in the peripheral cornea at a young age (i.e., before the age of 50 years) may be associated with hyperlipidemia. Arcus usually occurs as a normal aging change.

Cytomegalovirus Retinitis

See Chapter 10 for a discussion of ophthalmic disease associated with cytomegalovirus infection.

Hyperlipidemia

Symptoms

- Usually no symptoms are present.

Signs

The following signs may be associated with hyperlipidemia, but not invariably so:
- Heavy arcus of the cornea (especially in patients younger than 50 years of age) (Fig. 15–7)
- Xanthelasma (especially in those younger than 50), although in most cases the xanthelasma is not associated with increased lipids (see Fig. 4–11)

- Lipid deposition in the retina (lipemia retinalis)—a rare finding that may be seen when serum triglyceride levels exceed 2500 mg/mL

Treatment

- Systemic treatment of hyperlipidemia is given if indicated.
- Areas of xanthelasma may be excised for cosmetic purposes.
- Lipid deposition in the retina usually resolves when the triglyceride levels are normalized.

Hypertension

Symptoms

- Usually no symptoms are present.
- With malignant hypertension, blurred vision, blind spots, and visual loss are possible.

Signs

Ocular Manifestations

- Externally, no signs are noted.
- Retinal findings include focal narrowing of retinal arterioles or general vessel narrowing, light reflex changes, nerve fiber layer hemorrhages, and cotton-wool spots (see Chapter 10).

Additional Signs with Malignant Hypertension

- Papilledema is evident.
- Lipid exudates are found in a star configuration (Fig. 15–8).
- Macular edema occurs.

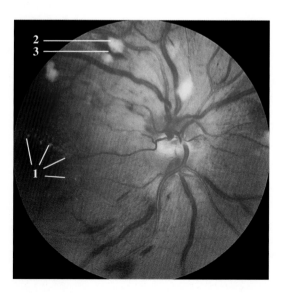

FIGURE 15–8 Advanced hypertensive retinopathy. Lipid deposits in the macula (1), cotton-wool spots (2), small flame hemorrhages (3), vascular light reflex changes, venous tortuosity, and early disc edema are present.

Treatment

- The elevated blood pressure is treated.

Inflammatory Bowel Disease

Inflammatory bowel disease, most notably Crohn's disease, and ulcerative colitis may be associated with ocular abnormalities in the anterior segment of the eye.

Symptoms

- Pain and redness are noted if episcleritis or scleritis is present.
- Pain, light sensitivity, and redness are noted if anterior uveitis is present.

Signs

- In cases of episcleritis and scleritis, local or diffuse scleral injection is observed.
- In cases of anterior uveitis, perilimbal injection, anterior chamber cell and flare, and corneal cellular precipitates are findings.
- Limbal corneal infiltrates may not stain with fluorescein and usually occur adjacent to an area of scleritis (Fig. 15–9).
- Cataracts are possible if the patient has been taking systemic corticosteroids for long periods.
- Dry eye and night blindness are possible findings in severe cases and are secondary to vitamin A deficiency with malabsorptive states.

Treatment

- Patients should be referred to an ophthalmologist.
- Topical corticosteroids and cycloplegics help control inflammation of the cornea or in the anterior chamber.
- Scleritis and associated limbal corneal infiltrates may respond to topical corticosteroids, but in some cases, systemic immunosuppression (e.g., with oral corticosteroids) is needed.

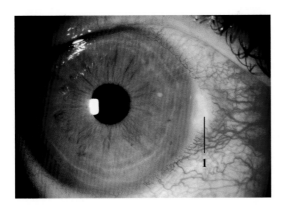

FIGURE 15–9 Sclerokeratitis (1) in a patient with Crohn's disease.

Marfan Syndrome

Marfan syndrome is a connective tissue disorder of autosomal dominant inheritance with ocular, skeletal, and cardiovascular manifestations. The basic defect is in collagen (fibrillin deficiency).

Symptoms

- Monocular diplopia occurs.
- A painless decrease in vision is noted.
- Fluctuating vision occurs.

Signs

- A subluxation or luxation of the lens, usually upward, occurs and is best seen on dilated examination (to allow visualization of the edge of the lens with a slit lamp) or occasionally on gross examination (Fig. 15–10). A tremulousness of the iris known as *iridodonesis* may indicate a lack of normal lens support.
- Glaucoma may be an associated finding.
- The axial length of the eye increases, resulting in myopia.

Treatment

- Contact lenses are prescribed if the luxated lens is out of the visual axis.
- Lens extraction is performed if the luxated lens obstructs the visual axis.

Mucopolysaccharidoses

The mucopolysaccharidoses are a group of lysosomal storage diseases caused by a deficiency of the enzymes that degrade glycosaminoglycans. Subtypes are categorized by enzyme deficit, inheritance pattern, and clinical features.

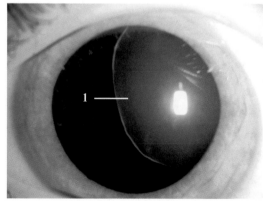

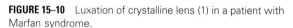
FIGURE 15–10 Luxation of crystalline lens (1) in a patient with Marfan syndrome.

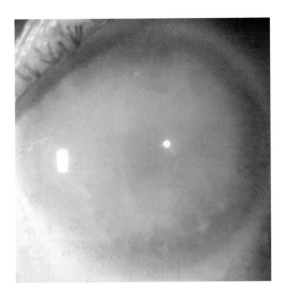

FIGURE 15–11 Diffuse corneal clouding in Maroteaux-Lamy syndrome, a disorder of mucopolysaccharide metabolism with an autosomal recessive pattern of inheritance.

Symptoms

- Central vision is poor.
- Night vision is poor.

Signs

- Corneal clouding is due to the presence of diffuse, fine punctate opacities in the stroma that are homogeneous and bilateral (Fig. 15–11).
- Depending on the type of storage disease, a pigmentary retinopathy may be manifested as a salt-and-pepper appearance of the retina.
- Papilledema and optic atrophy are possible findings.
- Glaucoma often is an associated disease.

Treatment

- No specific treatment for the eyes is prescribed.
- With extreme corneal clouding, corneal transplantation may be performed.
- Prognosis varies with the subtype of mucopolysaccharidosis.

Myotonic Dystrophy

Myotonic dystrophy is a disorder of autosomal dominant inheritance that involves body musculature with significant associated ophthalmic abnormalities.

Symptoms

- Foreign body sensation, tearing, and a burning sensation are noted with corneal drying and exposure due to the disease.

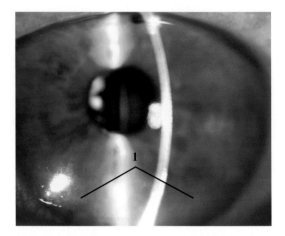

FIGURE 15–12 Exposure keratopathy (1) in a patient with myotonic dystrophy.

- Double vision results from extraocular muscle involvement.
- Vision is decreased if cataracts are present.

Signs

- Ptosis and weakness of the orbicularis muscles are characteristic ocular findings.
- Pupils are sluggishly reactive.
- The cornea may demonstrate fine punctate fluorescein staining caused by poor blinking, exposure, or decreased lacrimal secretions (Fig. 15–12).
- Iridescent flecks or metachromatic granules are found in the lens. Cortical cataracts also may be seen.
- Defective eye movements and ophthalmoplegia occur.
- Intraocular pressure is low.
- The macula and retinal periphery display fine pigmentary granules.

Treatment

- Ocular treatment includes lubrication with preservative-free artificial tears and ophthalmic lubricating ointments at bedtime.
- Surgery is performed for correction of ptosis and removal of cataracts when indicated.
- **Note:** Patients with myotonic dystrophy are at increased risk for complications from general anesthesia when muscle relaxants are used, and the anesthesia team should be made aware of the diagnosis.
- The prognosis for retention of vision is good.

Neurofibromatosis (von Recklinghausen's Disease)

Neurofibromatosis is a disorder of autosomal dominant inheritance that may be associated with significant ophthalmic involvement.

Symptoms

- Ocular symptoms typically are absent.
- Excessive tearing secondary to lid abnormalities may occur.
- A painless loss of vision is secondary to glaucoma or optic nerve glioma.

Signs

- Neuromas of the lid, often a plexiform neuroma, are found.
- Regional gigantism includes enlargement of the globe (buphthalmos) and also may be associated with congenital glaucoma.
- The iris may display an increased number of nevi or Lisch nodules, which are smooth, round, and translucent (Fig. 15–13).
- Optic atrophy may be caused by glaucoma or optic nerve glioma.

Treatment

- When the diagnosis of systemic disease is made, the patient should undergo a baseline ophthalmologic examination even if symptoms currently are absent.
- Elevated intraocular pressure is addressed if present.
- Plastic surgery may be indicated for disfiguring cosmetic problems.
- The ocular prognosis generally is good. Vision loss secondary to optic nerve glioma or glaucoma may occur.
- Neuroimaging should be performed with progressive optic atrophy to rule out optic nerve glioma.
- Excision of the tumor (and optic nerve) is indicated when the tumor enlarges in a blind eye without chiasmal involvement. When the tumor involves the chiasm, radiotherapy is used.

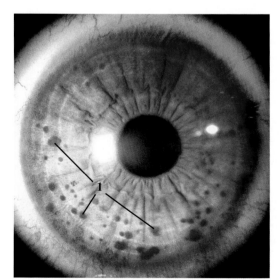

FIGURE 15–13 Lisch nodules (1) in a patient with neurofibromatosis.

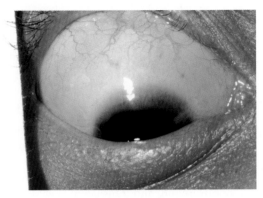

FIGURE 15–14 Osteogenesis imperfecta is an inherited disorder characterized by bone fractures, deafness, and blue sclerae.

Osteogenesis Imperfecta

Osteogenesis imperfecta is a heritable disorder of connective tissue with skeletal, ear, and eye manifestations. The several subtypes are classified by degree of involvement.

Symptoms

- No ocular symptoms occur.

Signs

- The major ocular sign is a blue sclera (Fig. 15–14). The color may be slate to dark blue, depending on the thickness of the sclera.
- Corneal thinning (keratoglobus) may occur.
- Congenital glaucoma may be associated with this disorder.
- Optic atrophy may be found secondary to skull fractures with nerve compression.

Treatment

- No specific ocular therapy is indicated.
- The ocular prognosis generally is very good.

Polycythemia Vera

Polycythemia vera is a blood disorder in which blood volume, blood viscosity, and the absolute number of red blood cells (RBCs) are increased, with resultant decreased blood flow.

Symptoms

- No symptoms may be present.
- Redness results from vascular congestion in the conjunctiva.
- Episodic blurring of vision is caused by retinal hemorrhages.
- A painless loss of vision may result from optic nerve involvement or central retinal vein occlusion.

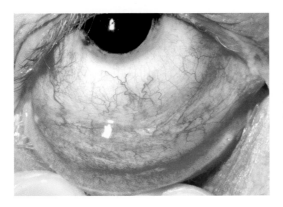

FIGURE 15–15 With polycythemia vera, engorged blood vessels of conjunctiva give rise to patient reports of redness of the eyes.

Signs

- Vascular congestion may be found, and prominent conjunctival vessels may mimic chronic conjunctivitis (Fig. 15–15).
- Hyperemia of the disc and a dark-purplish hue of the fundus may be seen.
- Scattered deep retinal hemorrhages and papilledema may be observed.
- In rare cases, the disorder is associated with central retinal vein occlusion.

Workup

- Retinal examination shows darkening, dilation, and tortuosity of the retinal veins; retinal arteries may appear normal.

Treatment

- Treatment is systemic, without any specific ocular therapy.

Reiter Syndrome

Reiter syndrome is defined by three associated problems: arthritis, urethritis, and eye inflammation (conjunctivitis and/or anterior uveitis). Mucocutaneous lesions frequently occur.

Symptoms

- Nonspecific irritation and a burning sensation are characteristic.
- Pain, redness, and light sensitivity are noted if anterior uveitis is present.
- Pain and redness are noted if episcleritis or scleritis is present.

Signs

- With conjunctivitis, a nonspecific conjunctival injection without a significant follicular or papillary response is found. A watery, mucoid discharge also may occur.
- With uveitis, perilimbal injection is noted, and cells and flare may be seen on slit lamp examination.

- With episcleritis or scleritis, which are extremely rare, sectoral or diffuse scleral injection is noted.

Treatment

- For conjunctivitis, no specific therapy is indicated. Artificial tears may be used for comfort.
- For iritis, cycloplegic agents and topical corticosteroids are administered.
- The ocular prognosis generally is excellent.

Rheumatoid Arthritis

Rheumatoid arthritis is a systemic, multisystem collagen-vascular disease associated with inflammatory joint pain. It also may cause infiltration and scarring of the salivary and lacrimal glands. The arthritis is polyarticular and usually symmetrical and affects adults in middle age, with a higher incidence in women than in men.

Symptoms

- A foreign body/burning sensation is noted if dry eye is present.
- Vision loss may occur.

Signs

- A dry eye with punctate staining of the corneal epithelium is noted (see Fig. 6–4).
- If present, scleral thinning is slow in onset and painless without inflammation (scleromalacia perforans; see Fig. 7–6), or with active inflammation and pain (necrotizing scleritis; Fig. 15–16).
- Corneal thinning may be found adjacent to the scleral inflammation (Fig. 15–17). These ulcerated areas may progress to perforation.

Treatment

- Lubricants, especially preservative-free artificial tears, are used.
- Punctal occlusion to increase tear film volume is performed by an ophthalmologist.

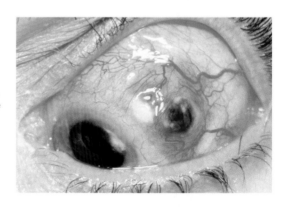

FIGURE 15–16 Necrotizing scleritis in rheumatoid arthritis. Active scleral inflammation surrounds an area of the tissue loss. Uveal tissue can be seen in the areas of scleral loss.

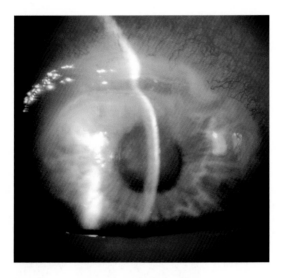

FIGURE 15–17   Peripheral corneal ulcer in rheumatoid arthritis. The cornea is markedly thinned, with corneal vascularization.

- Topical corticosteroids should not be prescribed because of the possibility of necrosis and perforation of the cornea.
- For corneal and scleral thinning, systemic immunosuppression usually is effective.
- Ocular perforation requires surgical repair.

Sarcoidosis

Sarcoidosis is a chronic granulomatous disease that is multisystemic and may directly or indirectly affect any part of the eye.

Symptoms

- Pain, redness, and light sensitivity accompany iritis if present.
- A foreign body sensation, dryness, and irritation are reported if dry eye is present.
- If the optic nerve is involved, if a vitreous hemorrhage is present (rare), or if a cataract is present, vision is decreased.
- Pain may be noted in the region of the lacrimal gland.

Signs

- A nodule (granuloma) may be present in the lids. Orbital inflammation may be manifested as lacrimal gland tenderness.
- Conjunctiva may display injection or nodules (Fig. 15–18).
- The cornea may show a fine punctate staining pattern after the instillation of fluorescein dye.
- Uveitis may manifest as cells on the endothelium or clumps of cells described as "mutton-fat" keratic precipitates (Fig. 15–19) and anterior chamber cell and flare. The iris may be adherent to the lens (posterior synechiae).
- Nodular lesions are possible on the iris.

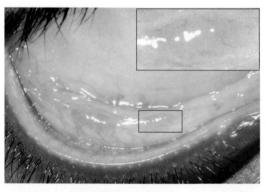
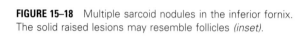

FIGURE 15–18 Multiple sarcoid nodules in the inferior fornix. The solid raised lesions may resemble follicles *(inset)*.

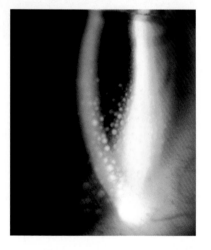

FIGURE 15–19 Granulomatous uveitis. "Mutton-fat" large keratic precipitates are seen on the corneal endothelium.

- The lens may have a cataract.
- The fundus may show inflammatory changes of the disc manifested as hyperemia or swelling.
- Candle wax–type drippings may be seen on the retinal surface in a linear pattern along the retinal veins.
- Retinal vasculitis with secondary retinal neovascularization may be a feature.
- Optic disc edema with infiltration of the optic nerve may be present.

Treatment

- This chronic disease requires ophthalmologist-monitored care.
- For uveitis, cycloplegia and topical and systemic corticosteroids are administered.
- The prognosis is good with mild to moderate inflammation. With severe or chronic involvement, however, band keratopathy, cataract, and glaucoma may lead to vision loss.
- Permanent vision loss usually is caused by glaucoma or optic neuropathy.

Sjögren Syndrome

Sjögren syndrome often is associated with rheumatoid arthritis and is the result of direct infiltration of inflammatory cells into the lacrimal and salivary glands. Dry eye (xerophthalmia) and dry mouth (xerostomia) are the dominant sequelae. This syndrome is seen most often with increasing age and is more common in women.

Symptoms

- Dry eye occurs.
- A foreign body sensation is reported.
- A burning sensation also is described.

Signs

- Mild conjunctival injection is noted.
- Keratoconjunctivitis sicca results in punctate fluorescein staining of the corneal epithelium (see Fig. 6–4).
- Mucous debris is found in the tear film.

Treatment

- Artificial tears, especially preservative-free preparations (e.g., hydroxypropyl methylcellulose [Bion Tears], polyvinyl alcohol [HypoTears PF], carboxymethyl-cellulose [Refresh Plus]) because they must be administered frequently, are used.
- Restasis, a low-dose cyclosporine (0.05%) in a preservative-free artificial tears solution, used twice a day, modulates inflammation in the lacrimal gland and may increase tear production. Many months of treatment may be required to see a benefit. Plasma cyclosporine levels need not be checked.
- Punctal occlusion is performed by an ophthalmologist.
- The eyelids are taped at night if a history of nocturnal lagophthalmos is reported. (**Note:** Sleeping with the eyes open is a relatively common phenomenon.)
- The ocular prognosis generally is good, but severe visual loss may occur with corneal necrosis. The patient's quality of life is significantly affected by the dryness, and continued attempts to maintain a moist environment are indicated (e.g., use of moisture chamber glasses or goggles).

Stevens-Johnson Syndrome

Stevens-Johnson syndrome (erythema multiforme) is an immunologically mediated syndrome that may occur in response to a microbial (e.g., herpes simplex virus) or pharmacologic (e.g., sulfonamide) agent. It is an immune complex vasculitis with inflammatory signs. When mucous membrane involvement dominates, Stevens-Johnson syndrome is the diagnosis.

Symptoms

- Eye pain is characteristic.
- Visual loss is noted.

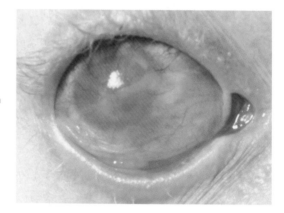

FIGURE 15–20 Conjunctival and corneal scarring are seen in this eye of a patient with Stevens-Johnson syndrome.

Signs

- Conjunctival hyperemia and eventually scarring are found.
- Eyelid closure is incomplete.
- The amount of tears decreases.
- Corneal epithelial defects stain readily with fluorescein and may progress to ulceration.
- Depending on the disease severity, the cornea may become dry and exposed because of conjunctival scarring and poor eyelid closure (Fig. 15–20).

Treatment

- Treatment includes eradication or cessation of the offending microbial or pharmacologic agent.
- In the acute stages, extremely frequent (i.e., every half to 1 hour) use of preservative-free tears (e.g., Bion Tears, HypoTears PF, Refresh Plus) is indicated. Even more effective and protective are lubricating, preservative-free ointments (e.g., Puralube, Refresh PM).
- Removal of offending eyelashes is indicated if trichiasis occurs.
- The use of topical and systemic corticosteroids is controversial.
- The disease usually resolves in 2 to 3 weeks.
- The visual prognosis is good unless severe corneal drying and ulceration have occurred.

Syphilis

The spirochete *Treponema pallidum*, which causes syphilis, leads to various systemic and ocular problems.

Symptoms

- Pain, light sensitivity, and redness are noted if iritis is present.
- Pain and redness are reported if episcleritis or scleritis is present.

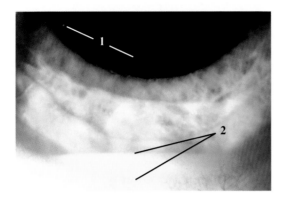

FIGURE 15–21 Syphilitic uveitis. Small cellular precipitates (1) on the posterior cornea and a layered hypopyon (2) are seen.

- Vision is decreased or visual field changes occur if the retina or optic nerve is involved.

Signs

- Iritis manifests as perilimbal injection, anterior chamber cells and flare, corneal cellular precipitates (Fig. 15–21), and a possibly engorged iris vasculature.
- Sectoral or diffuse scleral injection occurs with episcleritis and scleritis.
- Vasculitis may be seen in the retina with inflammatory changes adjacent to vessels.
- Swelling of the optic disc may ultimately lead to optic atrophy.
- An associated edema in a star-like pattern is found adjacent to the disc extending to the macula in cases of neuroretinitis.
- Classic Argyll Robertson pupils are noted. The pupils are poorly reactive or nonreactive to light but briskly reactive when the eye fixates on a near target.

Workup

- Rapid plasma reagin (RPR) and Venereal Disease Research Laboratory (VDRL) tests yield positive results early in the disease.
- The fluorescent treponemal antibody absorption (FTA-ABS) test is essential to detect active tertiary disease or previous infection. (**Note:** Most laboratories perform only the VDRL or RPR test unless the clinician insists on an FTA-ABS test.) If the result is positive and the patient has signs of tertiary disease, a neurologic evaluation with consideration of lumbar puncture is indicated. The HIV status should be checked in any patient with signs and symptoms of syphilis because syphilis is a frequent associated finding.

Treatment

- Systemic penicillin (or alternatives depending on patient allergy) is prescribed.
- Local ophthalmic treatment includes cycloplegia and topical corticosteroids for iritis, topical corticosteroids or oral nonsteroidal anti-inflammatory agents for episcleritis, and oral corticosteroids for scleritis.
- The ocular prognosis is excellent with early treatment.

Systemic Lupus Erythematosus

Systemic lupus erythematosus is a collagen-vascular disease that usually involves the skin, kidney, and eye but may affect any organ. Its manifestations result from immune-mediated vasculitis and necrosis of the small vessels and capillaries. Fibrin, immunoglobulins, and complement deposition take place in these structures.

Symptoms

- No ocular symptoms are present initially.
- Pain over the brow and redness are noted if scleritis is present.
- Foreign body sensation, burning, and dryness are noted if dry eye is present.

Signs

- Sectoral or diffuse injection and tenderness of the sclera occur with scleritis (Fig. 15–22).
- Dry eye displays fine punctate staining of the corneal epithelium with fluorescein dye.
- Usually no peripheral ulceration occurs in systemic lupus erythematosus, as is seen with rheumatoid arthritis.
- Retinopathy is manifested as cotton-wool spots.
- Blotchy retinal hemorrhages are found in the posterior pole.
- Roth spots, a retinal hemorrhage with a whitish center, are noted (see Fig. 10–26).

Treatment

- For surface ocular problems, artificial tears are used.
- For episcleritis, systemic nonsteroidal anti-inflammatory agents are administered. If no response occurs, topical corticosteroids may be used under the care of an ophthalmologist.
- For scleritis, systemic immunosuppression (primarily with corticosteroids) is used.

Thyroid Disease

For a discussion of thyroid-related eye disease, see Chapter 14.

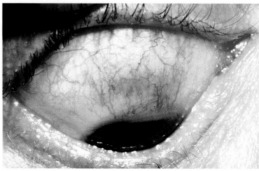

FIGURE 15–22 Focal episcleritis or scleritis in a patient with systemic lupus erythematosus.

Wegener's Granulomatosis

Wegener's granulomatosis is a necrotizing granulomatous vasculitis with multiorgan system involvement, affecting especially the eye, respiratory tract, and kidneys. The result of the cytoplasmic antineutrophil cytoplasmic antibody (c-ANCA) blood test often is positive.

Symptoms

- Pain, light sensitivity, and redness accompany iritis if present.
- Pain and redness are reported if scleritis or keratitis is present.

Signs

- In cases of iritis, perilimbal injection, anterior chamber cell and flare, and corneal cellular precipitates are found.
- In cases of scleritis, local or diffuse scleral injection or necrosis is present (Fig. 15–23). Keratitis and progressive marginal corneal inflammation and ulceration are additional findings (Fig. 15–24).

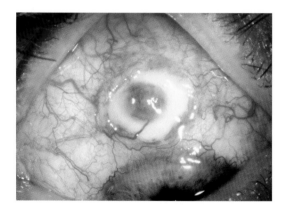

FIGURE 15–23 Wegener's granulomatosis: Necrotizing scleritis. A ring of avascular necrotic sclera surrounds an area of protruding uvea.

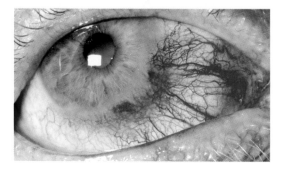

FIGURE 15–24 Wegener's granulomatosis: Peripheral sclerokeratitis.

Treatment

- Ocular treatment involves administration of cycloplegic agents and topical corticosteroids for associated iritis or episcleritis. Systemic nonsteroidal anti-inflammatory agents may be beneficial for scleritis. The mainstay of treatment involves administration of systemic corticosteroids and/or cytotoxic agents such as cyclophosphamide.
- This disorder is best managed by a team of physicians.
- The ocular prognosis is guarded because severe necrosis and vision loss may occur. Nevertheless, eye involvement often is controlled with aggressive systemic immunosuppressive therapy.

Wilson's Disease

Hepatolenticular degeneration results from a defect in copper metabolism that causes copper to be deposited in the liver and basal ganglia. A deficiency of ceruloplasmin in the blood leads to defective excretion of copper by the liver lysosomes.

Symptoms

- Normally, no eye complaints are reported.
- Blurred vision is possible in cases of advanced cataracts.

Signs

- The most notable ocular sign is presence of the Kayser-Fleischer ring, which is a gold-brown or blue-green peripheral corneal opacification resulting from the deposition of copper in Descemet's membrane (Fig. 15–25). Usually the superior and inferior aspects of the cornea are involved first. This feature may be seen in the absence of hepatic or neurologic disease, and gonioscopy may be required to identify early copper deposition.
- Copper deposition in the lens capsule causes a spokelike cataract ("sunflower cataract"). Usually no symptoms occur, and the cataract is best identified on dilated slit lamp examination.

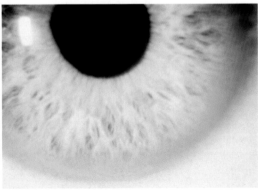

FIGURE 15–25 A Kayser-Fleischer ring in patient with Wilson's disease. The gold-yellow ring extends to the limbus without a clear interval.

Treatment

- Systemic penicillamine often is used. Ocular myasthenia may be a side effect of this treatment.
- With treatment, the ocular prognosis is excellent, and if the disease is diagnosed early, the systemic prognosis is vastly improved.
- The cataracts and Kayser-Fleischer ring may resolve with treatment.

Systemic Therapies

Use of any of various drugs may be associated with ophthalmic side effects.

Amiodarone Use

Amiodarone is used in the management of cardiac arrhythmias.

Symptoms

- No symptoms occur in the vast majority of patients.
- Vision loss or blurring may be noted if corneal changes are present.
- Rarely, sudden vision loss may occur with optic neuropathy.

Signs

- With long-term use, verticillate or stellate white-brown lines are found in the interpalpebral area of the corneal epithelium (Fig. 15–26).
- Rarely, disc edema with vision loss occurs.

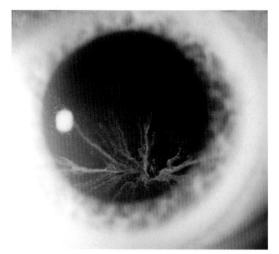

FIGURE 15–26 Amiodarone deposits in a typical serpiginous, whorl configuration in the corneal epithelium (cornea verticillata).

Differential Diagnosis

- Clinicians need to rule out any condition or use of any medication that produces a similar corneal epithelial line, such as Fabry's disease and use of chloroquine, hydroxychloroquine, indomethacin, and other nonsteroidal anti-inflammatory drugs (NSAIDs).
- See Chapter 12 for other causes of optic neuropathy.

Treatment

- With visual loss, a prompt ophthalmologic examination is recommended; the risk-to-benefit ratio may favor discontinuing the drug.
- The corneal changes are reversible, but some cases of optic neuritis may progress to permanent vision loss. The optic neuropathy may represent an ischemic optic neuropathy rather than a true toxic effect. The bilateral optic neuropathy has an insidious onset and slow progression and takes months to stabilize after the medication is discontinued. Regular ophthalmologic examinations (every 6 months) are recommended during amiodarone therapy.

Botox Use

Botulinum toxin type A (Botox), a neurotoxin derived from the organism *Clostridium botulinum*, acts at the neuromuscular junction to inhibit the release of acetylcholine. It is approved for use to treat essential blepharospasm, strabismus, and hemifacial spasm. It is widely used in plastic/cosmetic surgery for treating glabellar furrows and periorbital wrinkles. When injected in a muscle, it causes a functional denervation, inducing muscle relaxation. The duration of action typically is 3 to 4 months, but effects may last longer.

Symptoms

- Decreased visual acuity may result from ptosis of the eyelid and/or brow.
- Diplopia may occur.

Signs

- Ptosis may result.
- Extraocular muscle paresis is a possible effect.
- Loss of facial expression may occur.

Treatment

- The symptoms and signs resolve when the neuromuscular blockade wears off.
- Botox should be avoided in patients with neuromuscular disorders such as myasthenia gravis and myotonic dystrophy.

Chloroquine Use

Chloroquine hydrochloride is an antimalarial, amebicidal agent. In the past this drug was used for the treatment of collagen-vascular diseases, but at present it is seldom used because of the availability of hydroxychloroquine, which has much less ocular toxicity.

Symptoms

- No symptoms related to ocular discomfort are reported by the patient.
- Vision is blurred.
- Color vision defects are characteristic, initially in the blue-green region of color space and later in the red-green region.
- Focusing is difficult.
- Night blindness occurs.
- Blind spots (scotomata) are present in the visual field.
- Reading is difficult because words "disappear."

Signs

- Punctate or linear, whorl-shaped lesions are found in the corneal epithelium on slit lamp examination. These deposits may be seen early after treatment initiation. They usually are not visually significant.
- The retina displays mild pigment stippling of the macula, a decrease or loss of the normal foveal reflex, and if the disorder is progressive, a bull's-eye pattern maculopathy (Fig. 15–27). In extreme cases, optic atrophy with narrowing of the retinal arterioles and pigmentary changes in the retinal periphery may be seen.

Workup

- A baseline ophthalmologic examination, including visual acuity assessment, color vision testing, slit lamp examination, fundus examination, and examination of the central visual field, is needed.

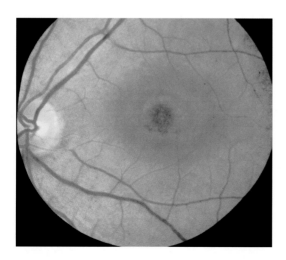

FIGURE 15–27 Chloroquine maculopathy, advanced. A well-defined bull's-eye pattern is evident.

Treatment

- The drug is immediately discontinued with any visual symptoms that are not explained by problems with accommodation.
- Chloroquine is thought to be safe at a dosage of 4.0 mg/kg lean body weight or less per day.

Follow-up

- An ophthalmologic evaluation is repeated every 3 months.

Corticosteroid Use

Symptoms

- Many patients are asymptomatic.
- Onset of blurred vision can be relatively acute, with refractive changes, or gradual, with cataractous changes.
- Headache and transient vision loss occur with pseudotumor cerebri.

Signs

- A refractive error change toward myopia results from corticosteroid-induced blood glucose changes (with systemic corticosteroids).
- Pseudotumor cerebri manifests as papilledema from increased intracranial pressure (systemic corticosteroids)
- Ptosis may occur.
- Intraocular pressure is increased (systemic and topical corticosteroids).
- A posterior subcapsular cataract is found (systemic and topical corticosteroids) (see Fig. 8–5).
- Corticosteroids may potentiate herpes simplex infection of the cornea or eyelids (systemic and topical corticosteroids).

Treatment

- A careful analysis of the risk-to-benefit ratio of topical and oral corticosteroids is needed.
- The intraocular pressure increase usually is reversible after discontinuation of corticosteroids. Cases of permanent increases in intraocular pressure have been reported, however.
- The cataractous changes are irreversible, and cataract surgery may be necessary.

Cytosine Arabinoside Use

Cytosine arabinoside (Cytarabine) is an inhibitor of DNA synthesis and when used systemically may be associated with ocular abnormalities.

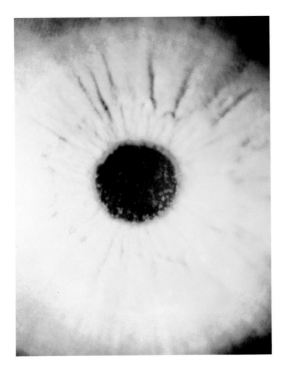

FIGURE 15–28 Magnified slit lamp view of multiple intra-epithelial cysts associated with use of the antimetabolite cytosine arabinoside (cytarabine).

Symptoms

- Vision is blurred.
- A foreign body sensation occurs.
- Light sensitivity is noted.

Signs

- Corneal epithelial cysts are found (Fig. 15–28).
- Hemorrhagic conjunctivitis is present.

Treatment

- Corneal lesions are reversible with cessation of medication.
- Administration of topical corticosteroid drops may prevent the hemorrhagic conjunctivitis and epithelial cysts, but their use should be regulated by an ophthalmologist.

Digoxin Use

Digoxin is a cardiac glycoside that causes ocular symptoms when blood levels of the drug are in the toxic range.

Symptoms

- Vision is blurred.
- Yellow-orange vision (xanthopsia) occurs.

Signs

- No signs are present.

Treatment

- The dosage is decreased to achieve proper therapeutic levels.

Ethambutol Use

Ethambutol is an antituberculosis medication that may have reversible or irreversible ocular toxicity.

Symptoms

- No symptoms related to ocular discomfort are reported by the patient.
- Visual acuity or visual field loss is noted.
- Color vision loss occurs.
- Paracentral blind spots (scotomata) are present.

Signs

- The optic nerve may appear normal.
- Optic atrophy occurs.

Workup

- A baseline ophthalmic examination should be performed before treatment and every 6 months thereafter.

Treatment

- The effects seem dose related, and ocular effects are almost never seen at dosages of 15 mg/kg per day and are rarely seen up to 25 mg/kg per day.
- The drug is immediately discontinued once changes in visual acuity, color vision, or visual field defects are documented. After discontinuation, the decrease in visual acuity may continue but often reverses after several months. The drug may be synergistic with isoniazid.

Isoniazid Use

Isoniazid (INH) is an antituberculosis medication that may produce reversible or irreversible ocular toxicity.

Symptoms

- No symptoms related to ocular discomfort are reported by the patient.
- Visual acuity or visual field loss is reported.
- Color vision loss occurs.
- Paracentral blind spots (scotomata) are present.
- Visual hallucinations (bright colors in bizarre patterns) or blurring of vision are early manifestations of overdosage.

Signs

- The optic nerve may appear normal.
- Optic atrophy occurs.

Workup

- A baseline ophthalmic examination is needed before treatment and every 6 months thereafter.

Treatment

- The effects seem dosage related, and ocular effects tend to occur when dosages exceed recommended levels (usually 300 mg/day).
- The drug is immediately discontinued once changes in visual acuity, color vision, or visual field defects are documented.

Phenothiazine Use

Virtually any phenothiazine can cause pigment deposition in the lens and cornea, although such changes are not visually significant. Thioridazine (Mellaril) is the most common phenothiazine associated with retinal findings, particularly at dosages greater than 800 mg/day.

Symptoms

- Dryness and photosensitivity may occur.
- Mild night visual dysfunction is possible.
- Vision is blurred.
- Color vision loss is reported.

Signs

- A fine, brown pigment dusting of the cornea or lens may be seen. This finding usually is subtle and requires experienced slit lamp–examination technique.
- Pigmentary retinopathy is found in the midperipheral retina. Advanced cases may involve the macula (Fig. 15–29).

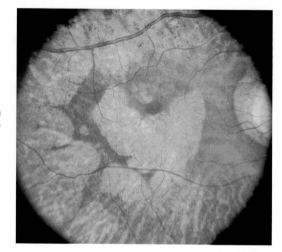

FIGURE 15–29 Advanced pigmentary changes in the macula and retinal periphery resulting from thioridazine (Mellaril) toxicity.

Treatment

- Pigment deposition in the cornea and lens is not visually significant and does not require a change in treatment.
- Thioridazine (Mellaril) is discontinued if signs or symptoms of retinal toxicity occur. Early retinal changes may be reversible.

Follow-up

- An annual ophthalmologic follow-up (every 6 months with Mellaril) is suggested.

Plaquenil Use

Hydroxychloroquine (Plaquenil) is used in the treatment of collagen-vascular disease. A host of ocular side effects have been reported with this drug, but in general, the incidence of ocular toxicity with Plaquenil is less than that with chloroquine. Most of the observable effects are in the cornea, which usually are reversible, and the retina, which may be reversible or permanent.

Symptoms

- No symptoms related to ocular discomfort are associated with Plaquenil use.
- Vision is blurred.
- Focusing is difficult.
- Night blindness occurs.
- Blind spots (scotomata) are present in the visual field.

Signs

- Punctate to linear, whorl-shaped lesions in the corneal epithelium may be seen on slit lamp examination. These deposits may be seen early after the patient begins medication but usually are not visually significant.

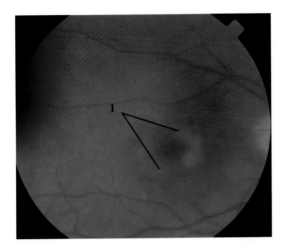

FIGURE 15–30   Plaquenil toxicity. Although rarely seen, retinal toxicity may occur with Plaquenil (hydroxychloroquine) use. In this case, a classic bull's-eye pattern of macular change (1) is evident. The daily dose used was greater than 7 mg/kg of lean body weight.

- The retina may show mild pigment stippling of the macula (Fig. 15–30) and a decrease or loss of the normal foveal reflex. If the effects are progressive, a bull's-eye pattern of maculopathy occurs in which pigment clumps are present centrally, surrounded by a ring of relative hypopigmentation encircled by a zone of relative hyperpigmentation. In extreme cases, optic atrophy, pallor of the disc with narrowing of the retinal arterioles, and pigmentary changes in the retinal periphery may be seen.

Workup

- A baseline ophthalmologic examination, including visual acuity assessment, color vision testing, slit lamp examination, dilated funduscopic examination, and examination of the central visual field, is indicated.

Treatment

- Ocular changes are virtually never seen with antimalarial prophylaxis but occur when the drug is used daily for treatment of systemic lupus erythematosus or rheumatoid arthritis. Recent evidence suggests that the *rate* of dosage is important; with a daily Plaquenil dose of 6.5 mg/kg (of ideal body weight) or less, retinopathy is virtually never seen.
- With early documented pigment changes on the retina or visual field changes, discontinuation of the drug may reverse any initial visual acuity or visual field effects. Rarely, visual field effects may progress after medication is discontinued. The frequency of retinal toxicity may increase in older age groups (60 years of age or older), but age-related macular degeneration changes also are more likely with increasing age.
- All patients should be advised to wear sunglasses (for ultraviolet light [UV] protection) and a hat with a brim in sunny climates, because light may play a role.
- Immediate evaluation of any patient with symptoms is indicated.

Follow-up

- The frequency of follow-up evaluations in patients taking Plaquenil is controversial. The manufacturer still recommends every 3 months. Many ophthalmologists, however, believe that the incidence of retinal findings is so rare with Plaquenil that every 6 months or even annual follow-ups are sufficient. Because the retinal changes may be reversible if found early and irreversible if found too late, a follow-up every 6 months appears reasonable in the usual patient who is symptom free.
- Thus, a recommended schedule for ophthalmic follow-up evaluation in a patient without symptoms who is taking Plaquenil is as follows:
  - *With low dosage* (e.g., 200 mg per day): once a year
  - *With usual dosage* (approaching but not exceeding 6.5 mg/kg [ideal body weight] per day): every 6 months
  - *With higher dosages* (greater than 6.5 mg/kg per day): every 3 to 4 months in most cases
  - *With decreased renal function:* downward adjustment of the dosage and evaluation of ocular status every 3 to 4 months
  - *With history of or concomitant gold or phenothiazine therapy:* adjustment of the dosage and monitoring of the ophthalmic status every 3 to 4 months, because the threshold for retinal toxicity may be lower

Tamoxifen Use

Tamoxifen is a nonsteroidal antiestrogen that may have asymptomatic or symptomatic ocular effects.

Symptoms

- No symptoms related to ocular discomfort occur.
- Vision is blurred or decreased.

Signs

- White subepithelial opacities are present in the cornea.
- Crystalline deposits are found in the retina, located in the paramacular area (Fig. 15–31).
- In rare cases, cystoid macular edema occurs.
- Optic neuritis, which may be dose related or idiosyncratic, may occur.

Treatment

- No treatment is indicated unless visual acuity changes are documented, in which case the drug is discontinued.
- Cornea lesions are reversible, but visual loss secondary to retinopathy may be permanent.
- Screening for retinopathy or optic neuropathy is not warranted, but any vision change should be evaluated by an ophthalmologist.

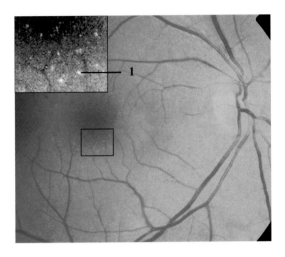

FIGURE 15–31   Tamoxifen deposition. White-yellow crystalline deposits are seen in the retina (1, *inset*).

Topomax Use

Topiramate (Topomax), a sulfa derivative, is used to treat epilepsy. It may idiosyncratically cause ciliary body swelling and forward movement of the lens and iris. The resultant bilateral angle-closure glaucoma is responsible for the ocular symptoms and signs.

Symptoms

- Acute onset of decreased visual acuity and/or ocular pain are important symptoms.
- The eye pain is often deep and periorbital.

Signs

- Sudden decrease in distance vision (acute myopia) is characteristic.
- Redness is observed.
- Pupils may be dilated and unreactive.
- Shallow anterior chamber is noted.
- Intraocular pressure is increased.

Treatment

- Discontinue Topomax as rapidly as possible.
- See treatment of acute angle-closure glaucoma in Chapter 11.

Viagra, Levitra, and Cialis Use

Viagra (sildenafil citrate), Levitra (vardenafil HCl), and Cialis (tadalafil) are selective inhibitors of phosphodiesterase 5 (PDE5) used to treat erectile dysfunction. PDE5 is the predominant phosphodiesterase in the smooth muscle cells of the corpus cavernosum. A closely related isozyme, phosphodiesterase 6 (PDE6), is present in high concentrations in the cone and rod cells of the retina.

Symptoms

- Transient impairment of blue-green discrimination may occur.
- Blue-color tinge to vision may be described by the patient.
- Sensitivity to light may be increased.

Signs

- No ocular signs are present.

Treatment

- No treatment is required, because all eye symptoms are transient.
- No evidence of ocular toxicity has been documented, nor have any effects on visual acuity or visual field.
- Because PDE5 does cross-react with PDE6, the theoretical risk of serious ocular side effects is increased in patients with retinitis pigmentosa, or other severe retinal diseases.

CHAPTER 16

Ocular Trauma

GEOFFREY BROOCKER • WAYNE A. SOLLEY

Periorbital or Ocular Contusion

Symptoms

- The patient relates a history of trauma to the eye or periorbital region.
- Periorbital erythema or ecchymosis is found superiorly and/or inferiorly and may involve the contralateral eye with dissection through tissue planes (Fig. 16–1).
- The patient reports minimal pain.
- The degree of periorbital edema varies.
- Vision is minimally decreased or blurred.

Signs

- Periorbital ecchymosis and edema are present.
- Uninflamed eye with no anterior chamber reaction is found unless iritis is present.
- Subconjunctival hemorrhage is possible.
- The eye shows full motility, with slight pain on eye movement possible.

Differential Diagnosis

Considerations in the differential diagnosis include the following:
- *In children*: child abuse
- *With bilateral ecchymoses in an infant*: child abuse or neuroblastoma
- Intraorbital neoplasm, such as hemangioma or lymphangioma, that has hemorrhaged
- *With mildly decreased visual acuity*: traumatic iritis or corneal abrasion
- *With markedly decreased visual acuity*: hyphema (an often-missed diagnosis if the hyphema is small), vitreous hemorrhage, traumatic optic neuropathy, or lens subluxation (Fig. 16–2)

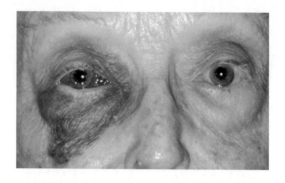

FIGURE 16–1 Periorbital contusion.

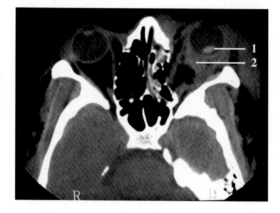

FIGURE 16–2 Orbital computed tomography scan showing sequelae of blunt orbital or ocular injury. The patient was struck with a can of soda, causing a dislocated lens (1), retrobulbar hemorrhage (2), and blow-out fracture of the medial orbital wall.

Workup

- A general examination is performed on both eyes; dilated examination is mandatory. The red reflex is examined through the dilated pupil to evaluate lens position and clarity.
- Plain x-ray films and/or computed tomography (CT) study of the orbit is needed if orbital fracture is suspected. Entrapment of orbital soft tissue in an orbital blow-out fracture often is seen clearly on CT scans.

Treatment

- If no severe ocular or periocular injury is evident, cool compresses are applied, and the patient is reassured. To avoid sports-related injury in a child, use of safety glasses or goggles should be encouraged.
- Nonemergency ophthalmologic follow-up is needed—specifically, a careful peripheral retinal examination. Trauma severe enough to cause substantial periorbital edema and ecchymosis can cause a tear in the retinal periphery that may not cause symptoms initially but may result in a delayed retinal detachment if not identified.
- Patients with evidence of hyphema should be immediately referred to an ophthalmologist.

Corneal Abrasion

Symptoms

- A history of mild trauma to the eye, possibly caused by a fingernail, tree branch, contact lens, make-up brush, or foreign body, is reported.
- Photophobia, conjunctival injection, and involuntary lid closure (blepharospasm) are characteristic.
- Pain and foreign body sensation may be quite severe.
- If the abrasion is in the central cornea, visual acuity is decreased (20/80 to 20/200).

Signs

- Conjunctival hyperemia, swollen eyelids, and tearing are noted.
- Slit lamp examination shows an epithelial defect but often an otherwise clear cornea. A surface irregularity may be identified with a penlight. Minimal cellular reaction is seen in the anterior chamber. If corneal haze or moderate to severe "flare and cell" is noted in the anterior segment, especially with an associated discharge, bacterial superinfection may be present.
- Fluorescein dye is absorbed by areas devoid of epithelium and outlines the defect (Fig. 16–3).
- Immediate relief is obtained with topical anesthesia (e.g., proparacaine, tetracaine). Topical anesthetics are used only to confirm the diagnosis and are not prescribed for long-term relief.

Differential Diagnosis

- Diagnostic considerations include the following:
  - Viral keratitis (herpes simplex or zoster), often with corneal dendrites (see Fig. 6–7)
  - Corneal or conjunctival foreign body, especially trapped on the conjunctiva under the upper lid, which can cause "ice-skate track" abrasions as the foreign body is repeatedly swept linearly over the corneal epithelium
  - Recurrent erosion, which is similar to a primary epithelial defect (abrasion) but occurs long after the initial corneal trauma, due to re-epithelialization healing problems (see Fig. 6–18)
  - Ultraviolet corneal injury (welder's flash, tanning booth exposure) (see Fig. 16–3)

Workup

- The area of denuded epithelium is documented. Location is important because any complications (infections) in the central portion of the cornea may have lasting visual consequences.
- The eyelids are everted to search for a foreign body, especially if the history is suggestive (e.g., glass from an automobile accident, vegetable matter from bark). Linear corneal abrasions should alert the examiner to flip the upper lid to look for the foreign body on the superior tarsal conjunctiva.

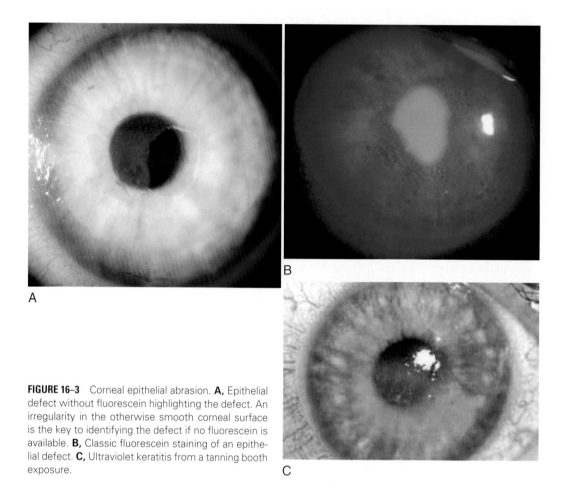

FIGURE 16–3   Corneal epithelial abrasion. **A,** Epithelial defect without fluorescein highlighting the defect. An irregularity in the otherwise smooth corneal surface is the key to identifying the defect if no fluorescein is available. **B,** Classic fluorescein staining of an epithelial defect. **C,** Ultraviolet keratitis from a tanning booth exposure.

Treatment

- For contact lens–associated corneal abrasions, see page 334.
- For non–contact lens–associated abrasions, the following apply:
  - A cycloplegic agent (e.g., homatropine 5% two to three times a day) is administered.
  - Antibiotic ointment appropriate for the injury is used. Polymyxin B/bacitracin (Polysporin) or erythromycin ophthalmic ointment twice a day and at bedtime is effective for most abrasions.
  - If the abrasion is large (more than 5 to 10 mm across) or the patient is in severe pain, cycloplegic drops and antibiotic ointment are instilled, followed by firm application of a pressure patch for 24 hours. (See Chapter 1 for proper patch application.) Although pressure patching promotes wound healing, the chance of infection is increased when a warm environment is created by the patching. In circumstances in which microbial contamination exists (especially in the setting of contact lens wear), use of a pressure patch is avoided.

○ Analgesia is given for pain; sometimes a narcotic analgesic is needed (e.g., acetaminophen plus codeine [Tylenol with Codeine]).
○ Under *no* circumstances should topical anesthetics be prescribed or given to the patient. Not only do anesthetics retard wound reepithelialization, but the loss of the cornea's normal pain response predisposes the patient to a much more severe injury.
○ Patients with a large central abrasion or high-risk abrasion should be referred to an ophthalmologist for management and follow-up care.

Follow-up

- All abrasions are monitored every day or two until they have completely resolved. If healing takes longer than 2 or 3 days, the patient should be referred to an ophthalmologist.
- Use of a pressure patch for more than 24 hours should be avoided. If patient compliance with follow-up is questionable, antibiotic ointment and cycloplegic drops are indicated to heal the abrasion without the added risk of patching.
- If visual acuity is markedly decreased (less than 20/400), more severe ocular injury needs to be ruled out, especially if the history suggests severe trauma.

Contact Lens Injury

Symptoms

- Pain, foreign body sensation, photophobia, tearing, and blepharospasm are noted immediately after insertion or removal of a contact lens.
- Blurred vision, conjunctival hyperemia, and pain during contact lens wear are characteristic. The presence of these symptoms on awakening suggests hypoxic corneal injury.

Signs

- Conjunctival hyperemia and ciliary flush, which is a manifestation of circumlimbal injection (redness around the corneoscleral junction), are noted.
- An epithelial defect is present if an abrasion exists.
- The contact lens is immobile and corneal edema is diffuse (in cases of tight lens syndrome or hypoxic corneal injury).

Etiology

- Direct trauma to the corneal epithelium with insertion or removal of the lens can result in injury.
- A foreign body between the lens and cornea can cause injury (Fig. 16–4).
- Hypoxic injury to the cornea results from improper contact lens fit, improper lens material for the patient's needs, or overwear by the patient (e.g., sleeping in a daily wear lens). While the patient sleeps, the oxygen available to the cornea is markedly decreased, and with a lens that is poorly oxygen-permeable, the corneal epithelium becomes hypoxic and edematous.
- Toxic product buildup in the contact lens can result in injury.

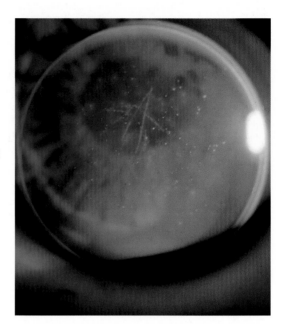

FIGURE 16–4 Foreign body between hard contact lens and cornea. Note the vertical "dust trails" or "ice skate tracks" caused by the vertically moving foreign body.

Differential Diagnosis

Diagnostic possibilities include the following:
- Early microbial keratitis (e.g., bacterial keratitis)
- Corneal or conjunctival foreign body
- Ultraviolet corneal injury

Workup

- A complete examination of both eyes, including slit lamp exam, fluorescein staining, and eversion of the lids to search for hidden foreign bodies, is indicated. Fluorescein is not used in an eye with the soft contact lens in place because the lens will absorb the fluorescein and turn green permanently. Hard or gas-permeable contact lenses do not turn yellow on fluorescein instillation.

Treatment

- The contact lens is removed; a specially designed suction cup can assist in removal of hard contact lenses. The patient is instructed not to wear the lens until the abrasion is completely healed (usually 10 to 14 days).
- If an abrasion exists, a topical ophthalmic solution/suspension/ointment that provides coverage for gram-negative organisms (e.g., gentamicin, tobramycin, ciprofloxacin) is administered frequently (e.g., four to six times a day with topical drops). Patients should be referred to an ophthalmologist for management, because a significant risk exists for gram-negative bacterial corneal infection (especially *Pseudomonas* infection) in soft contact lens wearers. Patches are not used, because

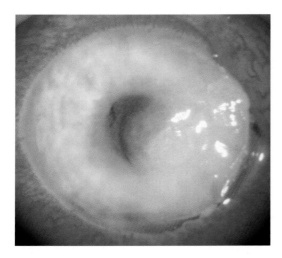

FIGURE 16–5 Extensive *Pseudomonas* bacterial corneal ulcer associated with soft contact lens wear.

any gram-negative infection can progress rapidly to corneal ulceration due to a more favorable microbial growth milieu.

- For overwear or tight lens syndrome, use of the contact lens is discontinued until the patient is assessed by an ophthalmologist; urgent referral may be indicated. Lens fit, oxygen permeability, and the overall health of the cornea must be addressed. Chronic hypoxia can lead to corneal neovascularization and scarring.

Follow-up

- For patients with abrasions, daily follow-up evaluation is mandatory.
- As a rule, contact lens–associated abrasions heal completely in a short time, although they may take longer than non–contact lens–associated abrasions. Management is fairly easy, but an error (e.g., patching in a contact lens wearer, inadequate follow-up, neglect of antibiotic coverage) can lead to severe corneal infection (ulceration) that threatens the ultimate visual outcome or even loss of the eye (Fig. 16–5).

Acute Ultraviolet Radiation Injury

Symptoms

- A history of welding or sunbathing (using an indoor sunlamp or tanning booth) without protective eyewear is reported.
- Moderate to severe pain is characteristic.
- Red eyes, tearing, blurred vision, photophobia, and blepharospasm are other complaints.
- Onset of symptoms occurs 6 to 12 hours after the activity; the patient often awakens with these symptoms the evening following the activity.

Signs

- Dense punctate staining of the cornea occurs on fluorescein instillation; the central cornea often is more involved than are the superior and inferior portions. (See Fig. 16–3.)
- Injection or edema of the eyelids is noted.
- Mild corneal edema or injected conjunctiva is evident.
- Minimal to no anterior chamber cell and flare may occur.

Differential Diagnosis

Considerations in the differential diagnosis include the following:
- Toxic epitheliopathy from drugs or chemicals, such as from overuse of ophthalmic solutions, even artificial tears, that contain preservatives; corneal anesthesia caused by topical anesthesic abuse (e.g., proparacaine, tetracaine); and exposure to crack cocaine smoke.
- Exposure keratopathy (e.g., thyroid eye disease, seventh nerve palsy, any lid abnormality causing poor closure), with particular attention to this possibility in obtunded/intubated patients in critical care units.
- Severe dry eye syndrome (usually sparing the upper portion of the cornea).

Workup

- A complete examination of both eyes, including fluorescein instillation and possibly lid eversion, is indicated.
- History should focus on recent welding or sunlamp use without eye protection.
- If no history of ultraviolet exposure is reported, use of topical medications or handling chemicals/drugs is addressed.

Treatment

- Cycloplegic agents (e.g., homatropine 5% two or three times a day) are administered.
- Antibiotic ointment (e.g., polymyxin B/bacitracin [Polysporin], erythromycin ointment two or three times a day) is applied.
- For severe ultraviolet keratopathy, pressure patching is bilateral if the patient has assistance. If this is not possible, the more affected eye is patched and antibiotic ointment is used in the less involved eye on a regular schedule.
- Systemic analgesics usually are needed.

Follow-up

- The patch is removed after 24 hours. If improvement is observed, antibiotic ointment use continues for an additional 2 to 3 days, and then symptoms should be resolved. If severe symptoms persist after 24 hours, the eye is repatched and reevaluated in 24 hours.
- Referral to an ophthalmologist usually is not needed unless the condition does not improve after 1 or 2 days.

- The prognosis is very good. The high absorption of ultraviolet rays in the corneal tissues usually protects the inner eye tissue from severe damage except with massive exposure. The lens is the next most susceptible tissue to injury but becomes cataractous only in cases of prolonged exposure to ultraviolet rays or markedly high levels of ultraviolet energy.

Subconjunctival Hemorrhage

Symptoms and Signs

- An acute, dense, "blood red" discoloration of the subconjunctival space often is noted on awakening (Fig. 16–6).
- The conjunctival appearance ranges from a flat, red, localized area with no chemosis of the conjunctiva to diffuse involvement (hemorrhagic discoloration completely covering the anterior sclera). Massive hemorrhagic conjunctival suffusion, possibly extending over the lid margin, is unusual unless there is associated significant trauma, tumor, or bleeding diathesis.
- The hemorrhage often appears after a Valsalva maneuver (e.g., coughing spells, straining with constipation, heavy lifting) is performed.

Etiology

- Blunt trauma that may seem insignificant can lead to the disorder.
- The disorder can result from rupture of small conjunctival vessels with a Valsalva maneuver.
- Microbial conjunctivitis (e.g., viral hemorrhagic conjunctivitis, adenoviral or pneumococcal conjunctivitis) is possible, especially if the disorder is associated with discharge or significant ocular discomfort.
- Hypertension, usually accelerated, can result in the disorder.
- The disorder can occur with a bleeding disorder, including those in patients using oral anticoagulants.
- Trauma to the globe and orbital periosteal injury are etiologic processes. Significant subconjunctival hemorrhage and a suggestive history should prompt inspection for

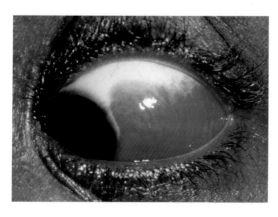

FIGURE 16–6 Subconjunctival hemorrhage. This usually results from minor trauma or Valsalva maneuvers and is benign. In the setting of severe traumatic injury, however, it may obscure a more significant injury to the globe.

possible orbital fracture. Zygomatic arch fracture should be suspected with a lateral subconjunctival hemorrhage that extends far posteriorly.

Differential Diagnosis

- Ruptured globe is considered, especially with trauma involving high-velocity projectiles (metal-on-metal or grinding injury) or a large subconjunctival hemorrhage, which may obscure a scleral rupture beneath the hemorrhage. A complete (360-degree) subconjunctival hemorrhage after blunt trauma may be a sign of retrobulbar blood that has progressed forward into the potential space between the conjunctiva and the globe. The posterior extent of the hemorrhage is therefore hidden. Fractures of the periorbital region or ruptured globe must be ruled out in these cases.
- Bleeding diathesis is a possible diagnosis, especially if multiple episodes of hemorrhage have occurred.
- Conjunctival or orbital neoplasm with associated hemorrhage is considered.
- Conjunctival Kaposi's sarcoma (reddish-purple subconjunctival mass) must be ruled out or confirmed.

Workup

- The history should focus on the possibility of abnormal bleeding/clotting, anticoagulant use, and any Valsalva maneuver (e.g., weightlifting, straining with constipation, severe coughing or strong sneezing [especially with chronic obstructive pulmonary disease or asthma]) or other cause of increased intraorbital venous pressure (e.g., scuba diving).
- If the history suggests the possibility of severe injury, a complete eye examination is needed; however, if globe rupture is suspected, only an ophthalmologist should attempt manipulation of the globe, including the measurement of the intraocular pressure.
- If the patient history details spontaneous, recurrent subconjunctival hemorrhage, complete blood count (CBC) and clotting studies are indicated.
- Blood pressure is measured.
- If a retrobulbar hemorrhage is suspected in a patient (usually in cases of blunt trauma), assessment of intraocular pressure, which can be markedly elevated, must be performed.

Treatment

- Reassurance of the patient is paramount; artificial tears help alleviate any surface discomfort. The patient is informed that the blood may take up to 2 weeks to clear.
- If clotting studies are abnormal (with recurrent spontaneous hemorrhage), referral for hematologic evaluation is necessary.
- If the hemorrhage is associated with trauma and a ruptured globe is possible, immediate referral to an ophthalmologist is indicated.

Follow-up

- The prognosis is excellent for a primary spontaneous subconjunctival hemorrhage. The patient is reevaluated in 2 to 3 weeks, if the hemorrhage does not clear or recurs.

Conjunctival Foreign Body

Symptoms

- A foreign body sensation, tearing, red eye, ocular irritation, and sharp pain are characteristic.
- A history of working underneath a car, boat, or machinery when a low-velocity foreign object strikes the eye is typical. Of note, high-speed missile injury (e.g., explosions, propelled foreign body from industrial equipment, lawn mowers, power tools) also may lodge a foreign body in the conjunctiva (but the object may have penetrated the globe).

Signs

- Conjunctival hyperemia, laceration, or obvious foreign body is found.
- Conjunctival or subconjunctival hemorrhage may obscure the foreign body.
- Linear, vertical corneal abrasions ("ice-skate track" abrasions) indicate retained foreign bodies on the superior tarsal conjunctiva under the upper lid (Fig. 16–7).

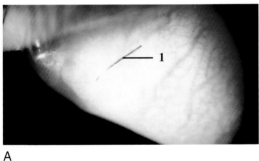

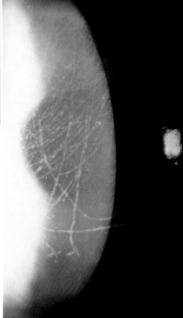

FIGURE 16–7   A, A grasshopper leg (1) embedded in the superior tarsal conjunctiva. **B,** "Dust trail" corneal linear abrasions are found in the same eye.

Differential Diagnosis

Diagnostic possibilities include the following:
- Ruptured globe and intraocular foreign body with ocular penetration, especially with high-speed missile injury
- Corneal foreign body, corneal abrasion, and contact lens–associated injury
- Other causes of ocular discomfort and redness (e.g., conjunctivitis, blepharitis, episcleritis, scleritis)

Workup

- Depending on the patient history, a complete examination of both eyes, including intraocular pressure measurement and slit lamp evaluation to assess anterior chamber depth and inflammation, iris defects, and lens clarity, is necessary.
- Lid eversion and dilated fundus examination are performed.
- If the patient history suggests a high-speed missile or metal-on-metal injury, a CT study of the orbits, which must specify scans obtained in axial and coronal planes with 1- to 2-mm cuts through the orbits, is needed to help detect an intraocular or intraorbital foreign body.
- If visual acuity is markedly decreased, the possibility of a more severe injury than superficial conjunctival foreign body should be investigated.

Treatment

- If globe penetration is suspected or undetermined, immediate referral to an ophthalmologist, shielding of the eye, and minimal manipulation of the globe are indicated.
- With suspected superficial foreign body and no ruptured globe, the foreign body is removed after topical anesthesia is ensured (e.g., with a drop of proparacaine or tetracaine). Irrigation with saline solution removes loosely adherent conjunctival foreign bodies. If the foreign material is slightly embedded in the conjunctiva and resistant to saline irrigation, it is removed at the slit lamp with a moistened cotton-tipped applicator, foreign body spatula, or a jeweler's forceps after anesthesia is achieved with a topical anesthesia pledget (a cotton-tipped applicator soaked in tetracaine or proparacaine and applied to the region for at least 30 seconds). The foreign body must be completely visible (i.e., it does not penetrate through the sclera and into the intraocular space) before removal. If it does extend further, immediate referral to an ophthalmologist and no manipulation of the globe are necessary steps.
- With multiple foreign bodies, the clinician irrigates with saline solution, removes the readily accessible objects with forceps, and sweeps the fornices with cotton-tipped applicators soaked in a topical anesthetic.
- After removal, a topical antibiotic (e.g., polymyxin B/bacitracin [Polysporin] ophthalmic ointment) and artificial tears are used as needed. If a significant number of foreign bodies remain, referral to an ophthalmologist is indicated.

Follow-up

- Follow-up evaluation is performed as needed, if a single or a few foreign bodies were easily removed and no further discomfort was experienced.

Conjunctival Laceration

Symptoms

- A history of trauma (especially with sharp objects) is reported.
- A red eye, mild foreign body sensation (less than with a corneal abrasion), and pain are characteristic.

Signs

- The conjunctival defect is noted on slit lamp examination, often with fluorescein pooling in the defect.
- Hemorrhage (subconjunctival) may obscure the injury (Fig. 16–8).
- White sclera may be visible in the base of the laceration, if it penetrates to the globe surface.

Differential Diagnosis

Diagnostic possibilities include the following:
- Serious injury to the globe (rupture) and orbital structures, including intraocular and intraorbital foreign bodies
- Subconjunctival foreign bodies

Workup

- As with all seemingly benign injuries of the periocular structures, a detailed history of the injury is imperative. The nature of the injury dictates the probability of severe ocular injury. For example, reports of a high-speed projectile or severe car accident with broken glass resulting in a conjunctival laceration raise suspicion of a more

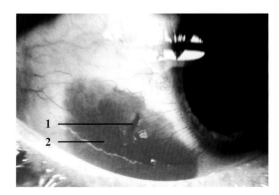

FIGURE 16–8 Note the small laceration in the conjunctiva (1) with surrounding subconjunctival hemorrhage (2). In this case, no associated subconjunctival foreign body or scleral injury occurred.

severe injury. A fingernail scratch or other less severe mechanism of injury is less likely to cause serious ocular injury.

- A complete examination of both eyes, including fluorescein staining to outline the defect, is needed. The base of the laceration is evaluated carefully to rule out the presence of retained foreign bodies in the subconjunctival space and to ensure that no scleral penetration or laceration has occurred. This area is explored with caution. If the globe is violated, even minimal pressure on the eye (even from the patient squeezing the lids together) can extrude intraocular contents and jeopardize the visual outcome. The clinician carefully examines the conjunctiva using topical anesthesia and a cotton-tipped applicator soaked in the anesthetic (e.g., tetracaine, proparacaine).
- The tetanus status of the patient is assessed.
- With suspicion of a ruptured globe or an intraocular or intraorbital foreign body, a CT scan with axial and coronal thin cuts (1 to 2 mm) through the orbits is indicated.

Treatment

- The patient is immediately referred to an ophthalmologist.
- For small lacerations (less than 1.0 cm in greatest dimension) in which a severe injury is not suspected, an antibiotic ointment (e.g., polymyxin B/bacitracin [Polysporin] two or three times a day) is administered for five to seven days.
- For large lacerations (greater than 1.0 cm across), sutures may be needed for closure. An ophthalmologist may perform this procedure with a microscope or loupes.

Follow-up

- A patient with a small laceration is referred to an ophthalmologist if the laceration does not heal properly or the foreign body sensation persists.
- The prognosis is excellent.

Corneal Foreign Body

Symptoms

- A history of acute foreign body sensation, red eye, tearing, and blurred vision is related. Often the patient can identify the moment the foreign body struck the eye.
- The pain is severe early and gradually becomes more tolerable. If the foreign body contains iron, rust will deposit in the surrounding cornea, inciting inflammation and causing pain.
- Blepharospasm (involuntary lid closure) is possible.

Signs

- Conjunctival injection, eyelid edema, and a mild anterior chamber reaction are seen.
- The foreign body usually is easily observed on the cornea with slit lamp or penlight examination (Fig. 16–9).

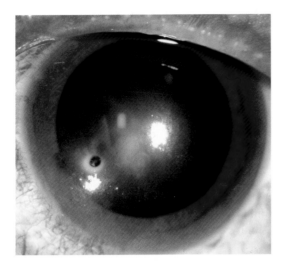

FIGURE 16–9 A small iron foreign body may be seen on external examination.

- A corneal stromal infiltrate usually is present if the foreign body has been present for more than 24 hours. The infiltrate may be noninfectious, but microbial keratitis must be suspected, especially if the foreign material is vegetable in origin (e.g., bark, thorn).
- Iron foreign bodies often form rust rings in the anterior corneal stroma, seen as reddish-orange circular opacities on slit lamp examination (even if the iron-containing foreign body has fallen out).
- A dense cellular reaction in the anterior chamber or hypopyon suggests microbial ulceration of the cornea or penetration of the globe by the foreign body and secondary endophthalmitis.

Differential Diagnosis

Considerations in the differential diagnosis include the following:
- Corneal abrasion or laceration
- Conjunctival foreign body

Workup

- **Note:** Use of topical anesthesia can greatly assist in determination of visual acuity and facilitates the patient's cooperation with the remainder of the examination.
- A complete examination of both eyes is indicated, including careful slit lamp examination of the cornea to assess the depth of penetration of the foreign body. If the foreign body is seen protruding into the anterior chamber, the globe is penetrated and at high risk for infection. No further manipulation of the foreign body should be attempted under any circumstances, to prevent dislodging it and decompressing the eye.
- Lid eversion is essential to rule out a hidden foreign body on the superior tarsal conjunctiva. The inferior conjunctival fornix also is examined carefully.

- With a suspected high-speed metal-on-metal or other projectile injury, a dilated fundus examination with indirect ophthalmoscopy by an ophthalmologist is essential. This evaluation will rule out globe penetration with intraocular foreign body. CT scanning or B-scan ultrasound examination also may be indicated.
- For deep foreign bodies, the *Seidel test* is performed to determine whether fluid (aqueous) is leaking from the eye:
    - The examiner places a drop of anesthetic (e.g., proparacaine) in the eye to be tested and on a sterile fluorescein strip. Excess anesthetic drips off the strip, which is then used to "paint" the area on the eye where the leak is suspected.
    - The examiner uses the cobalt-blue filter on the slit lamp to observe the area. Because of pH differences between the aqueous humor and the tear film, leaking aqueous manifests as a color change in the bright green stain as the aqueous dilutes the dye (Fig. 16–10). This finding is deemed *Seidel positive;* a *Seidel-negative* wound does not eliminate the possibility of intermittent leakage.

Treatment

- For globe penetration, the eye is shielded and the patient is immediately referred to an ophthalmologist.
- For superficial foreign material, simple irrigation often removes the material. If this procedure is unsuccessful, a cotton-tipped applicator can be used. The clinician instills a drop of topical anesthesia (e.g., proparacaine) into the eye and wets a sterile cotton-tipped applicator with saline solution or topical anesthetic. Most foreign bodies can be easily removed with minimal manipulation. If this procedure is also unsuccessful, the back of a sterile blade can be used to gently scrape the foreign body off the cornea. Use of a foreign body spud or sterile jeweler's forceps also may

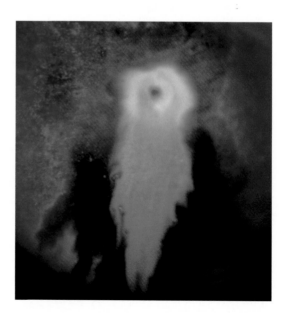

FIGURE 16–10   Seidel-positive wound.

be effective. Hypodermic needles should *not* be used for corneal foreign body removal, to prevent additional corneal injury or accidental perforation.

- For deep foreign material, referral to an ophthalmologist is indicated. Overaggressive manipulation or "digging" for a foreign body can cause more scarring and corneal damage. Similarly, overuse of an ophthalmic burr to remove a deep rust ring may cause extensive scarring that can compromise visual acuity. Removal in the operating room may be needed for deep, large, central, or infectious foreign bodies (such as vegetable matter). Also, uncooperative patients (especially young children) may require mask anesthesia.
- Corneal rust rings may be removed with an ophthalmic burr, a procedure probably best performed by an ophthalmologist. Patients with central rust rings should be referred to an ophthalmologist for management within 24 hours of the initial diagnosis. The natural propensity of corneal rust rings is for them to migrate superficially and become a white scar.
- Patients with numerous foreign bodies (as with an explosive injury) should be immediately referred to an ophthalmologist. If an attempt is made to remove each small object, undue scarring may result.
- After the foreign body is removed, the patient is given topical antibiotics (e.g., polymyxin B/bacitracin [Polysporin] ophthalmic ointment) until the epithelial defect has healed.

Follow-up

- The patient is seen daily until the epithelium heals; close follow-up reduces infectious complications.
- The residual corneal defect (epithelial defect) is treated as a corneal abrasion. If the corneal defect is large and central and associated with a discharge or other signs of infection (e.g., severe pain, corneal clouding, marked anterior chamber reaction), the patient should be immediately referred to an ophthalmologist. Topical corticosteroids are not used.
- Multiple, deep, central, iron-containing foreign bodies confer the worst visual prognosis. Patients with injuries caused by small, single, peripheral foreign bodies generally have excellent visual outcomes.

Corneal Laceration

A corneal laceration may be a full-thickness or partial-thickness injury. Depending on location and size, partial-thickness lacerations can be associated with an excellent visual prognosis and can be treated with patching and antibiotics, much as for corneal abrasions. Patients with deep or full-thickness lacerations should be urgently referred for ophthalmologic evaluation.

Symptoms

- A history of trauma with a sharp object or projectile (high velocity) is reported.
- Pain, decreased vision (depending on the depth and location of the laceration), involuntary lid closure (blepharospasm), and a red eye are characteristic.

- The patient may have observed a brief flow of fluid (aqueous) from the eye immediately after the injury.

Signs

- A positive result on Seidel's test is indicative of full-thickness corneal laceration.
- A corneal wound may be seen.
- More often, the iris prolapses out of the corneal wound, or the iris and cornea are in contact where the iris has plugged the corneal defect. A corneal laceration of this type is nearly always associated with a "peaking" or "teardrop" shape to the pupil, with the "peak" pointing in the direction of the corneal defect (Fig. 16–11).
- Other signs of a penetrated globe include an asymmetrical anterior chamber depth relative to that of the uninvolved eye, a hyphema, conjunctival injection and chemosis, reduced (in most cases) or normal or even elevated (in a few cases) intraocular pressure, lens injury, and pupillary asymmetry. Vision often is decreased.

Workup

- A complete examination of both eyes, including Seidel's test, is indicated. If rupture of the globe becomes evident (or rupture is suspected), the examination ends, the eye is shielded, and the patient is referred to an ophthalmologist immediately. Excessive manipulation of the globe or exertion of pressure on the eyelids during an examination may result in extrusion of intraocular contents.
- A CT scan of the orbits (in axial and coronal planes) is needed to evaluate possible intraocular or intraorbital foreign bodies.
- A slit lamp examination is performed to examine the extent and depth of the corneal injury. Distinguishing deep, nonpenetrating lacerations from penetrating, well-apposed wounds often is difficult. For this reason, if the extent of the injury is questionable, the patient should be referred to an ophthalmologist immediately.

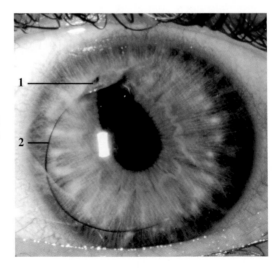

FIGURE 16–11 Acute corneal laceration with prolapsed iris (1) and resultant peaked pupil. An eyelash (2) has entered the anterior chamber.

Treatment

- To prevent extrusion of ocular contents, patients referred to the ophthalmologist must have a shield (without patch) over the eye with a suspected penetrating injury.
- Antibiotic ointment is not used in any patient with a suspected ruptured globe, because the medication may enter the eye.
- For a suspected or confirmed full-thickness laceration, operative intervention usually is necessary, and broad-spectrum intravenous antibiotics are administered preoperatively. Adults may receive 1 g of cefazolin (Ancef) every 8 hours. Children receive 25 to 50 mg/kg/day of cefazolin (Ancef) in three divided doses. Recent evidence shows better ocular penetration with third- and fourth-generation fluoroquinolones (even when given orally).
- The patient's tetanus immune status is addressed.

Scleral Laceration or Rupture

Symptoms

- A history of trauma, often with a high-velocity projectile or sharp object, is reported.
- Conjunctival swelling, red eye, pain, decreased vision, and possible inadvertent lid closure (blepharospasm) are characteristic.

Signs

- A defect may be noted in the conjunctiva or sclera, with or without subconjunctival hemorrhage (Fig. 16–12). Marked chemosis (clear swelling) or hemorrhagic suffusion may obscure the underlying scleral injury.
- Uveal or vitreous prolapse may occur through the scleral wound. Prolapsed uvea (iris, ciliary body, or choroid) may appear as a brownish discoloration beneath the conjunctiva, sometimes mistaken for blood. The pupil may be abnormally shaped (e.g., peaked), if the wound is close to the corneal limbus.

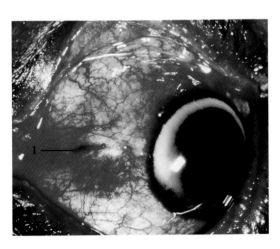

FIGURE 16–12 Scleral laceration. This lesion (1) was made with a sharp, penetrating object (a small knife). The clinician needs to ensure that no part of the object causing the injury is left in the eye.

- The intraocular pressure is low in most cases. Less commonly, the intraocular pressure is normal or elevated.

Etiology

- Usually, sharp objects or missiles (e.g., metal-on-metal projectile, broken glass, knife, bullet) cause the injury.
- Severe blunt trauma (e.g., from a fist, bottle, or club) is a common cause.

Differential Diagnosis

Diagnostic possibilities include the following:
- Conjunctival laceration without scleral injury
- Intraocular foreign body
- Clear or hemorrhagic chemosis without obvious scleral injury

Workup

- As with corneal and conjunctival lacerations, a complete examination of both eyes is indicated. If rupture of the globe is suspected, the eye is shielded, no antibiotic ointment or patching is used, and the patient is immediately referred to an ophthalmologist.
- A diagnosis of scleral rupture or laceration requires a high index of suspicion because these conditions often are obscured by chemotic or hemorrhagic conjunctiva. Minimal manipulation of the globe is prudent in cases in which the diagnosis is uncertain.
- A CT scan of the orbit (in axial and coronal planes) is indicated. If an intraocular foreign body is suspected, inform the radiologist to perform thin cuts.

Treatment

- In cases of partial-thickness laceration of the sclera (which is rare), the patient is referred to an ophthalmologist for evaluation and possible surgical repair.
- In cases of suspected or confirmed full-thickness laceration, the patient is immediately referred for ophthalmologic evaluation and surgical repair. Topical therapy is avoided. Prophylactic antibiotics are administered pre-operatively.
- The patient's tetanus immune status is addressed.

Follow-up

- The focus and frequency of follow-up evaluation vary depending on the extent of the injury.

Chemical Injury

Chemical injuries to the eye may be caused by acid, alkali, and other chemically active organic substances such as mace and tear gas. Acid and alkali injuries may cause profound visual loss. Organic agents (e.g., isopropyl alcohol) rarely cause severe vision loss, and exposures involving these agents are associated with a good prognosis.

Symptoms

- Severe pain, redness, blurred vision, and eyelid spasm are characteristic.
- A history of chemical exposure is reported.

Signs

- Signs vary depending on the severity of the injury and the time elapsed since the chemical exposure.

With Mild to Moderate Injuries

- Initial signs include corneal epithelial loss, chemosis and conjunctival hyperemia, subconjunctival hemorrhage, intact episcleral and conjunctival vessels, and mild periocular skin involvement (first-degree burns).
- Chronic signs include minimal corneal scarring.

With Severe Injuries

- Initial signs include severe chemosis; corneal edema and opacification; loss of conjunctival and episcleral vessels (limbal blanching), which causes a patchy avascular appearance to the sclera (Fig. 16–13); severe periocular skin involvement (second- or third-degree burns); and a marked anterior chamber reaction, which may not be visualized.
- Chronic signs include foreshortened fornices (loss of normal conjunctival cul-de-sac) with symblepharon formation (conjunctival and globe adhesions), cicatricial eyelid abnormalities such as trichiasis (misdirected eyelashes), entropion (in-turned lid), or ectropion (out-turned lid), severe tear film abnormalities (loss of mucin-producing cells in the conjunctiva); corneal scarring and opacification (Fig. 16–14); and phthisis bulbi (shrunken, nonseeing eye).

Etiology

- The most serious chemical burns to the eye are alkali burns such as from lye (NaOH), caustic potash (KOH), and ammonia (NH_3). Fresh lime ([$Ca(OH)_2$] and magnesium hydroxide [$Mg(OH)_2$]) also are alkaline but usually cause less severe

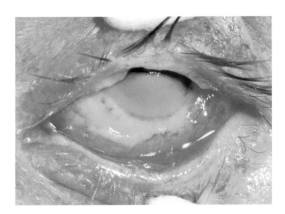

FIGURE 16–13 Acute, severe alkali burn with conjunctival and scleral ischemia and marked corneal edema.

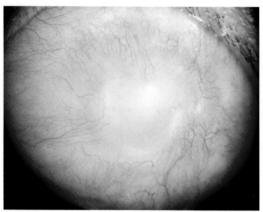

FIGURE 16–14 Severe alkali burn after 1 year. The cornea is scarred, and vascularization is extensive. The prognosis following corneal transplant surgery in patients with severe alkali burns to the eye is poor.

injury than other alkaline compounds. Household cleaners, fertilizers, and refrigerants contain ammonia. Plaster, cement, mortar, and whitewash contain fresh lime. "Sparklers" and flares contain magnesium hydroxide. Alkalis penetrate rapidly through the cornea and anterior chamber, causing disruption of the cell membrane lipids and secondary cellular necrosis. The degree of injury is correlated with the amount of chemical involved, as is the time from exposure to irrigation.

- Acid burns caused by strong acids in car batteries (sulfuric acid [H_2SO_4]), and swimming pool acid (hydrochloric acid [HCl]), do not penetrate the ocular tissues as readily because of the precipitation of tissue proteins. The protein precipitate acts as a barrier to further tissue penetration. An exception can be injuries from glass-etching chemicals (hydrofluoric acid [HF]).

Workup and Treatment

- As with other ocular injuries, the history guides the evaluation and treatment. It is important to ascertain the nature of the offending chemical agent.
- In cases of severe exposure, immediate treatment must precede the ocular evaluation. Copious irrigation with water on site should be followed with irrigation with at least 1 to 2 L of normal saline solution (0.9%) or lactated Ringer's solution over 1 hour in the emergency room. Topical anesthetic (e.g., proparacaine) is instilled initially and then every 10 to 15 minutes, to make this a much less painful procedure. Lid retractors are used if significant orbicularis spasm is present. Various contact lenses (e.g., Morgan lens) that connect to intravenous tubing are available commercially to assist in the irrigation.
- In cases of less severe exposure or questionable history (e.g., the patient reports getting a drop of cleaner in the eye but washing it out at home), less copious irrigation with pH measurement is performed initially.
- The clinician sweeps the conjunctival fornices with a moistened cotton-tipped applicator to remove any retained foreign matter, especially lime, which exists as particulate matter.
- The clinician everts the upper and lower lids to ensure that no retained chemical is present after sweeping the fornices.

- The possibility of early perforation is unlikely, but the globe is carefully assessed. Minimal pressure is placed on the globe during lavage when this diagnosis is a possibility or is indicated by the history.
- Irrigation continues until the conjunctival pH normalizes (i.e., 7.3 to 7.6); the pH is checked with the pH section of a urinalysis strip or pH paper. Two or three normal readings should be obtained at 15-minute intervals to ensure stability of the pH.
- Intraocular pressure may fluctuate widely and should be assessed. Broad areas of limbal blanching may be associated with markedly elevated intraocular pressure.
- Cycloplegic agents (e.g., homatropine 5%) and mydriatic agents (e.g., phenylephrine 2.5%) are instilled to dilate the pupil. **Note:** In severe injury, some researchers discourage instillation of phenylephrine because of the possibility of further vasoconstricting the conjunctival vessels.
- Antibiotics (e.g., polymyxin B/bacitracin [Polysporin], erythromycin ophthalmic ointment) are instilled and a pressure patch is placed over the eye.
- Immediate referral to an ophthalmologist is needed once the initial lavage is complete. Management of severe burns includes treatment of the intraocular pressure problems, exposure, scarring, and tear film dysfunction; therapy involves early topical corticosteroid administration, ascorbate or citrate supplementation (in cases of alkali burns only), and surgery (e.g., conjunctival grafting, corneal transplantation), if necessary.

Follow-up

- Patients usually are monitored daily for several days.
- The prognosis mainly depends on the type of injury.
- Even in the most severe alkaline injuries, the primary care physician can play a significant role in reducing the chronic sequelae by instructing the patient to irrigate at the place of injury (e.g., home, work) using a sink, shower, or garden hose, rather than immediately summoning the patient to the emergency room. As stated, the prognosis is directly affected by the adequacy of the lavage immediately after exposure.

Thermal Injury

Symptoms

- Pain, tearing, a foreign body sensation, a red eye, and decreased vision are characteristic.
- A history of exposure to a hot object (e.g., curling iron, tobacco ash, electrical arc, explosion) is reported.

Signs

- Corneal whitening indicates an epithelial or a stromal burn (Fig. 16–15).
- A corneal epithelial defect is evident.
- Conjunctival chemosis and injection occur.
- A minimal anterior chamber reaction is noted.
- Burns of the eyelids and periocular region are evident.

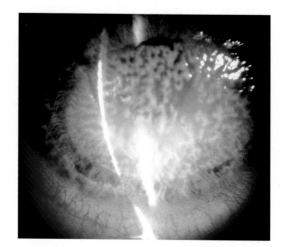

FIGURE 16–15   Corneal thermal injury from a curling iron.

Differential Diagnosis

Diagnostic possibilities include the following:
- Corneal abrasion or infection (especially if no history is available)
- Ultraviolet injury (welder's flash)

Workup

- A complete examination of both eyes, intraocular pressure evaluation, and careful notation of depth of burn (if corneal) are needed.
- Fluorescein instillation and a careful description or drawing of the epithelial defect should be performed.
- The diagnosis of globe perforation should be ruled out or confirmed if this condition is suggested by the history.
- Associated alkaline injury should be ruled out or confirmed if the thermal burn was caused by fireworks or flares (magnesium hydroxide).

Treatment

- In cases of mild injury involving only the superficial cornea, topical antibiotic ointment (e.g., polymyxin B/bacitracin [Polysporin]) is administered and a pressure patch is applied. Symptoms should resolve within 24 to 48 hours. The pressure patch is removed in 24 hours, and the cornea is reexamined.
- Cycloplegic agents (e.g., homatropine 5%) are administered before patching.
- In cases of deep burns of the cornea, patients are immediately referred to an ophthalmologist.
- Periocular burns are treated with ophthalmic antibiotic ointment preparations (e.g., polymyxin B/bacitracin [Polysporin], erythromycin ophthalmic ointment). Skin preparations may enter the ocular surface and cause irritation and corneal epithelial toxicity.

Follow-up

- An ophthalmologist or an oculoplastic surgeon is consulted if severe periocular injury accompanies the ocular injury. Cicatrization (scarring) of the eyelids from severe burns may lead to exposure and corneal scarring.

Hyphema

Hyphema, or blood in the anterior chamber of the eye, is an important indicator of the severity of trauma an eye has sustained. A microhyphema is a condition in which red blood cells are suspended in the aqueous fluid, not yet visibly layered in the dependent portion of the anterior chamber. Hyphemas require ophthalmologic management and follow-up evaluation because they can be associated with severe complications. The role of the primary care provider is to confirm the presence of vision, if possible, and to perform an initial examination with minimal manipulation of the globe, because concomitant ocular injury may be present, or the bleeding may be aggravated.

Symptoms

- A history of blunt trauma usually is reported; spontaneous hyphema is unusual.
- Pain, blurred vision, and a red eye are characteristic.
- Somnolence is noted, especially in children.

Signs

- Presence of red blood cells in the anterior chamber, either suspended (microhyphema) or layered along the dependent portion of the anterior chamber, is noted (Fig. 16–16). Isolated clots on the iris also may be seen.
- The red blood cells are not always found at the 6 o'clock position, because the patient may come for treatment after lying with the head in any position.
- Conjunctival injection, a sluggish or peaked pupil (resulting from a clot), pupillary sphincter or iris tears in some cases, and sometimes active bleeding from an iris vessel are other possible findings.

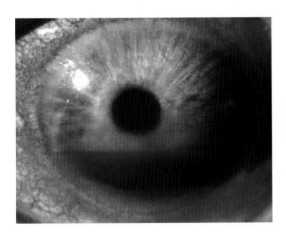

FIGURE 16–16 Hyphemas layer with time, much as with a hematocrit blood sample in a test tube. Here, a 30% hyphema is noted.

Etiology and Differential Diagnosis

- Concussive or sharp trauma to the iris or ciliary body can cause a hyphema.
- A hyphema may originate from the iris or a scleral wound after ocular surgery.
- A spontaneous occurrence is possible with intraocular neoplasms (seen in juvenile xanthogranuloma, malignant melanoma, retinoblastoma, and leukemia) and clotting disorders. Spontaneous hyphemas also may result from rubeosis iridis (neovascularization of the iris). This condition is seen in ocular ischemic states (e.g., vascular occlusions, proliferative diabetic retinopathy).
- If the hyphema is "spontaneous" in a child, child abuse also should be suspected.

Workup

- A history of the exact time and nature of the injury is needed. A ruptured globe must always be ruled out or confirmed.
- Both eyes and periorbital regions are examined. If the patient history suggests a projectile injury, the periorbital skin is assessed for possible entry wounds.
- The intraocular pressure needs to be measured; however, undue manipulation of the globe should be avoided to prevent rebleeding.
- The percentage of the anterior chamber that is layered with blood is measured (e.g., 10%, 20%, 50%), much as with determination of the hematocrit of red blood cells.
- All African American patients are screened for sickle cell disorders with a sickle dex test. If positive, hemoglobin electrophoresis testing may be necessary. Even patients with sickle trait (AS), in addition to full-blown disease (SS, SC), may be unable to clear the red blood cells from the anterior chamber, resulting in a markedly elevated intraocular pressure 1 to 2 days after injury. This finding is crucial in management because the intraocular pressure must be maintained at a much lower level (less than 25 mm Hg) in these patients due to the potential for optic nerve head perfusion compromise and subsequent optic atrophy.

Treatment

- Ophthalmologic consultation is mandatory. Accurate evaluation and management of the intraocular pressure are crucial in the care of these patients.
- Patients (especially children) with severe hyphemas and those in whom compliance with follow-up is questionable may require hospital admission.
- The involved eye is kept shielded with no patch, and bed rest, with careful ambulation, is instituted.
- A cycloplegic agent (e.g., atropine sulfate 1%) is administered twice a day unless the clot is well established (more than 24 to 48 hours old). An antiemetic (e.g., prochlorperazine [Compazine] 10 mg intramuscularly) and mild analgesia (e.g., acetaminophen [Tylenol]) can be used. Aspirin-containing compounds are avoided.

Follow-up

- Daily follow-up evaluation for 4 to 5 days is needed and should be performed by an ophthalmologist, who will monitor for intraocular pressure rise, corneal blood staining, and rebleeding. Because a hyphema is a manifestation of significant intraocular injury, regardless of whether the offending agent was sharp or blunt, evaluation for concomitant injury by the ophthalmologist also is crucial.

- The prognosis generally is good for patients with microhyphemas and small hyphemas without concomitant injury. In patients with large or total ("eight-ball") hyphemas, rebleeding, and sickle cell disease, the prognosis is more guarded. Long-term complications include glaucoma, corneal blood staining, and retinal injury.

Traumatic Iritis

Symptoms

- A history of ocular trauma (usually blunt) that occurred up to 2 to 3 days before the symptoms appeared is reported.
- Pain, marked photophobia, a red eye, tearing, and blurred vision are characteristic.

Signs

- Anterior chamber cell (white blood cells in the anterior chamber) and flare (proteinaceous leakage into the anterior chamber) are observed with the use of a thin, bright beam directed obliquely through the anterior chamber (before fluorescein instillation).
- Consensual pain (pain from ciliary body spasm in the involved eye) occurs with direct illumination in the uninvolved eye.
- Ciliary flush and conjunctival injection are noted. The pupil may display sluggish movement and may even be miotic (constricted).

Etiology

- Blunt trauma results in intraocular inflammation from a breakdown in the blood-aqueous barrier.

Workup

- A complete eye examination is needed, including a dilated fundus examination and intraocular pressure measurement, if the history suggests a significant ocular injury.

Treatment

- Cycloplegic agents (e.g., homatropine 5% three times a day) are administered.
- Corticosteroid drops may be used after consultation with an ophthalmologist. Before they are prescribed, ocular infection must be ruled out and arrangements for adequate follow-up must be in place.

Follow-up

- The patient is reevaluated 2 days to 1 week after the initial visit, depending on the severity of the patient's symptoms and visual acuity. Distance acuity should not be

markedly diminished after initial treatment; however, near vision will be poor because of the cycloplegic agent.
- As a rule, the prognosis is excellent. Symptoms should resolve in 7 to 10 days.

Traumatic Retrobulbar Hemorrhage

Symptoms

- A history of significant sharp or blunt trauma to the globe/periorbital region is reported.
- Pain, decreased vision, and marked swelling may be present.

Signs

- Proptosis of the involved globe occurs.
- Tense lids and chemosis or hemorrhagic suffusion of the conjunctiva are noted.
- A markedly elevated intraocular pressure and a tense orbit (significant resistance on retropulsion of the globe) are found.
- Diffuse and massive subconjunctival hemorrhage and/or chemosis are evident. The posterior border of the subconjunctival blood cannot be visualized.
- Eyelid and periorbital ecchymosis occurs (often delayed).
- Extraocular movements usually are limited.

Etiology

- Traumatic injury to the arteries within the confines of the orbit cause an abrupt rise in intraorbital pressure with consequent anterior displacement of the globe. The blood can dissect between tissue planes and be visible under the conjunctiva and Tenon's capsule. The elevated pressure is transmitted to the globe itself once the anterior displacement of the eye is limited by the surrounding periocular soft tissues.
- Complications result when the elevated intraorbital/intraocular pressure is not lowered, such as compromise to the optic nerve and central retinal artery circulation.

Differential Diagnosis

Diagnostic possibilities include the following:
- Orbital cellulitis, which often can be ruled out by the patient history
- Orbital fracture
- Carotid artery–cavernous sinus fistula, which is possible after severe head trauma

Workup

- Examination of the ocular fundus, with accurate assessment of the intraocular pressure, is indicated. The contralateral eye must always be examined in cases of trauma.
- If the orbit and globe are tense (from marked elevation in pressure), immediate referral to an ophthalmologist is indicated.

- The pupils and extraocular motility are evaluated carefully. The presence or development of a relative afferent pupillary defect may indicate optic nerve injury caused by compression or a traumatic optic neuropathy.
- CT scanning of the orbit (in axial and coronal planes) is indicated immediately unless the signs suggest a markedly elevated pressure, an impending vascular occlusion, or optic nerve dysfunction. CT study of the orbit is mandatory but should be delayed until the ophthalmologist has treated the elevated intraocular pressure.
- Intracranial penetration should be suspected in cases in which retrobular hemorrhage resulted from an orbital penetrating injury.

Treatment

- For significant retrobulbar hemorrhage, patients should be immediately referred to an ophthalmologist.
- Control of intraocular pressure is the first condition to be addressed. Carbonic anhydrase inhibitors (e.g., intravenous acetazolamide [Diamox] 500 mg) and topical beta blockers (e.g., timolol [Timoptic] 0.5%) help control the pressure in patients with limited hemorrhages or hematomas. For patients with active bleeding and worsening retrobulbar hemorrhages with elevated intraocular pressure (e.g., greater than 50 mm Hg), an ophthalmologist needs to perform a lateral canthotomy and possibly a cantholysis of the lateral canthal tendons (in upper and lower lids). This maneuver decreases the pressure on the globe by increasing the potential volume of the orbit.
- For persistently elevated intraocular pressure despite treatment and cantholysis, emergency orbital decompression by the ophthalmologist may be required. An anterior chamber tap also may decrease the intraocular pressure in an emergency, but this should also be performed by the consulting ophthalmologist.

Follow-up

- Daily follow-up evaluation is indicated, with careful monitoring of the intraocular pressure. If a cantholysis was performed, the lids may require surgical repair.

Glue Injury

Symptoms

- A history of ocular exposure to cyanoacrylate glue (e.g., Super Glue) is reported.
- Immediate closure of the eyelids (usually partial) occurs following exposure to the substance.
- A red eye, foreign body sensation, pain, and tearing are characteristic.

Signs

- Dried, hardened glue is found at the margin of the approximated eyelids or on the eye (Fig. 16–17).
- The epithelial defect displays diffuse fluorescein staining (with toxic epitheliopathy or direct abrasion from sharp glue edges).
- Conjunctival injection is evident.

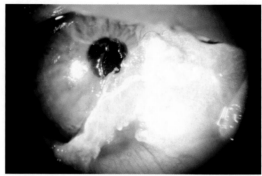

FIGURE 16–17 Epoxy glue injury to the cornea. Fortunately, the glue usually is stuck only to the epithelium, so that severe scarring does not result.

Workup

- The patient's visual acuity should be determined, and fluorescein staining is performed if possible.

Treatment

- Aggressively prying open the lids causes pain and further superficial injury to the lid margin and should not be attempted. Application of chemicals or solvents to try to break the bond is contraindicated because these substances can cause significant corneal toxic epitheliopathy.
- Warm compresses are applied, and the glued lids are gently massaged.
- Warmed topical antibiotic ointments (e.g., erythromycin, polymyxin B/bacitracin [Polysporin]) are placed in the eye three or four times a day or at least applied or rubbed on the lid margin. This treats any epithelial defects and mechanically facilitates lid separation. Artificial tears (e.g., hydroxypropyl methycellulose [Bion Tears, Tears Naturale], carboxymethylcellulose [Celluvisc], polyvinyl alcohol [Refresh]) are used as needed for comfort.
- The patient is reassured that the lids should become "unstuck" within several days of conservative treatment. If they do not, surgical separation of the lids may be required.

Follow-up

- The focus of follow-up evaluation is the same as for an epithelial defect. The patient is seen in 24 to 48 hours.

Intraocular Foreign Body

When the patient with a traumatic injury of the eye reports a history of striking metal on metal, grinding, or hammering, or if the injury was incurred during use of a lawn mower or edger or operation of industrial machinery or was from an explosion or gunshot, or with any other injury in which high-speed penetration of the globe with foreign material is possible, the primary care physician must be particularly alert. With small intraocular foreign bodies, the signs and symptoms may be minimal. Failure to consider the possibility of an intraocular foreign body in these patients, so that an incorrect diagnosis is made during the initial examination, often results in loss of a significant amount of vision and is a common cause of litigation. The possibility of an intraocular foreign body must always be considered in the differential diagnosis of traumatic eye injury evaluated by the primary care provider.

Symptoms

- Vision is decreased or may be normal in some patients.
- A history suggestive of penetration of the globe with foreign material is reported.
- Eye pain, photophobia, and a red eye are usual. In some patients, the eye may be relatively quiet.

Signs

- Conjunctival signs usually include chemosis, hemorrhage, and laceration. In some patients, the conjunctiva is normal.
- Scleral injury manifests as overlying subconjunctival hemorrhage. Laceration or perforation may be visible (but usually is obscured). The sclera can appear normal.
- A periocular entry site may be present (e.g., through the lids).
- Foreign material may be seen in the anterior segment of the eye (often in the iris or lens); gonioscopic evaluation by an ophthalmologist may be needed for visualization (Fig. 16–18).

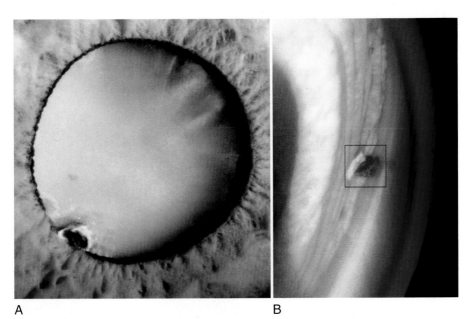

A   B

FIGURE 16–18   A, A traumatic cataract that developed in response to an iron foreign body that had penetrated the anterior lens capsule. **B,** Gonioscopic view of an iron foreign body that penetrated the globe during a metal-on-metal hammering injury.

Etiology

- Types of foreign bodies include metallic (e.g., iron, steel, nickel), nonmetallic (e.g., calcium, vegetable matter), and inert compounds (e.g., glass, plaster, lead, carbon, coal, rubber). "BB" shot may be composed of any of various metals, including lead, iron, and brass; these missiles are commonly found as intraocular foreign bodies after an injury. The physician should make every effort to determine the material/magnetic properties of the foreign body for surgical decision-making.

Workup

- Both eyes are examined carefully. A ruptured globe is suspected in cases in which uveal prolapse and a very soft eye are evident; a perforation site is noted; a conjunctival, corneal, or scleral laceration is seen; conjunctival chemosis and hemorrhage and pupillary or iris abnormalities are evident; or lens opacity or a projectile tract is found on slit lamp examination. With any of these findings, the examination is discontinued, the eye is shielded, and the patient is immediately referred to an ophthalmologist.
- A dilated fundus examination with indirect ophthalmoscopy and careful slit lamp examination are mandatory and should be performed by an ophthalmologist. Most anterior segment foreign bodies are visible on slit lamp examination or gonioscopy (which uses special examining lens with mirrors to see into the anterior chamber angle 360 degrees).
- Plain film imaging may help with the diagnosis, but in general, CT scanning (in axial and coronal planes with 1- to 2-mm cuts) is a much more effective tool to evaluate the globe (and adnexa) for foreign material (Fig. 16–19). Magnetic resonance imaging (MRI) should not be performed, because further injury to the globe

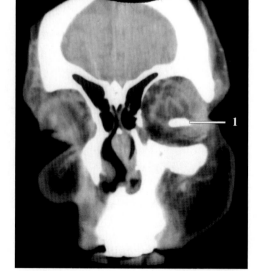

FIGURE 16–19   An intraocular metallic foreign body (1). In this case the globe was hypotonous and disorganized, as shown on computed tomographic imaging.

may rarely occur with movement of any magnetic objects during scanning. Cautious B-scan ultrasonography is extremely helpful in diagnosis and surgical planning but requires experienced ophthalmologic personnel.

Treatment

- The ophthalmologist should coordinate the patient's care. Surgical intervention is needed in most cases (especially with iron, steel, and copper foreign bodies). The patient is given nothing by mouth, tetanus status is addressed, the eye is shielded, and broad-spectrum intravenous antibiotics are administered preoperatively (e.g., cefazolin and gentamicin).
- Use of cycloplegic agents (e.g., homatropine 5%) enhances patient comfort and decreases the chance of formation of posterior adhesions of the iris to the lens (posterior synechiae) but may adversely affect uveal tissue that has prolapsed into a corneoscleral wound (i.e., may "unplug the hole").

Eyelid Trauma and Laceration

The role of the primary care physician in the evaluation of eyelid trauma is to answer several questions: Is the globe injured? Has the orbit been violated? Is the lid margin (or the body of the eyelid) affected? Has the canalicular system (proximal segment of the lacrimal drainage system) been compromised? Is eyelid closure adequate? If any of these conditions exist or are suspected, the ophthalmologist should be consulted immediately, with possible urgent patient referral.

Symptoms

- A history of sharp trauma to the eyelid or, in cases of avulsion of the lid, abrasive or contusive injury to the eyelid is reported.
- Periorbital pain, a foreign body sensation, and tearing are characteristic.

Signs

- Laceration through the lid margin occurs (Fig. 16–20).
- Conjunctival injection is evident.
- Orbital fat prolapse occurs if the orbital septum has been violated.
- Involvement of the eyelid medial to the superior and inferior puncta suggests canalicular laceration. (For lacrimal system anatomy, see Figs. 13–17 and 14–4.)

Workup

- A complete examination of both eyes is indicated. A ruptured globe is ruled out first; an object sharp enough to lacerate the eyelid can easily lacerate the globe as well.
- For injuries to the medial aspect of the eyelids, evaluation of the canalicular system, lacrimal sac, and medial canthal tendon is needed (Fig. 16–21). This is best performed by an ophthalmologist.

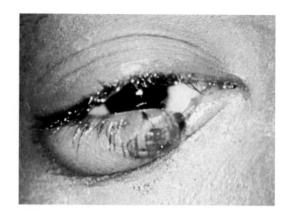

FIGURE 16–20 Eyelid margin laceration.

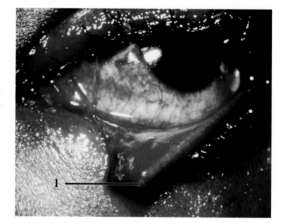

FIGURE 16–21 The lower punctum is evident at the extreme cut end of the medial aspect of the lower eyelid (1). Repair should be performed in the operating room, with reconstruction of the canalicular system. Careless repair of these injuries could leave the patient with globe exposure and chronic tearing (epiphora).

- For patients with injuries to the lateral eyelid, possible involvement of the lateral canthal tendons and lacrimal gland is addressed. Evaluation is best performed by an ophthalmologist.
- CT scanning is indicated in any patient in whom injury to the globe is possible or the orbital septum has been violated and the possibility exists for an orbital foreign body.
- The amount of ptosis (drooping of the eyelid) and excursion of the eyelid are evaluated to determine whether any levator muscle or tendon injury occurred.

Treatment

- Patients with vertical lid lacerations through the margin of the eyelid should be referred to an ophthalmologist for repair of the defects. The timing of repair for lid lacerations is immediate only with gross corneal exposure. Delay in repair with cool saline compresses for 1 to 2 days may improve visible anatomy and facilitate better cosmesis. Improper repair of the margin may result in corneal exposure, lagophthalmos (incomplete closure of the eyelids), corneal irritation from trichiasis, uneven edges of the margin, and poor cosmesis.

- Lid margin lacerations through the canalicular system (upper and/or lower eyelid) usually are repaired in the operating room using a microscope. The canalicular system is repaired and cannulated. Improper repair of the canalicular system can result in chronic tearing in addition to complications associated with improper margin repair.
- An avulsive injury of the eyelids necessitates complex surgical closure and reconstructive surgery.
- Horizontal lid lacerations with fat prolapse can be repaired by nonophthalmic staff. It is important to never pull on the prolapsed fat, because retrobulbar hemorrhage may result. For this repair, the fat is clamped and excised flush with the clamp; the end still in the clamp is cauterized and then gently released. Only the skin is closed in the surgical wound.

Follow-up

- The time of follow-up evaluation is determined by the ophthalmic surgeon but usually is within 5 to 7 days of repair. Oral broad-spectrum antibiotics may be necessary with complex or extensive injury/repair.
- The prognosis is very good if repairs have been performed properly. Even with proper repair, patients may need additional surgical procedures to revise scarring (cicatricial) changes and to improve cosmesis, or to correct exposure of the globe.

Orbital Blow-Out Fracture

Symptoms

- A history of significant blunt injury to the eye is reported.
- Pain, which may be aggravated with eye movements, is variable.
- Double vision (binocular) is noted (vertical diplopia).
- Swelling of eyelids occurs after sneezing or blowing the nose (orbital emphysema), which indicates that communication between orbit and sinus is present.

Signs

- Enophthalmos (posteriorly displaced globe) may occur and is manifested as a narrowing of the palpebral fissures in the involved eye relative to that of the contralateral side (pseudo-ptosis). More important, measuring the distance (from the side) from the lateral orbital rim to the corneal apex may show a significantly shorter distance on the involved side.
- Point tenderness or an irregularity in the orbital rim may be noted.
- Numbness or tingling of the upper lip and cheek on the ipsilateral side indicates an injury to the infraorbital nerve (which runs along the orbital floor).
- Subcutaneous and orbital emphysema and proptosis are seen if a one-way valve exists between the sinuses (maxillary or ethmoid) and the orbit, trapping air in the orbit. The air dissects anteriorly between the tissue planes.
- Extraocular movements, primarily upgaze, are restricted.

Etiology

- Orbital blow-out fractures occur in two forms: Direct fractures involve the orbital rim, with extension posteriorly involving the floor of the orbit. Indirect fractures result from compression of the soft tissues of the orbit (e.g., globe, extraocular muscles, fat), generating forces transmitted against the orbital walls. Thus, fractures of the walls of the orbit (often the floor and/or medial wall, which are extremely thin) may occur without a fracture of the orbital rim.

Workup

- A ruptured globe is ruled out, and the contralateral eye is examined. Extraocular motility is often unreliable in the early postinjury period because periorbital and extraocular muscle edema/hematoma can restrict motility and affect the position of the globe.
- The eyelids are examined for crepitus, which may be a sign that intraorbital air is present. The patient must be monitored for progressive proptosis and visual changes; if tension in the orbit rises because of the increasing orbital air, a compressive or an ischemic optic neuropathy or occlusions of the central retinal vessels may result.
- The ipsilateral cheek is checked for sensation; infraorbital nerve injury is commonly seen in inferior blow-out fractures.
- If entrapment of the inferior rectus and inferior oblique muscles is suspected, plain film imaging or preferably CT scanning of the orbits in the axial and coronal planes is performed to assist in the diagnosis (Fig. 16–22). In severe injuries, CT scanning also aids in evaluation of the anatomic and structural integrity of the globe and in management of injuries involving the relevant structures.

Treatment

- Referral is indicated for ophthalmologic examination in any case of an orbital blow-out fracture. Any possible injury to the globe is ruled out. The fracture is evidence

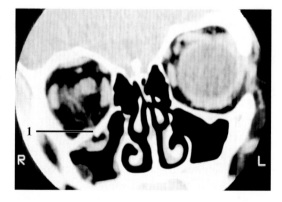

FIGURE 16–22 Entrapment of orbital soft tissue in an inferior blow-out fracture. A coronal computed tomographic scan shows orbital soft tissue protruding into the superior portion of the maxillary sinus (1).

of extreme shifts in intraocular pressure and force waves through the intraocular tissues. Chorioretinal injuries (tears, detachments, and edema), vitreous hemorrhage, lens subluxation, and damage to the anterior chamber structures (hyphema) are possible consequences of the blunt trauma.

- Nasal decongestants (e.g., Afrin) are administered twice a day on the involved side for 2 or 3 days.
- Antibiotic coverage is controversial, but should be considered if there is a previous history of sinus disease.
- Cold compresses or ice packs are applied to the periorbital region to help diminish edema.
- Instructions for gentle or minimally restricted nose blowing and sneezing are given.
- In most patients, surgical repair of the orbit floor is indicated for persistent entrapment, gross enophthalmos, diplopia (in primary gaze, distance and near) with motility limitation, and extremely large fractures of greater than or equal to one half of the orbital floor on CT evaluation, often associated with inferior displacement of the globe. An additional indication for repair is increased vagal tone from muscle entrapment stimulating the oculocardiac reflex. Patients may manifest persistent nausea, vomiting, and bradycardia.

Follow-up

- Follow-up evaluation is performed approximately 1 week after the initial injury. At this point, the acute edema should be decreased, so the position of the globe and motility can be more accurately assessed. The patient is instructed to watch for local changes, specifically periorbital erythema, an increase in pain, and fever, which can be signs of impending orbital cellulitis.

Traumatic Optic Neuropathy

Symptoms

- A history of traumatic injury to the globe or orbit, causing direct injury of the optic nerve, or to the forehead or temporal region, causing indirect injury of the optic nerve, is reported. Optic nerve injury manifests as a reduction in visual acuity not explained by refractive error or injury to the cornea, lens, or retina.
- Visual acuity can decrease immediately after injury or can be delayed.

Signs

- Color vision and red saturation are decreased and may be accompanied by a visual field defect.
- The optic disc appears normal initially. If an atrophic disc is seen on examination, a chronic process is ongoing or the nerve sustained injury at least 6 weeks previously.
- Signs of nerve injury such as disc hemorrhage and edema may be seen.
- A new relative afferent pupillary defect in the traumatized eye suggests the diagnosis (i.e., no concurrent retinal pathologic conditions or chiasmal damage).

Etiology

- Direct injury to the optic nerve from a sharp injury or compression by fragments of bone, foreign body, blood, or edema can lead to traumatic optic neuropathy.
- A shearing injury to the optic nerve in the optic canal from blunt trauma to the head also has been implicated (indirect traumatic optic neuropathy).

Differential Diagnosis

Diagnostic possibilities include the following:
- Widespread retinal injury, with detachment and/or massive subretinal hemorrhage
- Optic chiasm injury

Workup

- A ruptured globe is ruled out in the involved eye and the fellow eye is examined. A careful pupillary examination demonstrates a relative afferent defect if an optic neuropathy is present.
- Color vision (red saturation) and confrontation visual field testing are performed. Perceived loss of central red recognition in the involved eye is a strong sign of optic nerve compromise.
- CT scanning of the head and orbits should pay special attention to the optic chiasm and optic canal to rule out chiasm and compressive injuries if the history is suggestive of these conditions.

Treatment

- Once the diagnosis is suspected, the patient is immediately referred to an ophthalmologist/neuro-ophthalmologist for complete assessment and management. If a traumatic optic neuropathy is diagnosed, the patient can be hospitalized and given intravenous high-dose corticosteroids. A recommended regimen is Solu-Medrol 30 mg/kg loading dose, then 5.4 mg/kg/hr for 24 to 48 hours before reevaluating for further therapy. This is the same dosage of corticosteroids currently recommended for spinal cord trauma. Patients should be properly advised about the risks and benefits of this therapy, and appropriate consent should be obtained.
- Antacids or histamine H_2 blockers (e.g., oral ranitidine [Zantac] 150 mg every day) are administered in conjunction with the corticosteroids for prophylaxis against corticosteroid-induced gastrointestinal bleeding.
- The patient is reexamined after 2 or 3 days of the corticosteroid regimen. If the visual acuity, color vision (red saturation), and relative afferent defect are stable or improved, the patient begins an oral prednisone taper. If the signs are worse (or get worse after corticosteroid taper), surgical exploration of the orbit or unroofing of the optic canal may be indicated.
- If signs return during the oral prednisone taper, intravenous corticosteroid administration may be reinstituted.
- Serum electrolyte and glucose levels are carefully monitored during heavy corticosteroid administration.

Follow-up

- The prognosis depends on the mechanism of injury and the degree of damage sustained by the optic nerve. With a clinically evident relative afferent pupillary defect, the optic nerve must have sustained a fairly severe injury; therefore, ultimate visual functioning may be poor.

Pupil Asymmetry

See Anisocoria in Chapter 12 for a discussion of disorders potentially causing pupillary asymmetry.

CHAPTER 17

Guide to Ophthalmic Medications

GEOFFREY BROOCKER • MICHAEL D. BENNETT

This chapter describes commonly used and prescribed ophthalmic medications. The most common trade names, concentrations, and indications are included, but this is not an official therapeutic document. If discrepancies arise, the reader should obtain official and more complete information from the pharmaceutical manufacturer.

For ease of reference, this chapter has been divided into three main sections. The first section is an index of commonly used ophthalmic medications (Table 17–1) that refers the reader to specific tables for additional information on each listed drug. The second section reviews diagnostic medications, including stains, anesthetics, and mydriatic and cycloplegic agents (Table 17–2). The third section of this chapter comprises the different categories of therapeutic agents: lubricants (Table 17–3), antibiotics (Tables 17–4 and 17–5), antivirals (Table 17–6), antifungals (Table 17–7), anti-inflammatory medications (Tables 17–8 to 17–11), antiglaucoma medications (Tables 17–12 to 17–18), and agents for relief of seasonal allergic conjunctivitis (Table 17–19).

Index of Ophthalmic Medications

The following table guides the reader to additional information on ophthalmic agents.

Table 17–1 Ophthalmic Medications

Trade Name	Generic Name	Table(s) with Additional Information
Acular	Ketorolac	Tables 17–10, 17–11, 17–19
Adsorbotear	Hydroxyethyl cellulose, povidone	Table 17–3
Akarpine	Pilocarpine hydrochloride	Table 17–14
AK–Chlor	Chloramphenicol	Tables 17–4, 17–5
AK–Cide	Sulfacetamide/prednisolone	Table 17–9
AK–Dex	Dexamethasone sodium phosphate	Tables 17–8, 17–11
AK–Mycin	Erythromycin	Tables 17–4, 17–5
AK–Poly–Bac	Polymyxin B/bacitracin	Tables 17–4, 17–5
AK–Pred	Prednisolone sodium phosphate	Tables 17–8, 17–11
AK–Spore	Polymyxin B/neomycin/gramicidin	Tables 17–4, 17–5
AK–Sulf	Sulfacetamide sodium	Tables 17–4, 17–5
AK–Tracin	Bacitracin zinc	Tables 17–4, 17–5
Alamast	Pemirolast potassium	Table 17–19
Alomide	Lodoxamide	Table 17–19
Alocril	Nedocromil	Table 17–19
Alphagan-P	Brimonidine tartrate	Table 17–13
Alrex	Loteprednol etabonate	Tables 17–8, 17–11
Amphotericin B	Amphotericin B	Table 17–7
Ancobon	Flucytosine	Table 17–7
AquaSite	Polycarbophil, PEG-400, dextran 70	Table 17–3
AquaSite (multidose)	Polycarbophil, PEG-400, dextran 70	Table 17–3
Azopt	Brinzolamide	Table 17–16
Betagan	Levobunolol hydrochloride	Table 17–12
Betimol	Timolol hemihydrate	Table 17–12
Betoptic	Betaxolol hydrochloride	Table 17–12
Betoptic S	Betaxolol hydrochloride	Table 17–12
Bion Tears	Hydroxypropyl methylcellulose, dextran 70	Table 17–3
Bleph-10	Sulfacetamide sodium	Tables 17–4, 17–5
Blephamide	Sulfacetamide/prednisolone	Table 17–9
Celluvisc	Carboxymethyl cellulose	Table 17–3
Cetamide	Sulfacetamide sodium	Tables 17–4, 17–5
Chloramphenicol (generic)	Chloramphenicol	Tables 17–4, 17–5
Chloromycetin	Chloramphenicol	Tables 17–4, 17–5
Chloroptic	Chloramphenicol	Tables 17–4, 17–5
Ciloxan	Ciprofloxacin hydrochloride	Tables 17–4, 17–5
Comfort Tears	Hydroxyethyl cellulose	Table 17–3
Cosopt	Dorzolamide/timolol maleate	Table 17–16
Crolom	Cromolyn sodium	Table 17–19
Cytovene	Ganciclovir sodium	Table 17–6
Decadron	Dexamethasone sodium phosphate	Tables 17–8, 17–11
Defy	Tobramycin sulfate	Tables 17–4, 17–5
Dexacidin	Neomycin/polymyxin B/dexamethasone	Table 17–9
Diamox	Acetazolamide	Table 17–16
Econopred	Prednisolone acetate	Tables 17–8, 17–11
Econopred Plus	Prednisolone acetate	Tables 17–8, 17–11
Elestat	Epinastine hydrochloride	Table 17–19
Emadine	Emedastine difumarate	Table 17–19
Epifrin	Epinephrine hydrochloride	Table 17–15
Epinal	Epinephrine borate	Table 17–15

Table 17–1   Ophthalmic Medications—cont'd

Trade Name	Generic Name	Table(s) with Additional Information
Epitrate	Epinephrine bitartrate	Table 17–15
Eppy/n	Epinephrine borate	Table 17–15
Eserine	Physostigmine	Table 17–14
Famvir	Famciclovir	Table 17–6
Flarex	Fluorometholone acetate	Tables 17–8, 17–11
Fluor-OP	Fluorometholone	Tables 17–8, 17–11
FML	Fluorometholone	Tables 17–8, 17–11
FML Forte	Fluorometholone	Tables 17–8, 17–11
FML S.O.P.	Fluorometholone	Tables 17–8, 17–11
Foscavir	Foscarnet sodium	Table 17–6
Gantrisin	Sulfisoxazole diolamine	Tables 17–4, 17–5
Garamycin	Gentamicin sulfate	Tables 17–4, 17–5
Genoptic	Gentamicin sulfate	Tables 17–4, 17–5
Gentacidin	Gentamicin sulfate	Tables 17–4, 17–5
Gentak	Gentamicin sulfate	Tables 17–4, 17–5
Gentamicin (generic)	Gentamicin sulfate	Tables 17–4, 17–5
Glaucon	Epinephrine hydrochloride	Table 17–15
Glauctabs	Methazolamide	Table 17–16
Herplex	Idoxuridine	Table 17–6
HMS	Medrysone	Tables 17–8, 17–11
Humorsol	Demecarium bromide	Table 17–14
HypoTears	Polyvinyl alcohol, PEG-400, dextrose	Table 17–3
HypoTears PF	Polyvinyl alcohol, PEG-400, dextrose	Table 17–3
Ilotycin	Erythromycin	Tables 17–4, 17–5
Inflamase	Prednisolone sodium phosphate	Tables 17–8, 17–11
Inflamase Forte	Prednisolone sodium phosphate	Tables 17–8, 17–11
Iopidine	Apraclonidine	Table 17–13
Isopto Carbachol	Carbachol	Table 17–14
Isopto Carpine	Pilocarpine hydrochloride	Table 17–14
Isopto Cetamide	Sulfacetamide sodium	Tables 17–4, 17–5
Isopto Plain	Hydroxypropyl methylcellulose	Table 17–3
Isopto Tears	Hydroxypropyl methylcellulose	Table 17–3
Lacrisert	Hydroxypropyl cellulose	Table 17–3
Livostin	Levocabastine hydrochloride	Table 17–19
Lotemax	Loteprednol etabonate	Tables 17–8, 17–11
Lumigan	Bimatoprost	Table 17–17
Maxidex	Dexamethasone sodium phosphate	Tables 17–8, 17–11
Maxitrol	Neomycin/polymyxin B/dexamethasone	Table 17–9
Monistat	Miconazole nitrate	Table 17–7
Murine	Polyvinyl alcohol, povidone	Table 17–3
MZM	Methazolamide	Table 17–16
Naphcon-A	Naphazoline/pheniramine	Table 17–19
Natacyn	Natamycin	Table 17–7
Neodecadron	Neomycin/dexamethasone	Table 17–9
Neosporin	Polymyxin B/neomycin/bacitracin	Tables 17–4, 17–5
Neosporin	Polymyxin B/neomycin/gramicidin	Tables 17–4, 17–5
Neotal	Polymyxin B/neomycin/bacitracin	Tables 17–4, 17–5
Neptazane	Methazolamide	Table 17–16
Ocu-Chlor	Chloramphenicol	Tables 17–4, 17–5

Table 17–1   Ophthalmic Medications—cont'd

Trade Name	Generic Name	Table(s) with Additional Information
Ocufen	Flurbiprofen sodium	Tables 17–10, 17–11
Ocuflox	Ofloxacin	Tables 17–4, 17–5
Ocupress	Carteolol hydrochloride	Table 17–12
Ocusert-Pilo	Pilocarpine hydrochloride	Table 17–14
Opcon-A	Naphazoline/pheniramine	Table 17–19
Ophthacet	Sulfacetamide sodium	Tables 17–4, 17–5
Optipranolol	Metipropanolol	Table 17–12
Optivar	Azelastine hydrochloride	Table 17–19
Osmitrol	Mannitol	Table 17–18
Osmoglyn	Glycerin	Table 17–18
Patanol	Olopatadine hydrochloride	Table 17–19
Phospholine iodide	Echothiophate iodide	Table 17–14
Pilagan	Pilocarpine nitrate	Table 17–14
Pilocar	Pilocarpine hydrochloride	Table 17–14
Pilopine HS Gel	Pilocarpine hydrochloride	Table 17–14
Piloptic	Pilocarpine hydrochloride	Table 17–14
Pilostat	Pilocarpine hydrochloride	Table 17–14
Polysporin	Polymyxin B/bacitracin	Tables 17–4, 17–5
Polytrim	Polymyxin B/trimethoprim	Tables 17–4, 17–5
Pred-Forte	Prednisolone acetate	Tables 17–8, 17–11
Pred-G	Prednisolone/gentamicin	Table 17–9
Pred Mild	Prednisolone acetate	Tables 17–8, 17–11
Profenal	Suprofen	Tables 17–10, 17–11
Propine	Dipivefrin hydrochloride	Table 17–14
Quixin	Levofloxacin	Tables 17–4, 17–5
Refresh	Polyvinyl alcohol, povidone	Table 17–3
Refresh Plus	Carboxymethyl cellulose	Table 17–3
Rescula	Unoprostone	Table 17–17
Sodium Sulamyd	Sulfacetamide sodium	Tables 17–4, 17–5
Statrol	Polymyxin B/neomycin	Tables 17–4, 17–5
Storzine	Pilocarpine hydrochloride	Table 17–14
Sulf-10	Sulfacetamide sodium	Tables 17–4, 17–5
Sulfacetamide (generic)	Sulfacetamide sodium	Tables 17–4, 17–5
TearGard	Hydroxyethyl cellulose, polyvinyl alcohol	Table 17–3
Tearisol	Hydroxypropyl methylcellulose	Table 17–3
Tears Naturale II	Hydroxypropyl methylcellulose, dextran 70	Table 17–3
Tears Naturale Free	Hydroxypropyl methylcellulose, dextran 70	Table 17–3
Tears Plus	Polyvinyl alcohol, povidone	Table 17–3
Tears Renewed	Hydroxypropyl methylcellulose, dextran 70	Table 17–3
Terra-Cortril	Oxytetracycline/dexamethasone	Table 17–9
Terramycin	Polymyxin B/oxytetracycline	Tables 17–4, 17–5
Timoptic	Timolol maleate	Table 17–12
Tobradex	Tobramycin/dexamethasone	Table 17–9
Tobrex	Tobramycin	Table 17–4
Travatan	Travaprost	Table 17–17
Trusopt	Dorzolamide hydrochloride	Table 17–16
Ultra Tears	Hydroxypropyl methylcellulose	Table 17–3
Valtrex	Valacyclovir	Table 17–6
Vasocidin	Sulfacetamide/prednisolone	Table 17–9

Table 17–1   Ophthalmic Medications—cont'd

Trade Name	Generic Name	Table(s) with Additional Information
Vasocon-A	Naphazoline/antazoline	Table 17–19
Vexol	Rimexolone	Tables 17–8, 17–11
Vigamox	Moxifloxacin	Tables 17–4, 17–5
Vira-A	Vidarabine monohydrate	Table 17–6
Viroptic	Trifluridine	Table 17–6
Vitrasert	Ganciclovir implant	Table 17–6
Voltaren	Diclofenac sodium	Tables 17–10, 17–11
Xalatan	Latanoprost	Table 17–17
Zaditor	Ketotifen	Table 17–19
Zovirax	Acyclovir sodium	Table 17–6
Zymar	Gatifloxacin	Tables 17–4, 17–5

Diagnostic Medications

Diagnostic medications are agents used to facilitate the ophthalmic examination.

Stains

Stains used in eye examinations include fluorescein and rose bengal. These are topical agents used to highlight epithelial abnormalities.

Fluorescein. Helpful in diagnosing corneal abrasions, fluorescein stains epithelial basement membrane in areas where the epithelium has been removed. Fluorescein is supplied on sterile paper strips, which is the preferred modality, and as a 2% solution that contains benoxinate, a topical anesthetic. However, the bottle containing the 2% solution is easily contaminated in a clinical setting.

Rose Bengal. Rose bengal dye stains sick devitalized epithelial cells and may be helpful in the diagnosis of herpetic ulcers, which may mimic corneal abrasions. Rose bengal is supplied on sterile paper strips.

Anesthetics

Anesthetics are used with diagnostic stains and are essential for ensuring patient comfort and cooperation in intraocular pressure measurements. These agents facilitate ocular examination in the setting of trauma and hasten penetration of dilating agents. Tetracaine hydrochloride (Pontocaine) is available in 0.5% and 1.0% solutions, with a duration of effect of approximately 15 minutes, and stings. Proparacaine hydrochloride (Ophthetic, Ophthaine) is available in a 0.5% solution, with a duration of effect of 10 to 15 minutes, and is less irritating.

   Note: All anesthetics are toxic to epithelial cells and thus will delay or prevent epithelial wound healing when used repeatedly. Dispensing these agents to patients is a medical-legal risk and is strongly discouraged unless they are followed carefully.

Mydriatics and Cycloplegics

Mydriatic and cycloplegic agents can be used for diagnostic and therapeutic purposes. Mydriatics dilate the pupil, and cycloplegic agents additionally paralyze the ciliary muscle (preventing accommodation). Dilating the pupil is necessary for adequate examination of the internal ocular structures. Therapeutic benefits are numerous: Paralyzing the ciliary muscle reduces pain associated with iritis, prevents formation of posterior synechiae (adhesions between the iris and lens), and helps stabilize the blood-ocular barrier during bouts of intraocular inflammation. The containers for these medications usually have a red top.

The typical regimen for diagnostic evaluation of the ocular fundus using mydriatic and cycloplegic agents is as follows:

- *Adults:* Phenylephrine 2.5%, Tropicamide 0.5%; 1 drop of each; repeated if needed after 20 to 30 minutes
- *Children:* Phenylephrine 2.5%, Tropicamide 0.5%; 1 drop of each; repeated if needed after 20 to 30 minutes; Cyclopentolate 1% to 2% added if refraction to be performed
- *Term infants:* Cyclopentolate 0.5%, Phenylephrine 2.5%; 1 drop in each eye; repeated in 5 minutes
- *Preterm infants up to 3 months of age:* Cyclomydril (cyclopentolate and phenylephrine), 1 drop in each eye; repeated in 5 minutes

Dilating drops are contraindicated in patients with known angle-closure glaucoma. Dilating drops may be less effective in patients with dark irides (iris pigment absorbs product, reducing exposure to receptors) or intraocular inflammation. Administration of dilating drops to premature infants or children with cardiac disease or hypertension carries a high risk of adverse effects. These agents should be used cautiously in these patients.

Table 17–2   Dilating Drops

Agent	Approximate Maximum Effect	Approximate Duration
Mydriatic		
Phenylephrine 2.5%	20 minutes	3 hours
Cycloplegic/Mydriatic		
Tropicamide 0.5%, 1%	20-30 minutes	3-6 hours
Cyclopentolate, 0.5%, 1%, 2%	20-45 minutes	Up to 24 hours
Homatropine 2%, 5%	20-40 minutes	2-3 days
Scopolamine 0.25%	20-45 minutes	4-7 days
Atropine 0.5%, 1%, 2%	30-40 minutes	1-2 weeks

Therapeutic Medications

Ocular Lubricants

The tear film is a highly complex multi-layer responsible for vision (the primary ocular refractive surface) and ocular comfort. A large percentage of patients have tear film abnormalities and experience symptoms related to "dry eyes" (burning, itching, reflex tearing, and foreign body sensation). Patients with ocular surface abnormalities usually respond well to the "artificial tears" type of lubricant, although the symptomatic relief may be only temporary.

Restasis (cyclosporine 0.05% emulsion) is a newer agent for the topical treatment of severe dry eye associated with ocular inflammatory disorders.

Table 17–3   Artificial Tear Preparations

Generic Name	Trade Name	Preservative*
Carboxymethyl cellulose	Refresh Plus	None
	Celluvisc	None
Hydroxyethyl cellulose	Comfort Tears	Benzalkonium chloride, EDTA
Hydroxyethyl cellulose, polyvinyl alcohol	TearGard	Sorbic acid, EDTA
Hydroxyethyl cellulose, povidone	Adsorbotear	Thimerosal, EDTA
Hydroxypropyl cellulose	Lacrisert	None
Hydroxypropyl methylcellulose	Isopto Plain	Benzalkonium chloride
	Isopto Tears	Benzalkonium chloride
	Tearisol	Benzalkonium chloride, EDTA
	Ultra Tears	Benzalkonium chloride
Hydroxypropyl methylcellulose, dextran 70	Bion Tears	None
	Tear Naturale II	Polyquad
	Tears Naturale Free	None
	Tears Renewed	Benzalkonium chloride, EDTA
Polycarbophil, PEG-400, dextran 70	AquaSite	EDTA
	AquaSite (multidose)	EDTA, ascorbic acid
Polyvinyl alcohol, PEG-400, dextrose	HypoTears	Benzalkonium chloride, EDTA
	HypoTears PF	EDTA
Polyvinyl alcohol, povidone	Murine	Benzalkonium chloride, EDTA
	Refresh	None
	Tears Plus	Chlorobutanol

*Preparations containing preservatives should be used no more than 6 to 8 times a day, to prevent toxicity to the ocular surface.
EDTA, ethylenediaminetetra-acetic acid.

Antibiotics

The most common ocular pathogens usually are staphylococci, streptococci, and *Haemophilus* species. Empirical treatment generally is successful in eradicating most surface infections; however, resistant organisms are becoming more common. Appropriate culture and susceptibility testing should be addressed before the initiation of therapy when clinically indicated.

   In general, topical antibiotics are given 4 to 6 times a day for simple infections and during the postoperative period. Severe infections, however, may require the use of multiple fortified antibiotics or an appropriate topical fluoroquinolone every hour around the clock.

Fortified Antibiotics. Used by ophthalmologists for serious anterior segment and corneal infections when higher concentrations of drug are needed to fight unusually virulent pathogens, fortified antibiotics are easily prepared by most pharmacies. The most common examples are fortified tobramycin or gentamicin, fortified vancomycin, and fortified cefazolin.

Table 17–4 Antibiotics

Generic Name	Trade Name	Bacterial Coverage
Bacitracin zinc	AK-Tracin	Most gram-positive organisms, diphtheroids, *Haemophilus*, and *Actinomyces*
Chloramphenicol	AK-Chlor Chloramphenicol (generic) Chloromycetin Chloroptic Ocu-Chlor	Many gram-positive and gram-negative organisms, especially *Haemophilus*, *Moraxella* species, *Staphylococcus aureus*, beta-hemolytic streptococci, and diphtheroids
Ciprofloxacin hydrochloride	Ciloxan	Broad spectrum, particularly targeting staphylococci, streptococci, and *Pseudomonas aeruginosa*
Erythromycin	AK-Mycin Erythromycin (generic) Ilotycin	Most gram-positive organisms, diphtheroids, *Haemophilus*, *Actinomyces*, and *Neisseria* species
Gatifloxacin	Zymar	Fourth-generation fluoroquinolone with broader spectrum of coverage, but not as good for *Pseudomonas* species
Gentamicin sulfate	Garamycin Genoptic Gentacidin Gentak Gentamicin (generic)	Broad spectrum, particularly targeting staphylococci (when drug used in high concentrations), and *P. aeruginosa*
Levofloxacin	Quixin	Broad spectrum, particularly targeting staphylococci, streptococci, and *Haemophilus influenzae*
Moxifloxacin	Vigamox	Fourth-generation fluoroquinolone with broader spectrum of coverage, but not as good for *Pseudomonas* species
Ofloxacin	Ocuflox	Broad spectrum, particularly targeting staphylococci, streptococci, *Haemophilus*, and *P. aeruginosa*
Polymyxin B/bacitracin	AK-Poly-Bac Polysporin	Some gram-negative organisms and most gram-positive organisms, diphtheroids, *Haemophilus*, and *Actinomyces*

Table 17–4   Antibiotics—cont'd

Generic Name	Trade Name	Bacterial Coverage
Polymyxin B/ neomycin/bacitracin	AK-Spore Neosporin Neotal Polymyxin B (generic)	Gram-negative organisms and broad spectrum for gram-positive organisms, particularly targeting staphylococci, pseudomonads, diphtheroids, *Haemophilus*, and *Actinomyces*
Polymyxin B/ oxytetracycline	Terramycin	Most staphylococci, streptococci, gonococci, *Chlamydia* species, and few gram-negative organisms
Polymyxin B/ trimethoprim	Polytrim	Most staphylococci, streptococci, and *Haemophilus*
Sulfacetamide sodium	AK-Sulf Bleph-10 Cetamide Isopto Cetamide Ophthacet Sodium Sulamyd Sulf-10 Sulfacetamide (generic)	Wide range of gram-positive and gram-negative organisms; some staphylococci, pneumococci, *Haemophilus*, *Moraxella* and *Chlamydia* species
Sulfisoxazole diolamine	Gantrisin	Wide range of gram-positive and gram-negative organisms; some staphylococci, pneumococci, *Haemophilus*, *Moraxella* and *Chlamydia* species
Tobramycin sulfate	Defy Tobrex Tobramycin (generic)	Broad spectrum, including staphylococci, streptococci, *Haemophilus*, and *P. aeruginosa*

Table 17–5   Antibiotic Concentrations

Generic Name	Trade Name	Concentration of Solution	Concentration of Ointment
Bacitracin zinc	AK-Tracin	NA	50 units/g
Chloramphenicol	AK-Chlor	0.5%	1.0%
	Chloromycetin	0.5%	1.0%
	Chloroptic	0.5%	1.0%
	Ocu-Chlor	0.5%	1.0%
Ciprofloxacin hydrochloride	Ciloxan	0.3%	0.3%
Erythromycin	AK-Mycin	NA	0.5%
	Erythromycin (generic)	NA	0.5%
	Ilotycin	NA	0.5%
Gatifloxacin	Zymar	0.3%	NA
Gentamicin sulfate	Garamycin	0.3%	0.3%
	Genoptic	0.3%	0.3%
	Gentacidin	0.3%	0.3%
	Gentak	0.3%	0.3%
	Gentamicin (generic)	0.3%	0.3%

Table 17–5   Antibiotic Concentrations—cont'd

Generic Name	Trade Name	Concentration of Solution	Concentration of Ointment
Levofloxacin	Quixin	0.5%	NA
Moxifloxacin	Vigamox	0.5%	NA
Ofloxacin	Ocuflox	0.3%	NA
Polymyxin B/bacitracin	AK-Poly-Bac	NA	10,000 units, 500 units/g
	Polysporin	NA	10,000 units, 500 units/g
Polymyxin B/neomycin	Statrol	16,250 units, 3.5 mg/mL	10,000 units, 3.5 mg/g
Polymyxin B/neomycin/ bacitracin	Neotal	NA	5000 units, 5 mg, 400 units/g
	Neosporin	NA	NA
	Polymyxin B (generic)	NA	NA
Polymyxin B/neomycin/ gramicidin	AK-Spore	10,000 units in 1.75 mg or 0.025 mg/mL	NA
	Neosporin		NA
	Polymyxin B (generic)		NA
Polymyxin B/oxytetracycline	Terramycin	NA	10,000 units, 5 mg/g
Polymyxin B/trimethoprim	Polytrim	10,000 units, 1 mg/mL	NA
Sulfacetamide sodium	AK-Sulf	10.0%	10.0%
	Bleph-10	10.0%	10.0%
	Cetamide	NA	10.0%
	Isopto Cetamide	15.0%	NA
	Ophthacet	10.0%	NA
	Sodium Sulamyd	10%, 30%	10.0%
	Sulf-10	10.0%	NA
	Sulfacetamide (generic)	10%, 15%, 30%	10.0%
Sulfisoxazole diolamine	Gantrisin	4.0%	4.0%
Tobramycin sulfate	Defy	0.3%	0.3%
	Tobrex	0.3%	NA
	Tobramycin (generic)	0.3%	0.3%

NA, not applicable.

Antivirals

Advances in the pharmacology of chemotherapeutic agents used to fight viral diseases have progressed rather slowly compared with those in other areas of medicine, in part because of the more complex mechanisms of viral infection that must be addressed in developing such agents. Viruses are obligate intracellular pathogens that use the host's metabolic processes for their survival and replication. Thus, antiviral agents need to target the pathogen while leaving uninfected host cells essentially unaffected from their toxic side effects. To date, the most effective antiviral agents target viral enzymes and proteins that are essential for viral assembly.

Table 17–6   Antiviral Agents

Generic Name	Trade Name	Concentration	Indication
Idoxuridine	Herplex	0.1% solution	HSV infection
	Stoxil	0.5% ointment	HSV infection
Trifluridine	Viroptic	1.0% solution	HSV infection
Vidarabine monohydrate	Vira-A	3.0% ointment	HSV infection
Acyclovir sodium	Zovirax	Systemic preparation only	HSV, HZV infection
Foscarnet sodium	Foscavir	Systemic preparation only	CMV infection in immunocompromised patients
Famciclovir	Famvir	Systemic preparation only	HZV infection
Ganciclovir sodium	Cytovene	Systemic preparation only	CMV infection in immunocompromised patients
	Vitrasert	Intraocular implant	
Valacyclovir hydrochloride	Valtrex	Systemic preparation only	HSV, HZV infection

CMV, cytomegalovirus; HSV, herpes simplex virus; HZV, herpes zoster virus.

Antifungal Agents

Deciding on the appropriate ophthalmic antifungal usually depends on several variables, including the site of primary infection, route of administration, organism involved, and drug sensitivities. Currently, Diflucan (fluconazole) and Sporanox (itraconazole) are oral/systemic agents that show good ocular penetration as an adjunct in these difficult to treat infections.

Table 17–7   Antifungal Agents

Generic Name	Trade Name	Topical Concentration	Spectrum
Amphotericin B	Amphotericin B	0.1-0.5% solution	Blastomycetes; *Candida*, *Coccidioides*, and *Histoplasma* species
Flucytosine	Ancobon	1.0% solution	*Candida* species
Natamycin*	Natacyn	5% suspension	*Candida* species, aspergilli, and *Cephalosporium*, *Fusarium*, and *Penicillium* species
Miconazole nitrate	Monistat	1% solution	*Candida* and *Cryptococcus* species, aspergilli

*Often the drug of choice for most mycotic corneal infections and the only ocular formulation commercially available. The others need to be prepared by the pharmacy.

Anti-inflammatory Agents

Anti-inflammatory agents are used most frequently to suppress immunologic mechanisms of all types, both externally and within the eye. Suppression of severe external inflammation is necessary to prevent corneal scarring and permanent tear film abnormalities. Within the eye, these agents help prevent synechiae (scarring), some forms of glaucoma, and postoperative inflammation. Topical administration allows excellent penetration into the anterior chamber. Some agents penetrate easier (e.g., suspensions) than others depending on the chemical composition. Topical corticosteroids should be used with caution because they can cause cataracts and glaucoma used chronically and may acutely potentiate herpes simplex viral replication or microbial infection.

Table 17-8 Anti-inflammatory Agents

Generic Name	Trade Name	Formulation	Topical Concentration
Dexamethasone	Maxidex	Suspension*	0.1%
Dexamethasone sodium phosphate	AK-Dex	Ointment	0.05%
	Decadron	Ointment	0.05%
	Maxidex	Ointment	0.05%
	Dexamethasone (generic)	Ointment	0.05%
Dexamethasone sodium phosphate	AK-Dex	Solution	0.1%
	Decadron	Solution	0.1%
	Dexamethasone (generic)	Solution	0.1%
Fluorometholone	Fluor-OP	Suspension*	0.1%
	FML	Suspension*	0.1%
	FML Forte	Suspension*	0.25%
	FML S.O.P.	Ointment	0.1%
Fluorometholone acetate	Flarex	Suspension*	0.1%
Loteprednol etabonate	Alrex	Suspension*	0.2%
	Lotemax	Suspension*	0.5%
Medrysone	HMS	Suspension*	1.0%
Prednisolone acetate	Econopred	Suspension*	0.125%
	Econopred Plus	Suspension*	1.0%
	Pred-Forte	Suspension*	1.0%
	Pred Mild	Suspension*	0.125%
Prednisolone sodium phosphate	AK-Pred	Solution	0.125%, 1.0%
	Inflamase	Solution	0.125%
	Inflamase Forte	Solution	1.0%
	Prednisolone (generic)	Solution	0.125%, 1.0%
Rimexolone	Vexol	Suspension*	1.0%

*Suspensions need to be shaken before instillation.

Anti-inflammatory and Antibiotic Combinations. Generally, anti-inflammatory medications are indicated for steroid-responsive inflammatory ocular conditions for which a corticosteroid is indicated and bacterial infection or risk of bacterial ocular infection exists. These medications may be contraindicated in any condition in which an epithelial defect exists, including patients with epithelial herpes simplex keratitis and those who have recently undergone uncomplicated removal of a corneal foreign body.

Table 17–9   Anti-inflammatory and Antibiotic Combinations

Generic Name	Trade Name	Formulation and Amount	Typical Dosage
Gentamicin sulfate/ prednisolone acetate	Pred-G	Suspension (5 mL) Ointment (3.5 g)	1 drop 4 times a day Up to 4 times a day
Neomycin/polymyxin B/ dexamethasone	Dexacidin Maxitrol	Suspension (5 mL) Ointment (3.5 g)	1 drop 4 times a day Up to 4 times a day
Neomycin/dexamethasone	NeoDecadron	Suspension (5 mL) Ointment (3.5 g)	1 drop 4 times a day Up to 4 times a day
Oxytetracycline/dexamethasone	Terra-Cortril	Suspension (5 mL)	1 drop 3 times a day
Sulfacetamide sodium/ prednisolone acetate	AK-Cide Blephamide Vasocidin	Suspension (5 mL) Ointment (3.5 g)	1 drop 4 times a day Up to 4 times a day
Tobramycin/dexamethasone	Tobradex	Suspension (5 mL) Ointment (3.5 g)	1 drop 4 times a day Up to 4 times a day

Nonsteroidal Anti-inflammatory Agents. Nonsteroidal anti-inflammatory drugs (NSAIDs) also are used to suppress inflammatory mechanisms, both externally and within the eye. They differ from corticosteroids in their mechanisms of action and effectiveness; however, they do not cause cataracts or glaucoma or potentiate herpes simplex viral replication.

Table 17–10   Nonsteroidal Anti-inflammatory Agents

Generic Name	Trade Name	Formulation	Topical Concentration
Diclofenac	Voltaren	Solution	0.1%
Flurbiprofen	Ocufen	Solution	0.03%
Ketorolac	Acular	Solution	0.5%
Suprofen	Profenal	Solution	1.0%

Table 17–11   Comparison of Selected Anti-inflammatory Agents

Generic Name	Trade Name	Comment
NSAIDs	Ocufen Voltaren Acular	Interference with prostaglandin-induced operative miosis, other inflammations (e.g., iritis, cystoid macular edema), and allergy-related irritation; no causation of cataracts or glaucoma; no potentiation of herpes simplex infection
Loteprednol	Alrex Lotemax	Used for ocular surface allergy control Higher strength, better for intraocular inflammation Fewer side effects than with prednisolone and dexamethasone
Medrysone	HMS	Weak steroid, useful for surface allergy, very few side effects
Fluorometholone	FML	More potent than medrysone, excellent for external inflammation, fewer side effects than with prednisolone and dexamethasone
Prednisolone acetate	Pred-Forte	Potent steroid, highly effective for anterior segment inflammation, higher risk of side effects (IOP elevation, infection, HSV activation)
Dexamethasone sodium phosphate	Decadron	Highly potent and effective, very high risk of side effects
Rimexolone	Vexol	Potent steroid, with somewhat fewer ocular side effects (similar to those with FML)

HSV, herpes simplex virus; IOP, intraocular pressure; NSAIDs, nonsteroidal anti-inflammatory drugs.

Antiglaucoma Medications

Antiglaucoma medications are used to reduce optic nerve damage and visual loss associated with elevated introcular pressure. The seven classes of these medications, which differ in their mechanisms of action, are as follows:

1. Beta-blocking agents (Table 17–12)
2. Adrenergic agonists (Table 17–13)
3. Cholinergic agonists (Table 17–14)
4. Sympathomimetics (Table 17–15)
5. Carbonic anhydrase inhibitors (Table 17–16)
6. Prostaglandins (Table 17–17)
7. Hyperosmotic agents (Table 17–18)

Beta Blockers. A class of drugs commonly used as first-line agents for treatment of open-angle glaucoma and ocular hypertension, beta blockers work mostly by reducing aqueous humor secretion by the ciliary body. Because of some systemic absorption, they may be contraindicated in some patients with heart and respiratory conditions. More selective beta blockers appear to have less severe side effects, but are not as efficacious. Ocular side effects include stinging and burning.

Table 17–12   Antiglaucoma Medications: Beta Blockers

Generic Name	Trade Name	Typical Dosage	Comments
Betaxolol hydrochloride	Betoptic-S (0.25%) 1 drop 2 times a day	Generic (0.5%) 1 drop 2 times a day	Beta-2 selective; use cautiously in patients with respiratory conditions
Carteolol hydrochloride	Ocupress (1.0%)	1 drop 2 times a day	Nonselective beta blocker
Levobunolol hydrochloride	Betagan (0.25%, 0.5%) Generic (0.25%, 0.5%)	1 drop 2 times a day 1 drop 2 times a day	Nonselective beta blocker
Metipranolol	Optipranolol (0.3%)	1 drop 2 times a day	Nonselective beta blocker
Timolol maleate	Timoptic (0.25%, 0.5%)	1 drop 2 times a day	Nonselective beta blocker
Timolol maleate	Timoptic XE (0.25%, 0.5%)	Once a day	Nonselective beta blocker; solution becomes a gel once in contact with the eye, increasing period of drug delivery
Timolol hemihydrate	Betimol (0.25%, 0.5%)	1 drop 2 times a day	Nonselective beta blocker

Alpha Agonists. Alpha agonists reduce intraocular pressure by decreasing aqueous production and increasing uveoscleral outflow. This class may prove to be effective at reducing intraocular pressure without the cardiac side effects of beta blockers. Currently, two drugs are on the market. The most common side effect is an allergic reaction developing with long-term use.

Table 17–13   Antiglaucoma Medications: Alpha Agonists

Generic Name	Trade Name	Typical Dosage	Comments
Apraclonidine	Iopidine (0.5%, 1%)	1 drop 3 times a day	Short-term adjuvant for patients on maximal medical therapy; approximately 1 month to be effective
Brimonide tartrate	Alphagan-P (0.15%)	1 drop 3 times a day	Agent with seemingly better toleration than its predecessor; less tachyphylaxis noted
	Generic (0.2%)	1 drop 3 times a day	High allergy incidence

Cholinergics. Parasympathomimetic agents are divided into direct-acting (cholinergic) and indirect-acting (anticholinesterase) agents. Used primarily for glaucoma and control of accommodative esotropia, they reduce intraocular pressure by causing contraction on the ciliary muscle. This contraction pulls on the trabecular meshwork and facilitates aqueous outflow. Acute poisoning with these agents (unusual with topical application) can produce the cholinergic crisis syndrome, which includes sweating, gastrointestinal disturbances, bradycardia, and paralysis of the respiratory muscles.

Table 17–14   Antiglaucoma Medications: Cholinergic Agents

Generic Name	Trade Name	Typical Dosage	Concentrations
Cholinergic Agents			
Carbachol	Isopto Carbachol	1 drop 3 times a day	1.5%, 3%
Pilocarpine	Akarpine	1 drop 4 times a day	1%, 2%, 4%
hydrochloride	Isopto Carpine	1 drop 4 times a day	0.5%, 1%-6%, 8%, 10%
	Ocusert-Pilo	1 insert a week	20-40 mg/hr/week
	Pilocar	1 drop 4 times a day	0.5%, 1%-4%, 6%
	Pilopine HS Gel	½ inch at bedtime	4%
	Piloptic	1 drop 4 times a day	0.5%, 1%-4%, 6%
	Pilostat	1 drop 4 times a day	1%, 2%, 4%
	Storzine	1 drop 4 times a day	1%, 2%, 4%
	Generic	1 drop 4 times a day	0.5%, 1%-4%, 6%
Pilocarpine nitrate	Pilagan	1 drop 4 times a day	1%, 2%, 4%
Anticholinesterase Agents			
Physostigmine	Eserine	1 drop 4 times a day	0.25%
	Generic (ointment)	½ inch 3 times a day	0.25%
Demecarium	Humorsol	1 drop 2 times a day to 1 drop a week	0.125%, 0.25%
Echothiophate iodide	Phospholine iodide	1 drop 2 times a day	0.125%, 0.25%

Sympathomimetics. Sympathomimetics have been of limited usefulness in the general population due to the numerous side effects (surface allergy, tolerance) associated with their use. However, a certain subset of the population tolerates these medications. These agents reduce intraocular pressure by mostly increasing aqueous outflow.

Table 17–15   Antiglaucoma Medications: Sympathomimetics

Generic Name	Trade Name	Typical Dosage	Concentration
Epinephrine bitartrate	Epitrate	1 drop every day or 2 times a day	2%
Epinephrine borate	Epinal	1 drop 2 times a day	0.5%, 1%
	Eppy/n	1 drop 2 times a day	0.5%, 1%, 2%
Epinephrine hydrochloride	Epifrin	1 drop every day or 2 times a day	0.5%, 1%, 2%
	Glaucon		1%, 2%
Dipivefrin hydrochloride	Propine	1 drop 2 times a day	0.10%

Carbonic Anhydrase Inhibitors. Carbonic anhydrase inhibitors (CAIs) reduce aqueous formation by direct inhibition of carbonic anhydrase within the ciliary body. Oral CAIs are highly effective but can also result in serious side effects such as paresthesias, anorexia, gastrointestinal disturbances, headaches, altered taste and smell, and sodium and potassium depletion. Kidney stone formation may be facilitated in certain patients. Topical CAIs appear to be much better tolerated, with a lower side-effect profile, but are not as effective.

Table 17–16   Antiglaucoma Medications: Carbonic Anhydrase Inhibitors

Generic Name	Trade Name	Typical Dosage	Comments
Topical			
Brinzolamide	Azopt (1%)	1 drop 3 times a day	Not as effective as oral preparations
Dorzolamide hydrochloride	Trusopt (2%)	1 drop 3 times a day	Not as effective as oral preparations
	Cosopt	1 drop twice a day	Combined with timolol maleate
Oral			
Acetazolamide	Diamox	250 mg tablet 4 times a day	Numerous systemic side effects
	Diamox Sequel	500 mg tablet 2 times a day	Slightly better tolerated
Methazolamide	Neptazane	50 mg tablets 2 times a day	Not as effective as Diamox but appears to be better tolerated by some patients

Prostaglandins. This newer class of agents is used to treat open-angle glaucoma and ocular hypertension. The mechanism of action is to increase uveoscleral outflow, thus reducing intraocular pressure. The most common side effects are hyperemia, an increase in iris pigmentation, and lash growth. These agents have become heavily prescribed, even as monotherapy, due to lack of autonomic side effects and once-daily dosing.

Table 17–17   Antiglaucoma Medications: Prostaglandins

Generic Name	Trade Name	Typical Dosage	Comments
Bimatoprost	Lumigan (0.03%)	1 drop daily (evening)	Note effects on iris color, lashes
Latanoprost	Xalatan (0.005%)	1 drop daily (evening)	
Travoprost	Travatan (0.004%)	1 drop daily (evening)	
Unoprostone	Rescula (0.15%)	1 drop 2 times a day	Not as efficacious

Hyperosmotic Agents. Given systemically, hyperosmotic agents increase the osmolality of the blood. This creates an osmotic gradient between the intravascular space and vitreous cavity and effectively pulls fluid from the vitreous into the bloodstream. These medications are used to acutely lower the intraocular pressure in an attack of angle-closure glaucoma and to reduce eye pressure for certain ocular procedures.

Table 17–18   Antiglaucoma Medications: Hyperosmotic Agents

Generic Name	Trade Name	Typical Dosage	Comments
Glycerin	Osmoglyn (50%)	1-1.5 g/kg	Antiemetic often required to prevent side effect of vomiting
Mannitol	Osmitrol (5%-20%)	0.5-2 g/kg	Intravenous drug; adult dose ranges from 20 to 200 g/24 hr

Agents for Relief of Allergy Symptoms (Seasonal Allergic Conjunctivitis)

Ocular allergy encompasses a broad spectrum of diseases characterized by a marked type I hypersensitivity response. Exposure to environmental allergens such as animal dander, pollens, and dust can cause symptoms in sensitized individuals. An allergic response is typically characterized by conjunctival injection, chemosis (swelling of the conjunctiva), tearing, eyelid swelling, burning, and ocular and periocular itching. Treatment of allergic ocular disease ideally entails removing the offending agent or modifying the patient's environment and treating the patient topically to provide symptomatic relief.

Table 17–19   Agents for Relief of Allergy Symptoms

Generic Name	Trade Name	Typical Dosage	Mechanism of Action
Azelastine hydrochloride	Optivar	1 drop 2 times a day	Histamine H_1 antagonist
Cromolyn	Crolom	1 drop 4 times a day	Mast cell inhibitor
Emedastine difumurate	Emadine	1 drop up to 4 times a day	H_1 antagonist
Epinastine hydrochloride	Elestat	1 drop 2 times a day	Antihistamine and mast cell stabilizer
Ketorolac	Acular	1 drop 4 times a day	NSAID
Ketotifen	Zaditor	1 drop 2 times a day	Antihistamine and mast cell stabilizer
Levocabastin	Livostin	1 drop 4 times a day	H_1 antagonist
Lodoxamide	Alomide	1 drop 4 times a day	Mast cell inhibitor
Naphazoline/antazoline	Vasocon-A	1 drop 4 times a day	Antihistamine/decongestant
Naphazoline/pheniramine	Naphcon-A Opcon-A	1 drop 4 times a day	Antihistamine/decongestant
Nedocromil	Alocril	1 drop 2 times a day	Mast cell stabilizer
Olopatadine hydrochloride	Patanol	1 drop 2 times a day	Antihistamine and mast cell stabilizer
Pemirolast potassium	Alamast	1 drop 4 times a day	Mast cell stabilizer

NSAID, nonsteroidal anti-inflammatory drug.

Index

Note: Page numbers followed by f refer to figures (illustrations); page numbers followed by t refer to tables.

A

Abducens nerve (sixth cranial nerve), 7, 222

Abducens nerve (sixth cranial nerve) palsy, 32, 222-223
signs of, 222, 222f

Abrasion, of cornea, 331-333, 332f
due to conjunctival foreign body, 331, 339, 339f

Abscess. See Cellulitis.

Abuse (child abuse), ocular signs of, 261-262, 262f

Acanthamoeba infection, keratitis due to, 44f

Accommodation, 127, 129f
age-related changes in, 30, 230, 230f

Accommodative esotropia, 268, 269f

Acid injury, to eye, 350

Acquired immunodeficiency syndrome (AIDS), 298
ocular lesions associated with, 177, 298, 299f

Acquired nystagmus, 226-227

Actinic keratosis, 74
eyelid involvement in, 74-75, 75f

Acuity (visual acuity), 2
measurement of, 2-4
Snellen charts in, 3f, 4f
refractive power and, 4-6

Acute angle-closure glaucoma. See Angle-closure glaucoma.

Adenoviral conjunctivitis, 56
in children, 259-260

Adie's syndrome, 216, 217f

After-cataract, 136, 136f

Aging
and cataract formation, 128-131, 130f, 131f
and changes in accommodation, 30, 230, 230f

Aging—cont'd
and loss of lens elasticity, 128
and macular degeneration, 173-176, 174f, 175f
and thinning of orbital septum, 67

AIDS (acquired immunodeficiency syndrome), 298
ocular lesions associated with, 177, 298, 299f

Alkali injury, to eye, 349f, 349-350, 350f

Allen figures, in vision testing of children, 236, 236f

Allergic conjunctivitis, 58, 58f, 59f, 96, 97f
treatment of, 59, 96-97
medications used in, 386t
vs. other conjunctivitides, 36t

Alpha agonists, for glaucoma, 383, 383t

Amaurosis fugax, 30

Amblyopia, 269-271

Amiodarone therapy, 317
ocular problems associated with, 317, 317f, 318

Amsler grid testing, 10-11, 11f

Anesthetics, 373

Angiography, 153

Angioid streaks, in retina, 297
Ehlers-Danlos syndrome and, 297, 297f, 298

Angle-closure glaucoma, 28, 39-40, 195-197
treatment of, 196
laser iridectomy in, 193f, 196

Anisocoria, 216-218

Ankylosing spondylitis, 293
anterior uveitis associated with, 141f, 293-294

Anterior chamber of eye, 1
blood in, 39, 40f, 353f, 353-355
impaired clearance of, in sickle cell disease, 354

Anterior chamber of eye—cont'd
inflammatory cells in
as postoperative finding, 181, 182f
as sign of corneal ulcer, 111, 112f
as sign of uveitis, 141, 142f
shallow, penlight demonstration of, 194f
slit lamp examination of, 13

Anterior ischemic optic neuropathy, 201-205
arteritic, 203-205, 204f
nonarteritic, 201-203, 202f

Anterior scleritis, 47f, 121, 121f, 122f

Anterior uveitis, 140-145
ankylosing spondylitis and, 141f, 293-294
Behçet's disease and, 294
hypopyon accompanying, 141, 142f
iridal nodules in, 142, 143f
keratic precipitates associated with, 141, 141f
synechiae as signs of, 141, 143f

Antibiotic ocular medications, 375-378, 376t-378t, 381t

Antifungal ocular medications, 379, 379t

Antiglaucoma medications, 194, 196, 382-385, 383t-385t

Anti-inflammatory ocular medications, 380-381, 380t-382t

Antiviral ocular medications, 378, 379t

Applanation tonometry, 14f, 14-15

Aqueous humor
flow of, 189, 190f
blockage of. See Angle-closure glaucoma.
leakage of, Seidel test for, 344, 344f

Arcus, of cornea, 299, 299f

Arteritis, giant cell, 203-205
optic neuropathy in, 204, 204f

Arthritis, rheumatoid, 308
   ocular problems associated with,
      308f, 308-309, 309f
Artificial tears, 106-107, 375t
Astigmatism, 5, 5f
Atrophic ("dry") age-related macular
      degeneration, 29, 174, 174f,
      175

B

Bacterial conjunctivitis, 55, 55f, 91f, 92,
      93f, 94
   discharge associated with, 55, 55f,
      92, 92f, 93f
   pediatric cases of, 260
   vs. other conjunctivitides, 36t
Bacterial corneal ulcer, 111, 112f, 113f
   in contact lens wearers, 334, 335f
Basal cell carcinoma, of eyelid, 77f,
      77-78
Behçet's disease, 294
   ocular lesions in, 294-295
Benign essential blepharospasm, 86-87,
      87f
Beta blockers, for glaucoma, 382,
      383t
Binocular diplopia, causes of, 31-33
Blepharitis, 34, 51, 79-81, 98f
   conjunctivitis and, 97-98
   facial sebaceous gland dysfunction
      (rosacea) and, 98, 98f
   infection and, 51, 52f, 80, 80f, 84,
      85f
   meibomian gland dysfunction and,
      51, 52f, 81
   pediculosis and, 52, 53f
   seborrheic, 51, 51f, 80, 80f
Blepharospasm, 86-87, 87f
Blindness. See Visual loss.
Blood cells, in anterior chamber of eye,
      39, 40f, 353f, 353-355
   impaired clearance of, in sickle cell
      disease, 354
Blood loss. See Hemorrhage.
Blow-out fracture, orbital, 33, 363-365,
      364f
Blue sclera(e)
   in Ehlers-Danlos syndrome, 297f
   in osteogenesis imperfecta, 306, 306f
Botox therapy, 318
   management of blepharospasm via,
      87
   ocular problems associated with,
      318

Bowel disease, inflammatory, 301
   ocular lesions associated with, 301,
      301f
Brain
   infarct in, and visual loss, 27
   tumor of, and visual loss, 29
Branch retinal artery occlusion, 162. See
      also Retinal artery, occlusion
      of.
Branch retinal vein occlusion, 167, 168,
      168f, 169
Buckling, scleral, in retinal surgery, 186,
      187f
Bull's-eye maculopathy
   in patients receiving chloroquine,
      319, 319f
   in patients receiving
      hydroxychloroquine, 325,
      325f
Burn(s), ocular, 348-353, 349f, 350f,
      352f
Burning sensation, ocular, 34
Busacca nodules, 142, 143f

C

Calcium accumulation, on cornea, 115,
      115f
Canalicular injury, 361, 362t
Canaliculitis, 284f, 284-285
Carbonic anhydrous inhibitors, for
      glaucoma, 384, 385t
Carcinoma, of eyelid, 77f, 77-79, 79f
Carotid artery–cavernous sinus fistula,
      223-224
   red eye associated with, 65, 65f,
      224f
Cataract(s), 29
   congenital, 245-246
   and leukocoria, 245, 246f
   cortical, 130, 130f
   dense white, 131, 131f
   diabetes mellitus and, 296, 296f
   laser therapy for, 136, 137f
   nuclear, 130, 130f
   posterior subcapsular, 131, 131f
   senile, 128-131, 130f, 131f
   surgery for, 132-136, 133f-135f
      opacification following, 136-137
   traumatic, 359f
   Wilson's disease and, 316
Cavernous sinus, fistula between carotid
      artery and, 223-224
   red eye associated with, 65, 65f,
      224f

Cellulitis
   orbital, 48f, 279f, 279-281, 280f
      pediatric cases of, 263-264
   preseptal, 49, 275-276, 278-279
      pediatric cases of, 263-264
Central retinal artery occlusion, 162,
      162f. See also Retinal artery,
      occlusion of.
Central retinal vein occlusion, 167,
      167f, 168, 169
Chalazion, 50, 51f, 82-83
   in children, 266, 267
Chemical injury, to eye, 348-351, 349f,
      350f
Chemosis, allergen-induced, 96, 97f
Cherry-rod spot, in fovea of retina, as
      sign of arterial occlusion, 17,
      163, 163f
Children. See Pediatric patients.
Chlamydial conjunctivitis, 56-57,
      94-95, 95f
   laboratory findings in, 95, 96f
   treatment of, 57-58, 95
   vs. other conjunctivitides, 36t
Chloroquine therapy, 318-319
   ocular problems associated with, 319,
      319f
Cholinergics, for glaucoma, 383, 384t
Choroid, 2, 139, 140f
Chronic conjunctivitis, in children, 260
Cialis (tadalafil) therapy, 327
   ocular effects of, 328
Ciliary body, 2, 139, 140f
Ciliary muscle paralysis, agents
      inducing, 374, 374t
Coloboma, 254-255, 255f
Color vision, 11-12
Confrontation visual field test, 10, 11f
Congenital eye anomalies, 245-259
Conjunctiva(e), 89, 90f. See also
      Conjunctivitis.
   chemosis of, allergen-induced, 96,
      97f
   examination of, 7, 13
   foreign body in, 339f, 339-341
      corneal abrasion due to, 331, 339,
         339f
   growth(s) on or in, 60-62, 62f,
      98-102, 99f-101f
      extension of, onto cornea, 61, 62f,
         113, 114f
      HIV infection and, 298, 299f
   hemorrhagic discoloration of, 337f,
      337-339
   laceration and, 341, 341f

Conjunctiva(e)—cont'd
  inflammation of. *See* Conjunctivitis.
  injection (congestion) of
    as manifestation of infection, 89,
      90f, 92f, 95f
    as sign of uveitis, 141, 141f
  laceration of, 341f, 341-342
  scarring of, in Stevens-Johnson
      syndrome, 312, 312f
  slit lamp examination of, 13
Conjunctivitis, 35, 36t, 54-58, 89-98
  adenoviral, 56
    in children, 259-260
  allergic, 58, 58f, 59f, 96, 97f
    treatment of, 59, 96-97
      medications used in, 386t
    vs. other conjunctivitides, 36t
  bacterial, 55, 92, 94
    discharge associated with, 55, 55f,
      92, 92f, 93f
    pediatric cases of, 260
    vs. other conjunctivitides, 36t
  blepharitis and, 97-98
  chlamydial, 56-57, 94-95, 95f
    laboratory findings in, 95, 96f
    treatment of, 57-58, 95
    vs. other conjunctivitides, 36t
  chronic, in children, 260
  drug allergy and, 58, 59f
  eye-rubbing and, 59
  herpes simplex virus infection and,
    36t
    in children, 260
  molluscum contagiosum and, 60, 61f
  Neisseria gonorrhoeae infection and, 48,
    49f, 92, 93f
    in infants, 239, 240, 240f
  Neisseria meningitidis infection and, 92
  pediatric cases of, 56, 238-240, 240f,
    259-261
  vernal, 58, 58f
    in children, 260
  viral, 55-56, 89, 90f, 91, 91f
    follicular lesions in, 55, 55f, 91,
      91f
    pediatric cases of, 259-260
    subepithelial corneal infiltrates
      associated with, 91, 92f
    vs. other conjunctivitides, 36t
  vs. nasolacrimal duct obstruction, in
    infants, 241, 242f
Contact dermatitis, 86
  eyelid involvement in, 85-86, 86f
Contact lens injury, 40, 43f, 333-335,
  334f, 335f

Contusion, periorbital/ocular, 329-330,
  330f
Copper deposition, sites and signs of,
  in Wilson's disease, 316, 316f
Cornea, 1, 103, 104f
  abrasion of, 331-333, 332f
    due to conjunctival foreign body,
      331, 339, 339f
  arcus of, 299, 299f
  calcium accumulation on, 115, 115f
  chemical injury to, 349f, 350f
  clouding of, mucopolysaccharidosis
    and, 303, 303f
  contact lens injury to, 40, 43f,
    333-335, 334f, 335f
  copper deposition in, 316
  cysts of, in patients receiving
    cytosine arabinoside, 321,
    321f
  drying of. *See* Dry eye.
  dystrophies of, 273
  erosion of, recurrent, 28, 62, 63f,
    114f, 114-115
  examination of, 13
  excess exposure of, 326
    myotonic dystrophy and, 304,
      304f
  extension of conjunctival growth
    onto, 61, 62f, 113, 114f
  foreign body in or on, 63, 64f,
    342-345
    movement of, under contact lens,
      334f
  glue injury to, 358f
  hyopic injury to, from contact lens,
    333
  infectious lesions of, 40, 43f, 44f,
    107-112
    in contact lens wearers, 334, 335f
  infiltrates in
    infectious ulcer and, 111, 112f
    subepithelial, secondary to viral
      conjunctivitis, 91, 92f
  inflammation of, 44f, 107-108, 108f
    Wegener's granulomatosis and,
      315, 315f
  laceration of, 345-347, 346f
  opacity of, white, 255-257
  precipitates on
    in iritis, 46f
    in sarcoidosis, 309, 310f
    in syphilis, 313f
    in uveitis, 141, 142f
  recurrent erosion of, 28, 62, 63f,
    114f, 114-115

Cornea—cont'd
  refractive surgery of, 116, 117f
  ring in
    as sign of embedded iron foreign
      body, 63, 64f
    as sign of Wilson's disease, 316,
      316f
  scarring of
    from herpes simplex virus
      infection, 108f
    from herpes zoster ophthalmicus,
      109f
    in Stevens-Johnson syndrome,
      312, 312f
  slit lamp examination of, 13
  thermal injury to, 351, 352, 352f
  thickness of, 105f
    glaucoma risk in relation to, 191
  transplantation of, 116
    sutures used in, 116, 116f
  ulcer of, 28
    bacterial infection and, 111, 112f,
      113f
      in contact lens wearers, 334,
        335f
    fungal infection and, 111, 113f
    herpes simplex virus infection and,
      44f
    Pseudomonas infection and, in
      contact lens wearers, 334,
      335f
    rheumatoid arthritis and, 308,
      309f
  ultraviolet radiation injury to, 332f,
    336
  vascularization of
    blepharoconjunctivitis and, 97, 97f
    herpes simplex virus infection and,
      107, 108f
  verticillate lines on, in patients using
    amiodarone, 317, 317f
Cortical cataract, 130, 130f
Corticosteroids
  as anti-inflammatory agents, 380,
    380t, 381
  as source of ocular problems, 320
Cotton-wool spots, on retina, 152,
  152f, 167f
  in AIDS patients, 298
Cranial nerve palsies. *See ordinal cranial*
  nerve entries, e.g., Third cranial
  nerve (oculomotor nerve)
  palsy.
Craniopharyngioma, chiasmal
  compression by, 215f

Crystalline deposition, retinal, in
    patients using tamoxifen, 326,
    327f
Crystalline lens, 1, 127, 128f
    accommodation by, 127, 129f
        age-related changes in, 30, 230,
        230f
    copper deposition in, 316
    examination of, 13
    loss of elasticity of, with aging, 128
    opacity of. See Cataract(s).
    subluxation of
        syndrome-associated occurrence
        of, 302, 302f, 373
        traumatic, 330f
Cupping, of optic disc, in glaucoma,
    189, 191f
Cycloplegics, 374, 374t
Cyst(s)
    corneal, in patients receiving
        cytosine arabinoside, 321,
        321f
    epithelial inclusion, of eyelid, 76f,
        76-77
Cytarabine (cytosine arabinoside)
    therapy, 320
    ocular abnormalities correlated with,
        321, 321f
Cytomegalovirus infection, retinitis due
    to, 177-180, 178f
Cytosine arabinoside (Cytarabine)
    therapy, 320
    ocular abnormalities correlated with,
        321, 321f

D

Dacryoadenitis, 282-283, 283f, 291,
    291f
Dacryocele, in infants, 243, 243f
Dacryocystitis, 49, 49f, 281-282,
    282f
Degeneration, macular, 26, 29
    age-related, 173-176
        drusen in, 174, 174f, 175f
        retinal hemorrhage in, 175, 175f
Dense white cataract, 131, 131f
Dermatitis, eyelid involvement in,
    84-86, 85f, 86f
Dermatomyositis, 295
    ocular problems associated with, 295,
        295f
Dermoid
    corneal, 256, 256f
    eyebrow area as site of, 257f

Descemet's membrane, 103
    copper deposition in, 316
Detachment
    posterior vitreous, 183
    retinal, 26, 183-185
        diabetes mellitus and, 155, 155f
        surgery for, 186
            scleral buckling in, 186, 187f
        tear leading to, 183, 184f
Diabetes mellitus, 296
    cataract as complication of, 296,
        296f
    macular edema associated with,
        157-159, 158f
    retinopathy in, 153-157
        extra-retinal neovascularization
        characterizing, 154, 154f
        complications associated with,
        154, 155, 155f
Diagnostic medications, 373-374
Diffuse anterior scleritis, 47f, 121, 121f
Digoxin toxicity, ocular symptoms of,
    321-322
Diplopia, 31
    causes of, 31-33
Dislocation, of lens
    syndrome-associated occurrence of,
        273, 302, 302f
    traumatic, 330f
Distance acuity chart, 3f
Distorted vision (metamorphopsia), 30
Double vision, 31
    causes of, 31-33
Droopy eyelids. See Eyelid(s), drooping
    of.
Drug allergy, and conjunctivitis, 58, 59f
Drug-induced ocular lesions, 317-328
Drusen, 174, 174f, 175f, 211, 212f
"Dry" (atrophic) age-related macular
    degeneration, 29, 174, 174f,
    175
Dry eye, 54, 54f, 103-107, 105f,
    106f
    artificial tears for, 106-107, 375t
    punctal plugs in treatment of, 107,
        107f
    severe, in patients with Sjögren
        syndrome, 40, 41f, 42f
    tear test for, 18, 106
Dystrophy(ies)
    corneal, 273
    myotonic, 303, 304
        ocular lesions associated with,
        303-304, 304f
    retinal, 273

E

Ectropion, 52, 53f, 67-68, 69f
Edema
    macular, diabetes mellitus and,
        157-159, 158f
    optic disc, 208, 209f, 210, 266f
Ehlers-Danlos syndrome
    angioid streaking of retina in, 297,
        297f, 298
    blue sclera(e) in, 297f
Embolus (emboli), retinal artery
    occlusion by, 162, 163f, 164,
        165, 165f
    treatment of, 166
Emmetropia, 4, 5f
Endophthalmitis, 28, 140
    endogenous, 183
    foreign body as cause of, 45, 47f,
        182, 182f
    postoperative, 181
    trauma and, 182
Entropion, 52, 53f, 68, 69, 70f
Epidemic keratoconjunctivitis, 56, 57f
Epiretinal membrane, 185f, 185-186
Episclera, 119
Episcleritis, 42, 46f, 120-124, 121f
    lupus erythematosus and, 314, 314f
Epithelial cyst(s)
    of cornea, in patients receiving
        cytosine arabinoside, 321,
        321f
    of eyelid, 76f, 76-77
Erectile dysfunction, drugs for, 327
    ocular effects of, 328
Erosion, corneal, recurrent, 28, 62, 63f,
    114f, 114-115
Erythema, of eyelid(s), 35
    in viral conjunctivitis, 89, 91f
Erythema multiforme, 311
    ocular lesions associated with,
        311-312, 312f
Esodeviation, 8, 10f
Esotropia, 234, 235f, 267, 268
    accommodative, 268, 269f
    congenital, 251-252
Essential blepharospasm, 86-87, 87f
Ethambutol-induced visual loss, 322
Exodeviation, 8, 10f
Exophthalmometry, 19, 20f
Exophthalmos (proptosis), 37t
    thyroid disease and, 285, 285f,
        286f
Exotropia, 234, 235f, 267, 268
    congenital, 251-252

Exposure, excessive, of cornea, 326
 myotonic dystrophy and, 304, 304f
Extracapsular cataract extraction, 134
Extraocular muscles, 7, 9f, 277f
Exudative ("wet") age-related macular
  degeneration, 26, 174, 175,
  175f, 176
Eye(s). *See* Ocular *entries and structure-
  specific citations.*
Eyedrop-related hazards, 20-21
Eyelash(es), rubbing of, against globe,
  52, 54f, 70, 71f
Eyelid(s), 67, 68f, 69f
 actinic keratoses on, 74-75, 75f
 basal cell carcinoma of, 77f, 77-78
 carcinoma of, 77f, 77-79, 79f
 contact dermatitis involving, 85-86,
  86f
 cyst of, 76f, 76-77
 dermatitis involving, 84-86, 85f, 86f
 drooping of, 37t, 67, 72, 72f
  congenital, 247f, 247-248
  third cranial nerve palsy and, 67,
   219, 219f
 epithelial inclusion cyst of, 76f,
  76-77
 erythema of, 35
  in viral conjunctivitis, 89, 91f
 examination of, 7, 8f, 11
  eversion and, 7, 8f, 60f
 floppy, 72-73, 73f
 glue injury to, 357, 358
 heliotrope discoloration of, in
  patients with
  dermatomyositis, 295, 295f
 hemangioma of, in infants, 249, 249f
 herpes simplex virus dermatitis
  involving, 84-85, 85f
 inflammation of, 35, 51, 79-81, 98f
  conjunctivitis and, 97-98
  facial sebaceous gland dysfunction
   (rosacea) and, 98, 98f
  infection and, 51, 52f, 80, 80f, 84,
   85f
  meibomian gland dysfunction and,
   51, 52f, 81
  pediculosis and, 52, 53f
  seborrhea and, 51, 51f, 80, 80f
 keratoses on, 73-75, 74f, 75f
 laceration of, 361-363, 362f
 louse infestation of, 52, 53f
 meibomian glands of, 67, 69f
  lesions due to blockage or
   dysfunction of, 50, 51, 51f,
   52f, 81, 82, 83f

Eyelid(s)—cont'd
 molluscum contagiosum on, 83-84,
  84f
 port-wine stain on, 250
 seborrheic keratoses on, 73-74,
  74f
 spasm of, 86-87, 87f
 squamous cell carcinoma of, 78-79,
  79f
 swelling of, 35
 turning in of, 52, 53f, 68, 69, 70f
 turning out of, 52, 53f, 67-68, 69f
 twitching of, 35
 xanthomas on, 75-76, 76f

F

Facial nerve (seventh cranial nerve)
  palsy, as factor in
   lagophthalmos, 71, 71f
 and dry eye, 106f
Farsightedness (hyperopia), 5, 5f
Fields of vision, 10
 effects of glaucoma on, 189, 192f
 flashes in, 30
 relation between defects in, and
  lesions of optic nerve or optic
  chiasm, 199, 200f, 201
 testing of, 10-11, 11f, 20, 21f
Fistula, carotid artery–cavernous sinus,
  223-224
 red eye associated with, 65, 65f,
  224f
Fixation, assessment of, in pediatric
  patients, 234, 234f
Flashes, in visual fields, 30
Flashlight test, of pupillary function,
  6-7
Floaters, 31
Floppy eyelid syndrome, 72-73, 73f
Fluorescein stain, 153, 373
Foreign body
 conjunctival, 339f, 339-341
  abrasion of cornea by, 331, 339,
   339f
 corneal, 63, 64f, 342-345
  movement of, under contact lens,
   334f
 intraocular, 45, 182f, 358-361, 359f,
  360f
  endophthalmitis associated with,
   45, 47f, 182
Foreign body sensation, 34
Fourth cranial nerve (trochlear nerve),
  7, 220

Fourth cranial nerve (trochlear nerve)
  palsy, 32, 220-222
 signs of, 220, 221f
Fovea of retina, 150. *See also* Macula.
 cherry-rod spot in, as sign of arterial
  occlusion, 17, 163, 163f
Fracture, orbital, 33, 363-365, 364f
Funduscopy, 15-17
 color and structural details on, 16,
  17, 149, 150, 150f, 151f
Fungal corneal ulcer, 111, 113f

G

Giant cell arteritis, 203-205
 optic neuropathy in, 204, 204f
Glaucoma, 189-197
 angle-closure, 28, 39-40, 195-197
  treatment of, 196
   laser iridectomy in, 193f, 196
 congenital, 248-249
 medications for, 194, 196, 382-385,
  383t-385t
 neovascular, 154
 open-angle, 29, 190-195
  treatment of, 194-195
   filtering bleb in, 195, 195f
 optic disc cupping in, 189, 191f
 pupillary dilation in, 41f, 196f
 retinal vein occlusion and, 168
 risk of, in relation to corneal
  thickness, 191
 visual fields in, 189, 192f
Glue injury
 to cornea, 358f
 to eyelids, 357, 358
Gonioscopy, 18, 18f
Gonococcal infection, and
  conjunctivitis, 48, 49f, 92,
  93f
 in infants, 239, 240, 240f
Granulomatosis, Wegener's, 315
 ocular lesions associated with, 315f,
  315-316
Granulomatous uveitis, sarcoidosis and,
  309, 310f

H

Halos, around lights, perception of,
  31
Headache
 migraine, 265
  visual symptoms of, 30
 pediatric cases of, 264-265

Heliotrope discoloration, of eyelid, in patients with dermatomyositis, 295, 295f
Hemangioma, in infants, 249f, 249-250
Hemorrhage. *See also* Hyphema.
  retinal, 17, 152-153
    cytomegalovirus infection and, 178, 178f
    macular degeneration and, 175, 175f
    posterior uveitis and, 146, 146f
    Roth spot, 176-177, 177f
    shaken baby syndrome and, 261, 262f
    sickle cell disease and, 170, 170f
    venous occlusion and, 167, 167f, 168f
  retrobulbar, 356-357
  subconjunctival, 60, 61f, 337f, 337-339
    around conjunctival laceration, 341, 341f
  vitreous, 26, 186
Herpes simplex virus infection
  and blepharitis, 84, 85f
  and conjunctivitis, 35t
    in children, 260
  and dermatitis, 84
    eyelid involvement in, 84-85, 85f
  and iritis, 40, 45f
  and keratitis, 107-108, 108f
  and ulceration of cornea, 44f
Herpes zoster ophthalmicus, 108-111, 109f, 110f
  HIV infection and, 298
Hertel exophthalmometry, 19, 20f
Heterochromia iridis, 258-259
HIV (human immunodeficiency virus) infection, 298
  ocular lesions associated with, 177, 298, 299f
Hordeolum (stye), 50, 50f, 81-82, 82f
  in children, 266-267
Horner syndrome, 218, 218f
Human immunodeficiency virus (HIV) infection, 298, 299f
  ocular lesions associated with, 177, 298, 299f
Hutchinson's sign, 108-109, 109f
Hydroxychloroquine (Plaquenil) therapy, 324
  ocular toxicity of, 324-326, 325f
Hyopic injury, to cornea, from contact lens, 333

Hyperlipidemia, ocular lesions associated with, 299f, 299-300
Hyperopia (farsightedness), 5, 5f
Hyperosmotic medications, for glaucoma, 385, 385t
Hypertension
  intracranial, 208, 210
    and headache, in children, 265
    and papilledema, 208, 209f, 266f
  systemic, and retinopathy, 159-161, 300
    with arteriolar narrowing, 159, 160, 160f
Hypertropia, 269
Hyphema, 39, 353, 353f. *See also* Hemorrhage.
  impaired clearance of, in sickle cell disease, 354
  traumatic, 39, 40f, 353-355
Hypopyon
  corneal ulcer and, 111, 112f
  postoperative occurrence of, 181, 182f
  uveitis and, 141, 142f

I

Idiopathic intracranial hypertension (pseudotumor cerebri), 208, 210
  papilledema associated with, 208, 209f
In situ keratomileusis, via excimer laser, 116, 117f
Inclusion cyst, of eyelid, 76f, 76-77
Indocyanine green angiography, 153
Infants. *See* Pediatric patients.
Inflammatory bowel disease, 301
  ocular lesions associated with, 301, 301f
Inflammatory cells
  in anterior chamber of eye
    as postoperative finding, 181, 182f
    as sign of corneal ulcer, 111, 112f
  in anterior chamber of eye or vitreous, as sign of uveitis, 141, 142f, 145, 146f
Inherited ocular dystrophies, in pediatric patients, 273
Inherited pigmentary retinopathy, 171-173, 172f
Intracranial hypertension, 208, 210
  and headache, in children, 265
  and papilledema, 208, 209f, 266f

Intraepithelial neoplasia, conjunctival, 99-100, 100f
Intraocular pressure
  measurement of, 14f, 14-15, 15f, 191-192
  normal to high, in glaucoma. *See* Glaucoma.
Intrauterine infections, and ocular pathology, 245
Involutional ectropion, 68, 69f
Involutional entropion, 53f, 68, 70f
Iridectomy, via laser, for glaucoma, 193f, 196
Iridodonesis, in Marfan syndrome, 302
Iris (irides), 1, 139, 140f. *See also* Iritis.
  differences between colors of, 258-259
  examination of, 13
  neovascularization of, in diabetic retinopathy, 154, 154f
  nodules on
    in anterior uveitis, 142, 143f
    in neurofibromatosis, 305, 305f
  tremulousness of, in Marfan syndrome, 302
Iritis, 40, 45f, 46f
  pediatric cases of, 260
  traumatic, 355-356
Ischemic optic neuropathy, 27, 201-205
  anterior, 201-205
    arteritic, 203-205, 204f
    nonarteritic, 201-203, 202f
Isoniazid-induced visual loss, 323
Itching, of eyes, 34

K

Kaposi's sarcoma, on conjunctiva, 298, 299f
Kayser-Fleischer ring, 316, 316f
Keratic precipitates
  in iritis, 46f
  in sarcoidosis, 309, 310f
  in syphilis, 313f
  in uveitis, 141, 141f, 142f
Keratitis
  infection and, 44f, 107-108, 108f
  Wegener's granulomatosis and, 315, 315f
Keratoconjunctivitis, epidemic, 56, 57f
Keratoconjunctivitis sicca. *See* Dry eye; Sjogren syndrome.
Keratomileusis, laser in situ, 116, 117f

Keratosis
    actinic, 74
        eyelid involvement in, 74-75, 75f
    seborrheic, eyelid involvement in,
        73-74, 74f
Koeppe nodules, 142, 143f

L

Laceration
    of conjunctiva, 341f, 341-342
    of cornea, 345-347, 346f
    of eyelid, 361-363, 362f
    of sclera, 347f, 347-348
Lacrimal apparatus, 275, 277f, 278f. *See
    also* Nasolacrimal duct *entries
    and citations beginning with the
    prefix Dacryo-.*
    dye test of, 18-19
Lagophthalmos, 70-71, 71f
    and dry eye, 106f
Large pupil, discrepant in size from
        other pupil, 36, 216-218
Laser in situ keratomileusis, 116, 117f
Laser therapy
    for cataract, 136, 137f
    for glaucoma, 193f, 194, 196
    for refractive error, 116, 117f
Leber's optic neuropathy, 211
Lens (contact lens), injury from, 40,
        43f, 333-335, 334f, 335f
Lens (crystalline lens), 1, 127, 128f
    accommodation by, 127, 129f
        age-related changes in, 30, 230,
            230f
    copper deposition in, 316
    examination of, 13
    loss of elasticity of, with aging, 128
    opacity of. *See* Cataract(s).
    subluxation of
        syndrome-associated occurrence
            of, 302, 302f, 373
        traumatic, 330f
Leukocoria, congenital cataract and,
        245, 246f
Leukoma, 255-257
Levitra (vardenafil) therapy, 327
    ocular effects of, 328
Lice, infestation of eyelids by, 52, 53f
Light(s)
    intolerance of, 31
    perception of halos around, 31
Lisch nodules, 305, 305f
Louse infestation, of eyelids, 52, 53f
Lubricant tears, artificial, 106-107, 375t

Lupus erythematosus, systemic, 314
    ocular lesions associated with, 314,
        314f
Luxation, of lens
    syndrome-associated occurrence of,
        273, 302, 302f
    traumatic, 330f

M

Macula, 151
    bull's-eye appearance of
        in patients receiving chloroquine,
            319, 319f
        in patients receiving
            hydroxychloroquine, 325,
            325f
    degeneration of, 26, 29
        age-related, 173-176
            drusen in, 174, 174f, 175f
            retinal hemorrhage in, 175, 175f
    edema of, in diabetic patients,
        157-159, 158f
Marfan syndrome, 302
    ocular lesions associated with, 302,
        302f
Meibomian glands, 67, 69f
    lesions due to blockage or
        dysfunction of, 50, 51, 51f,
        52f, 81, 82, 83f
Melanoma, conjunctival, 101f
Melanosis, racial, 102
    conjunctival lesion associated with,
        101f, 102
Mellaril (thioridazine) toxicity, and
        pigmentary retinopathy, 323,
        324f
Metamorphopsia (distorted vision), 30
Migraine, 265
    visual symptoms of, 30
Molluscum contagiosum, 83
    conjunctivitis associated with, 60,
        61f
    eyelid involvement in, 83-84, 84f
    HIV infection and, 298
Monocular diplopia, causes of, 32
Motor system problems, and neuro-
        ophthalmic disorders,
        218-227
Mucopolysaccharidoses, 302-303
    ocular lesions associated with, 303,
        303f
"Mutton-fat" keratic precipitates
    in sarcoidosis, 309, 310f
    in uveitis, 141, 142f

Myasthenia gravis, 33
    ocular, 33, 225f, 225-226
Mydriatics, 374, 374t
Myopia (nearsightedness), 4-5, 5f
    severity of, risk of vitreous
        detachment correlated with,
        183
    syndrome-associated occurrence of,
        273
Myositis, orbital, 290, 290f
Myotonic dystrophy, 303, 304
    ocular lesions associated with,
        303-304, 304f

N

Nasolacrimal duct, 275
Nasolacrimal duct obstruction, 48-49,
        281
    pediatric cases of, 241f, 241-244
        treatment of, 242-244, 243f
        vs. congenital glaucoma, 248
        vs. conjunctivitis, 241, 242f
Near acuity chart, 4f
Nearsightedness (myopia), 4-5, 5f
    severity of, risk of vitreous
        detachment correlated with,
        183
    syndrome-associated occurrence of,
        273
Necrotizing scleritis, 122, 122f
    rheumatoid arthritis and, 308, 308f
    Wegener's granulomatosis and,
        315f
Neisseria gonorrhoeae infection, and
        conjunctivitis, 48, 49f, 92,
        93f
    in infants, 239, 240, 240f
Neisseria meningitidis infection, and
        conjunctivitis, 92
Neovascular glaucoma, 154
Neovascularization, of optic disc and
        iris, in diabetic retinopathy,
        154, 154f
    complications associated with, 154,
        155, 155f
Nerve, optic. *See* Optic nerve *entries and*
        Optic disc.
Nerve fiber layer, of retina, 152, 152f
Nerve palsies. *See ordinal cranial nerve
        entries, e.g.,* Third cranial nerve
        (oculomotor nerve) palsy.
Neurofibromatosis, 304
    ocular lesions associated with, 305,
        305f

Neuro-ophthalmic disorders, 199-227
  disc pathology in, 201. *See also* Optic
      nerve disorders.
  motor system problems and,
      218-227
  sensory pathway problems and, 199,
      200f, 201
Nevus (nevi), conjunctival, 100, 101f
Night blindness, 30
Nodular anterior scleritis, 47f, 121,
      122f
Nodular episcleritis, 121f
Nodule(s)
  iridal
    in anterior uveitis, 142, 143f
    in neurofibromatosis, 305, 305f
  sarcoid, ocular, 309, 310f
Nonarteritic anterior ischemic optic
      neuropathy, 201-203,
      202f
Nonsteroidal anti-inflammatory ocular
      medications, 381, 381t
Nuclear cataract, 130, 130f
Nystagmus
  acquired, 226-227
  pediatric cases of, 252-254

O

Ocular disorders. *See also particular lesion
      types and site-specific entries.*
  drug-induced, 317-328
  pediatric, 238-273. *See also specific
      conditions under* Pediatric
      patients.
  signs and symptoms of, 25-38
  syndrome-associated occurrence of,
      273
  systemic disease–related, 293-317
  traumatic, 182, 329-367. *See also
      specific types, e.g.,* Laceration.
    in children, 261-263, 262f
Ocular examination, 1-23
  pediatric, 230-238
    lid speculum as aid to, 239f
    timing of, 23, 231, 232
Ocular medications, 369-386,
      370t-386t
  problems with patients' consumption
      of, 20, 21
Ocular trauma, 182, 329-367. *See also
      specific types, e.g.,* Laceration.
  pediatric cases of, 261-263, 262f
Oculomotor nerve (third cranial nerve),
      7, 218-219

Oculomotor nerve (third cranial nerve)
      palsy, 32, 219-220
  and ptosis, 67, 219, 219f
Open-angle glaucoma, 29, 190-195
  treatment of, 194-195
    filtering bleb in, 195, 195f
Ophthalmoscopy. *See* Funduscopy.
Optic chiasm, lesions of, 213, 215f,
      215-216
  visual field defects due to, 201
Optic disc, 201
  cupping of, in glaucoma, 189, 191f
  edema of, 208, 209f, 210, 266f
  neovascularization of, in diabetic
      retinopathy, 154, 154f, 155f
  pallor of, 211
Optic nerve, 2, 149
Optic nerve disorders, 201-213
  correlation between visual field
      defects and, 199, 200f
  disc pathology in, 201. *See also specific
      abnormalities under* Optic disc.
  infiltrative, 210, 211
  inflammmatory, 27, 205-208, 207f
  ischemic, 27, 201-205, 202f, 204f
  neoplastic, 213, 214f
  thyroid disease and, 287, 287f
  toxic, 211
  traumatic, 211, 365-367
Orbit, 275, 276f
  effects of disease of, 45, 48f
Orbital blow-out fracture, 33, 363-365,
      364f
Orbital cellulitis, 48f, 279f, 279-281,
      280f
  pediatric cases of, 263-264
Orbital myositis, 290, 290f
Orbital pseudotumor, 33, 288-291
  classification of, 288-291, 288f-291f
Orbital septal thinning, age-related, 67
Osteogenesis imperfecta, 306
  blue sclerae in, 306, 306f

P

Pain, ocular, 34
Pallor, optic disc, 211
Palsy(ies), cranial nerve. *See ordinal
      cranial nerve entries, e.g.,* Third
      cranial nerve (oculomotor
      nerve) palsy.
Panuveitis, 140
Papilledema, 208, 209f, 210, 266f
Patching, of eye, 20, 22f
  in pediatric vision testing, 237, 237f

Peaked (teardrop) pupil, 254, 255f,
      346, 346f
Pediatric patients, 229
  amblyopia in, 269-271
  cataracts in, 245-246
  chalazion in, 266-267
  coloboma in, 254-255
  congenital eye anomalies in, 245-259
  conjunctivitis in, 56, 238-240, 240f,
      259-261
  esotropia in, 251, 252, 267, 268
  exotropia in, 251, 252, 267, 268
  glaucoma in, 248-249
  headache in, 264-265
  hemangioma in, 249-250
  heterochromia iridis in, 258-259
  hordeolum (stye) in, 266-267
  inherited ocular dystrophies in,
      273
  iritis in, 260
  leukoma in, 255-257, 256f
  nasolacrimal duct obstruction in,
      241f, 241-244, 248
  nystagmus in, 252-254
  ocular disorders in, 238-273
  ocular examination in, 230-238
    lid speculum as aid to, 239f
    timing of, 23, 231, 232
  ocular trauma in, 261-263, 262f
  orbital/preseptal cellulitis in,
      263-264
  port-wine stain in, 250
  ptosis in, 247f, 247-248
  refractive errors in, 273-275
  retinoblastoma in, 257-258
  retinopathy of prematurity in, 231,
      244-245
  strabismus in, 251-252, 267-269
  stye (hordeolum) in, 266-267
  syndrome-associated occurrence of
      ocular disorders in,
      273
  visual development in, 229
  visual loss in, 269-271
Pediculosis, blepharitis due to, 52,
      53f
Penlight demonstration, of shallow
      anterior chamber, 194f
Perimetry, 20, 21f
Periorbital contusion, 329-330, 330f
Phacoemulsification, 133f, 133-134,
      134f, 135f
Phenothiazine-induced pigment
      deposition, in eye, 323
Photophobia, 31

Pigmentary retinopathy
  hereditary, 171-173, 172f
  thioridazine (Mellaril) toxicity and, 323, 324f
Pinguecula, 60-61, 62f, 98-99, 99f
Pinhole testing, 6
Plaquenil (hydroxychloroquine) therapy, 324
  ocular toxicity of, 324-326, 325f
Polycythemia vera, 306-307
  red eye associated with, 65, 65f, 307, 307f
Port-wine stain, 250
Posterior subcapsular cataract, 131, 131f
Posterior tenonitis, 289, 289f, 290f
Posterior uveitis, 145-148, 146f
  toxoplasmosis and, 146, 147f
Posterior vitreous detachment, 183
Poxvirus infection, and molluscum contagiosum. See Molluscum contagiosum.
Premature infants
  pupillary membrane in, 231, 231f
  retinopathy in, 231, 244-245
Presbyopia, 4, 30, 127-128
Preseptal cellulitis, 49, 275-276, 278-279
  pediatric cases of, 263-264
Proliferative diabetic retinopathy, 153-157
  neovascularization of optic disc and iris in, 154, 154f
  complications associated with, 154, 155, 155f
Proptosis (exophthalmos), 37t
  thyroid disease and, 285, 285f, 286f
Prostaglandins, for glaucoma, 385, 385t
Pseudoesotropia, 235f
Pseudomonas infection, and corneal ulcer, in contact lens wearers, 334, 335f
Pseudo–retinitis pigmentosa, 173
Pseudotumor, orbital, 33, 288-292
  classification of, 288-291, 288f-291f
Pseudotumor cerebri (idiopathic intracranial hypertension), 208, 210
  papilledema associated with, 208, 209f
Pterygium, 61-62, 62f, 113, 114f
Ptosis, 37t, 67, 72, 72f
  congenital, 247f, 247-248
  third cranial nerve palsy and, 67, 219, 219f

Punctal plugs, in treatment of dry eye, 107, 107f
Pupil(s), 139. See also Iris (irides).
  agents dilating, 374, 374t
  examination of, 6-7
  inequality in size of, 36, 216-218
  membrane over, in premature infants, 231, 231f
  mid-dilation of, in glaucoma, 41f, 196f
  teardrop (peaked), 254, 255f, 346, 346f
  white, congenital cataract and, 245, 246f
Pupillary light reflex, assessment of, in pediatric patients, 234, 234f

R

Racial melanosis, 102
  conjunctival lesion associated with, 101f, 102
Recurrent corneal erosion, 28, 62, 63f, 114f, 114-115
Red blood cells, in anterior chamber of eye, 39, 40f, 353f, 353-355
  impaired clearance of, in sickle cell disease, 354
Red eye, 39-65
  non–vision-threatening causes of, 48-65, 307, 307f
  vision-threatening causes of, 39-48
Red reflex, assessment of, 232-233, 233f, 238
Refractive errors, 4-5, 5f
  in children, 271-273
Refractive power, 4-6
  improvement of, via laser in situ keratomileusis, 116, 117f
Reiter syndrome, 307
  ocular lesions in, 307-308
Relative afferent pupillary defect, 6, 6f
Retina, 2, 149-152, 152f. See also entries beginning with the prefix Retino-.
  angioid streaks in, 297
    Ehlers-Danlos syndrome and, 297, 297f, 298
  cotton-wool spots on, 152, 152f, 167f
    in AIDS patients, 298
  crystalline deposition in, tamoxifen use and, 326, 327f
  cytomegaloviral infection of, 177-180, 178f

Retina—cont'd
  detachment of, 26, 183-185
    diabetes mellitus and, 155, 155f
    surgery for, 186
      scleral buckling in, 186, 187f
    tear leading to, 183, 184f
  dystrophies of, 273
  fovea of, 150. See also Retina, macula of.
    cherry-red spot in, as sign of arterial occlusion, 17, 163, 163f
  hemorrhages in, 17, 152-153
    cytomegalovirus infection and, 178, 178f
    macular degeneration and, 175, 175f
    posterior uveitis and, 146, 146f
    Roth spot, 176-177, 177f
    shaken baby syndrome and, 261, 262f
    sickle cell disease and, 170, 170f
    venous occlusion and, 167, 167f, 168f
  macula of, 151
    bull's-eye appearance of
      in patients receiving chloroquine, 319, 319f
      in patients receiving hydroxychloroquine, 325, 325f
    degeneration of, 26, 29
      age-related, 173-176
        drusen in, 174, 174f, 175f
        hemorrhage in, 175, 175f
    edema of, in diabetic patients, 157-159, 158f
    membrane on, 185f, 185-186
    nerve fiber layer of, 152, 152f
    occlusion of vasculature of, 26, 162-169. See also under Retinal artery and Retinal vein.
    in Behçet's disease, 294f
    surgery of, 186-187
      scleral buckling in, 186, 187f
    systemic diseases compromising. See specifics under Retinopathy.
Retinal artery, occlusion of, 26, 162-167
  cherry-red spot in fovea as sign of, 17, 163, 163f
  emboli causing, 162, 163f, 164, 165, 165f
    methods of dislodging, 166

Retinal vein, occlusion of, 26, 167f, 167-169, 168f
  glaucoma associated with, 168
Retinitis, cytomegalovirus infection and, 177-180, 178f
Retinitis pigmentosa, 171-173, 172f
Retinoblastoma, 257-258
Retinopathy
  diabetic, 153-157
    neovascularization of optic disc and iris in, 154, 154f
      complications of, 154, 155, 155f
  hypertensive, 159-161, 300
    arteriolar narrowing in, 159, 160, 160f
  pigmentary
    hereditary, 171-173, 172f
    thioridazine (Mellaril) toxicity and, 323, 324f
  prematurity and, 231, 244-245
  sickle cell disease and, 169-171, 170f
Retrobulbar hemorrhage, 356-357
Rheumatoid arthritis, 308
  ocular problems associated with, 308f, 308-309, 309f
Ring
  Kayser-Fleischer, 316, 316f
  rust, in cornea, 63, 64f
Rosacea, 98, 98f, 99f
Rose bengal stain, 373
Roth spots, 176-177, 177f
Rubbing, of eyes, 59, 63
  conjunctivitis due to, 59
Rubeosis iridis, 154, 154f
Rupture, scleral, 347-348

S

Sarcoidosis, 309
  ocular lesions accompanying, 309-310, 310f
Sarcoma, Kaposi's, on conjunctiva, 298, 299f
Schirmer tear test, 18, 19f, 106
Sclera(e), 1, 119
  blue
    in Ehlers-Danlos syndrome, 297f
    in osteogenesis imperfecta, 306, 306f
  inflammation of. See Scleritis.
  trauma to, 347f, 347-348
Scleral buckling, in retinal surgery, 186, 187f
Scleritis, 42, 119, 124-125
  anterior, 47f, 121, 121f, 122f
  classification of, 121f, 121-122, 122f

Scleritis—cont'd
  diffuse anterior, 47f, 121, 121f
  herpes zoster ophthalmicus and, 110f
  inflammatory bowel disease and, 301, 301f
  lupus erythematosus and, 314, 314f
  necrotizing, 122, 122f
    rheumatoid arthritis and, 308, 308f
    Wegener's granulomatosis and, 315f
  nodular anterior, 47f, 121, 122f
  rheumatoid arthritis and, 308, 308f
  systemic lupus erythematosus and, 314, 314f
  Wegener's granulomatosis and, 315, 315f
Scleromalacia perforans, 122, 123f, 308
Seborrheic blepharitis, 51, 51f, 80, 80f
Seborrheic keratosis, eyelid involvement in, 73-74, 74f
Seidel test, for leakage of aqueous humor, 344, 344f
Senile cataract(s), 128-131, 130f, 131f
Sensory pathway problems, and neuro-ophthlamic disorders, 199, 200f, 201
Seventh cranial nerve (facial nerve) palsy, as factor in lagophthalmos, 71, 71f
  and dry eye, 106f
Shaken baby syndrome, 261
  ocular signs of, 261-262, 262f
Sickle cell disease, 170
  impaired clearance of hyphema in, 354
  retinopathy in, 169-171, 170f
Sight. See Vision.
Sildenafil (Viagra) therapy, 327
  ocular effects of, 328
Sixth cranial nerve (abducens nerve), 7, 222
Sixth cranial nerve (abducens nerve) palsy, 32, 222-223
  signs of, 222, 222f
Sjögren syndrome, 40, 41f, 42f, 104, 311
Skin inflammation, eyelid involvement in, 84-86, 85f, 86f
Slit lamp examination, 12f, 12-14
Small pupil, discrepant in size from other pupil, 36, 218
Snellen acuity charts, 3f, 4f
Spasm, of eyelids, 86-87, 87f
Spondylitis, ankylosing, 293
  anterior uveitis associated with, 141f, 293-294

Squamous cell carcinoma, of eyelid, 78-79, 79f
Staphylococcal blepharitis, 51, 52f, 80, 80f
Steroids
  as anti-inflammatory agents, 380, 380t, 381, 381t
  as source of ocular problems, 320
Stevens-Johnson syndrome, 311
  ocular lesions associated with, 311-312, 312f
Storage diseases, 302-303
  ocular lesions associated with, 303, 303f
Strabismus, 234, 235f, 267-269
  amblyopia due to, 271
Strain (eyestrain), 63, 65
  and red eye, 64f
Stress headache, in children, 265
Stye (hordeolum), 50, 50f, 81-82, 82f
  in children, 266-267
Subcapsular cataract, 131, 131f
Subconjunctival hemorrhage, 60, 61f, 337f, 337-339
  around conjunctival laceration, 341, 341f
Subluxation, of lens
  syndrome-associated occurrence of, 273, 302, 302f
  traumatic, 330f
Sunsetting, 233, 233f
Swinging flashlight test, of pupillary function, 6-7
Sympathomimetic agents, for glaucoma, 384, 384t
Synechiae, formation of
  in iritis, 42, 46f
  in uveitis, 141, 143f
Syphilis, 312
  ocular problems associated with, 312-313, 313f
Systemic disease–related ocular lesions, 293-317

T

Tadalafil (Cialis) therapy, 327
  ocular effects of, 328
Tamoxifen use, and retinal crystalline deposition, 326, 327f
Tear(s), artificial, 106-107, 375t
Tear test (Schirmer tear test), 18, 19f, 106
Teardrop (peaked) pupil, 254, 255f, 346, 346f

Tearing, excessive, 34
Tenon's capsule, 119
   inflammation of, 289, 289f
Tension headache, in children, 265
Thermal injury, to eye, 351-353, 352f
Thioridazine (Mellaril) toxicity, and
      pigmentary retinopathy, 323,
      324f
Third cranial nerve (oculomotor nerve),
      7, 218-219
Third cranial nerve (oculomotor nerve)
      palsy, 32, 219-220
   and ptosis, 67, 219, 219f
Thyroid ophthalmopathy, 33, 285f,
      285-287, 286f
   optic neuropathy in, 287, 287f
   orbital inflammation accompanying,
      48f
Tonometers, 14f, 14-15, 16f
Tonometric mires, 15, 15f
Topiramate (Topomax) therapy, 327
   ocular problems associated with, 327
Toxoplasmosis, 180
   ocular, 146, 147f, 180f, 180-181
Transient visual loss, 30
Transplantation, corneal, 116
   sutures used in, 116, 116f
Trauma, ocular, 182, 329-367. *See also*
      specific types, e.g., Laceration.
   pediatric cases of, 261-263, 262f
Treponema pallidum infection, 312
   ocular problems associated with,
      312-313, 313f
Trichiasis, 52, 54f, 70, 71f
Trochlear nerve (fourth cranial nerve),
      7, 220
Trochlear nerve (fourth cranial nerve)
      palsy, 32, 220-222
   signs of, 220, 221f
Twitching, of eyelids, 35

U

Ulcer(s), corneal, 28
   bacterial infection and, 111, 112f,
      113f
      in contact lens wearers, 334, 335f
   fungal infection and, 111, 113f
   herpes simplex virus infection and,
      44f
   Pseudomonas infection and, in contact
      lens wearers, 334, 335f
   rheumatoid arthritis and, 308, 309f
Ultraviolet radiation injury, ocular,
      332f, 335-337

Usher syndrome, 173
   "bone spicule" pigmentary
      retinopathy in, 172, 173f
Uveal tract, 139, 140f
Uveitis, 28, 139-148
   anterior, 140-145
      ankylosing spondylitis and, 141f,
         293-294
      Behçet's disease and, 294
      hypopyon accompanying, 141,
         142f
      iridal nodules in, 142, 143f
      keratic precipitates associated
         with, 141, 141f
      synechiae as signs of, 141, 143f
   granulomatous, sarcoidosis and, 309,
      310f
   herpes zoster ophthalmicus and,
      110f
   keratic precipitates accompanying,
      141, 141f, 142f
   posterior, 145-148, 146f
      toxoplasmosis and, 146, 147f
   syphilitic, 313f

V

Vardenafil (Levitra) therapy, 327
   ocular effects of, 328
Vernal conjunctivitis, 58, 58f
   in children, 260
Verticillate lines, on cornea, in patients
      using amiodarone, 317,
      317f
Viagra (sildenafil) therapy, 327
   ocular effects of, 328
Viral conjunctivitis, 55-56, 89, 90f, 91,
      91f
   follicular lesions in, 55, 55f, 91,
      91f
   pediatric cases of, 259-260
   subepithelial corneal infiltrates
      associated with, 91, 92f
   vs. other conjunctivitides, 36t
Viral dacryoadenitis, 283f
Vision. *See also* Visual acuity; Visual
      fields; Visual loss.
   aids to testing of, in children, 236f,
      236-237, 237f
   color, 11-12
   development of, 229-230
      stimuli to, 229, 232, 232f
   distorted, 30
   double, 31
      causes of, 31-33

Visual acuity, 2
   measurement of, 2-4
      Snellen charts in, 3f, 4f
   refractive power and, 4-6
Visual fields, 10
   effects of glaucoma on, 189,
      192f
   flashes in, 31
   relation between defects in, and
      lesions of optic nerve or optic
      chiasm, 199, 200f, 201
   testing of, 10-11, 11f, 20, 21f
Visual loss, 25-30
   conditions potentiating risk of, as
      cause of red eye, 39-48
   neuropathology of, 199, 200f
   night-time, 30
   pediatric cases of, 269-271
   transient, 30
Vitrectomy, 187
Vitreous, 1
   slit lamp examination of, 14
Vitreous detachment, 183
Vitreous floaters, 31
Vitreous hemorrhage, 26, 186
von Recklinghausen's disease, 304
   ocular lesions associated with, 305,
      305f

W

Wegener's granulomatosis, 315
   ocular lesions associated with, 315f,
      315-316
"Wet" (exudative) age-related macular
      degeneration, 26, 174, 175,
      175f, 176
White cataract, dense, 131, 131f
White corneal opacity, 255-257
White pupil(s), congenital cataract and,
      245, 246f
White-centered hemorrhages, in retina,
      176-177, 177f
Wilson's disease, 316-317
   sites and signs of copper deposition
      in, 316, 316f

X

Xanthelasma, 75, 76f
Xerophthalmia. *See* Dry eye.

Z

Zonules of lens, 127, 128f